AF615905

Butterworths International Medical Reviews

Gastroenterology 2

Small Intestine

Butterworths International Medical Reviews

Gastroenterology 2

Published in this Series
Volume 1 Foregut
Edited by J. H. Baron and Frank G. Moody

Future volumes to include
Large Intestine

Butterworths International Medical Reviews

Gastroenterology 2

Small Intestine

Edited by
V. S. Chadwick, MA, MSc, MD, FRCP
Senior Lecturer and Honorary Consultant Physician
Department of Medicine
Royal Postgraduate Medical School
Hammersmith Hospital
London, UK

and

Sidney F. Phillips, MD, FRACP, FACP
Professor of Medicine
Mayo Medical School and
Director, Gastroenterology Unit
Mayo Clinic
Rochester
Minnesota, USA

Butterworth Scientific
London Boston Durban
Singapore Sydney Toronto Wellington

First published 1982

British Library Cataloguing in Publication Data

Small intestine. – (Gastroenterology; 2). –
(Butterworths international medical reviews,
ISSN 0260-0110)
1: Intestines – Diseases
I. Chadwick, V. S. II. Phillips, Sidney F.
III. Series
616.3′4 RC806

ISBN 0-407-02288-0

Photoset by Butterworths Litho Preparation Department
Printed and bound in England by Robert Hartnoll Ltd, Bodmin, Cornwall

Preface

Butterworths International Medical Reviews – *Small Intestine* is the second volume in the Gastroenterology series. The coeditors have followed the general philosophy of selecting subjects for inclusion in which there have been definite advances in the past decade and have not tried to be all-inclusive.

The first part of the volume consists of eight chapters which review basic knowledge of aspects of intestinal anatomy and function providing a foundation upon which to develop an understanding of disease. In the second part, four disease areas were selected which exemplified some clinical correlations of the basic topics in Part A.

The emphasis in this volume on immunology, endocrinology, gut motility and micro-organism–host interactions is justified, we believe, by the rapid expansion in knowledge in these areas. Similarly in the areas of gut anatomy and physiology we have selected topics on ultrastructure, cell organelle biochemistry, *in vitro* methods and functional development of the small intestine.

The authorship is multinational with contributions from the UK, USA, Canada, France, Belgium, Algeria and Australia and the editors are grateful to all the authors who have contributed with enthusiasm and to Butterworths who have provided expert help at all stages.

Vinton S. Chadwick
Sidney F. Phillips

List of Contributors

T. E. Adrian, PhD, MIBiol
Senior Research Officer, Department of Medicine, Royal Postgraduate Medical School, Hammersmith Hospital, London, UK

C. Hocine Asselah, MD
Docent en Médecine, Institut des Sciences Médicales, Université d'Alger, Alger, Algérie

Fatima Asselah, MD
Docent en Histopathologie, Institut des Sciences Médicales, Université d'Alger, Alger, Algérie

Jean-Jacques Bernier, DM
Professeur de Clinique Gastroentérologique, Unité de Recherches sur la Physiopathologie de la Digestion, INSERM U54, Hôpital Saint-Lazare, Paris, France

Ruth F. Bishop, DSc
Principal Research Fellow, Department of Gastroenterology, Royal Children's Hospital, Melbourne, Victoria, Australia

S. R. Bloom, MA, MD, FRCP
Reader in Medicine and Consultant Physician, Department of Medicine, Royal Postgraduate Medical School, Hammersmith Hospital, London, UK

Raymond Calvert, PhD
Professeur Agrégé, Département d'Anatomie et de Biologie Cellulaire, Faculté de Médecine, Université de Sherbrooke, Sherbrooke, Québec, Canada

M. Camilleri, MD, MRCP
Registrar, Department of Medicine, Royal Postgraduate Medical School, Hammersmith Hospital, London, UK

V. S. Chadwick, MA, MSc, MD, FRCP
Senior Lecturer and Honorary Consultant Physician, Department of Medicine, Royal Postgraduate Medical School, Hammersmith Hospital, London, UK

C. Richard Fleming, MD
Associate Professor of Medicine, Mayo Medical School, Rochester, Minnesota, USA

Gary Gitnick, MD
Professor of Medicine, UCLA School of Medicine, University of California at Los Angeles, California, USA

Richard J. Grand, MD
Chief, Division of Gastroenterology and Nutrition, The Children's Hospital Medical Center, Boston; Associate Professor of Pediatrics, Harvard Medical School, Boston, Massachusetts, USA

Kristin Henry, MRCP, FRCPath
Reader in Pathology, Department of Histopathology, Westminster Medical School, London, UK

J. S. Hugon, MD
Chairman, Department of Anatomy and Cell Biology, Faculty of Medicine, University of Sherbrooke, Sherbrooke, Quebec, Canada

J. Janssens, MD, AggHO
Associate Professor of Medicine, Division of Gastroenterology, Departments of Medicine and Medical Research, St. Rafaël University Hospital, University of Leuven, Leuven, Belgium

Keith A. Kelly, MD
Professor of Surgery, Mayo Medical School, Rochester, Minnesota, USA

George B. McDonald, MD
Associate Professor of Medicine, University of Washington School of Medicine, Seattle, Washington, USA

Daniel Menard, PhD
Professeur Agrégé, Département d'Anatomie et de Biologie Cellulaire, Faculté de Médecine, Université de Sherbrooke, Sherbrooke, Québec, Canada

Hugh R. P. Miller, BVMS, PhD
Principal Veterinary Research Officer, Department of Pathology, Moredun Research Institute, Edinburgh, UK

Robert Modigliani, DM
Professeur Agrégé de Gastroentérologie, Unité de Recherches sur la Physiopathologie de la Digestion, INSERM U54, Hôpital Saint-Lazare, Paris, France

Robert K. Montgomery, PhD
Research Associate, Harvard Medical School; Research Associate, Children's Hospital Medical Center, Boston, Massachusetts, USA

John H. Pemberton, MD
Surgical Fellow, Mayo Medical School, Rochester, Minnesota, USA

J. Pepys, MD, FRCP, FRCPE, FRCPath, FCCP, MD, Hon. CAUSA CLERMONT FERRAND
Emeritus Professor of Clinical Immunology, University of London, London, UK

T. J. Peters, MSc, PhD, FRCP, MRCPath
Head of Division of Clinical Cell Biology; Consultant Physician, Clinical Research Centre, Northwick Park Hospital, Harrow, Middlesex, UK

Sidney F. Phillips, MD, FRACP, FACP
Professor of Medicine, Mayo Medical School; Director, Gastroenterology Unit, Mayo Clinic, Rochester, Minnesota, USA

J. M. Polak, DSc, MD, MRCPath
Senior Lecturer (Consultant) in Histochemistry, Department of Histochemistry, Royal Postgraduate Medical School, Hammersmith Hospital, London, UK

C. D. Pusey, MA, MRCP
Senior Registrar, Department of Medicine, Royal Postgraduate Medical School, Hammersmith Hospital, London, UK

A. J. Rees, MSc, MRCP
Consultant Physician and Honorary Senior Lecturer, Department of Medicine, Royal Postgraduate Medical School, Hammersmith Hospital, London, UK

Roy G. Shorter, MD, FACP
Professor of Medicine and Pathology, Mayo Medical School, Rochester, Minnesota, USA

Thomas B. Tomasi, Jr, MD, PhD
Professor and Chairman, Department of Cell Biology; Director of the Cancer Center, University of New Mexico Medical Center, Albuquerque, New Mexico, USA

G. Vantrappen, MD, AggHO
Professor of Medicine, University of Leuven; Head, Department of Medicine and Division of Gastroenterology, University Hospitals of Leuven; Head, Laboratory of Gastrointestinal Pathophysiology, Department of Medical Research, University of Leuven, Leuven, Belgium

P. D. Walker, DSc, PhD, FRCPath, FIBiol
Head, Bacteriology Research and Development, Wellcome Research Laboratories, Beckenham, Kent

David L. Wingate, DM, FRCP
Senior Lecturer (Consultant) in Gastroenterology and Director, Gastrointestinal Science Research Unit, London Hospital Medical College, London, UK

Contents

Part A

1 Functional development of the small intestine 1
Richard J. Grand and Robert K. Montgomery

2 Ultrastructure of the small intestine 19
Kristin Henry

3 Biochemical anatomy of the enterocyte 40
T. J. Peters

4 *In vitro* methods and their applications 58
J. S. Hugon, R. Calvert and D. Menard

5 Immune mechanisms in the small intestine 73
Roy G. Shorter and Thomas B. Tomasi, Jr

6 Endocrine functions and disorders of the small intestine 97
T. E. Adrian, J. M. Polak and S. R. Bloom

7 Motility of the small intestine 119
David L. Wingate

8 Interactions among micro-organisms and the host 142
P. D. Walker

Part B

Immunologically related diseases

9 Intestinal parasites 162
H. R. P. Miller

10 Alpha-chain disease and intestinal lymphoma 174
C. Hocine Asselah and Fatima Asselah

11 Graft-versus-host disease: effects on the intestine 203
George B. McDonald

12 Vasculitis and the intestine 227
M. Camilleri, C. D. Pusey, V. S. Chadwick and A. J. Rees

13 'Atopy' and the gut 249
J. Pepys

Neuroendocrine disorders

14 Pathophysiology of hormonal diarrhea 265
R. Modigliani and J. J. Bernier

15 Motility disorders in small bowel diseases 280
G. Vantrappen

16 Surgical aspects of small bowel motility 292
John H. Pemberton and Keith A. Kelly

Micro-organisms in disease

17 Infectious agents and inducers of cytotoxicity in Crohn's disease and ulcerative colitis 302
Gary Gitnick

18 Spectrum of infectious agents in acute diarrhoea 319
Ruth F. Bishop

Nutritional disorders

19 Response of the small intestine to nutritional deficiencies 332
C. Richard Fleming and Sidney F. Phillips

Index 345

1
Functional development of the small intestine

Richard J. Grand and Robert K. Montgomery

INTRODUCTION

In the process of development, the gastrointestinal tract acquires a large surface area which becomes a major interface between the organism and its environment. Simultaneously, molecular mechanisms of digestion and absorption are established and elaborated. For example, in the four-week human embryo, the small intestine is a simple tube a few millimeters long; between five weeks and birth, the intestine increases its length one thousand times, while the small intestine becomes six times the length of the large intestine.

The factors mediating the digestive and absorptive functions of the small intestine reside in the columnar epithelial cells which line the intestinal villi. Functional development of the small intestine is initiated immediately after the appearance of this columnar epithelium. In humans, this occurs during the second trimester, beginning at approximately the tenth week of gestation, and, in the 22-week fetus, the proximal intestinal morphology largely resembles that of adults. The anatomical development of the small intestine is described in detail in a number of works[24, 29, 30, 37, 48, 75] and will only be discussed briefly. This review will focus upon the ontogenesis of intestinal functions integrating prenatal and postnatal developmental patterns.

MORPHOGENESIS

Morphogenesis of the intestine has been described in detail in a number of standard works[7, 33, 60], and will, therefore, only be outlined here. During the 5–9 mm stage, the intestine elongates more rapidly than the embryo as a whole, and begins to form a loop which protrudes into the umbilical cord. Between the 8 and 16 mm stages, the small intestine increases rapidly in length and rotates around the axis of the superior mesenteric artery, moving counterclockwise (viewing the embryo from the ventral surface). Subsequently, further rapid elongation and coiling, beyond the capacity of the slower growing abdominal cavity, force the bulk of the developing intestine into the umbilical cord (physiological umbilical herniation). Thick mesenteric bands fix the duodenum and splenic flexure of the colon and prevent their entrance into the cord. The small intestine continues to elongate and coil inside the cord.

At about the 40 mm stage (10 weeks' gestation), the intestine re-enters the abdominal cavity. The control of re-entry has not been elucidated, but it occurs rapidly, with the jejunum returning first and filling the left half of the abdominal cavity, and the ileum filling the right half. The colon enters last, with fixation of the cecum close to the iliac crest and the ascending and transverse colon slanting upwards across the abdomen to the splenic flexure. Later development of the colon leads to elongation and establishment of the hepatic flexure and loose transverse colon. The earlier concept of the cecum descending after re-entry and during further colonic development has been discarded[70].

Auerbach's plexus in the small intestine appears at 9 weeks of gestation and Meissner's plexus at 13 weeks[36]. Peristalsis can be detected at about this time.

Lymphopoiesis is found at the 110 mm stage (15 weeks), and Peyer's patches may be well developed by the 160 mm stage (20 weeks)[7,19]. The latter have been quantitated by Cornes[19], and, in the jejunum and ileum, increase in number with gestational and postnatal age, reaching a plateau at approximately 10 years. Meconium appears at approximately 16 weeks, first in the terminal ileum, and later throughout the ileum.

CYTODIFFERENTIATION

During the period of extensive growth in length, the small intestine consists of a simple tube whose inner wall is a stratified epithelium approximately four cell layers thick. Shortly before the initiation of villus formation, this epithelium contains three cell types: undifferentiated epithelial cells, goblet cells, and enteroendocrine cells. By the beginning of the second trimester, following one to two weeks of cytodifferentiation, all of the cell types known to occur in adult human small intestine have appeared. Between 8 and 12 weeks of gestation, as the small intestine returns to its intra-abdominal position, the occluded duodenal lumen again becomes patent (a recent study indicates that only the region of the duodenal papilla is actually occluded),[67] and mucosal folds develop.

By the 10th to 11th week, well-defined villi develop, while primordial crypts are first seen between the 11th and 12th week. Thirteen distinct types of enteroendocrine cells have been identified in the fetal small intestine by 12 weeks of gestation[61]. By 22 weeks, fetal epithelial cells closely resemble those of adult human intestine[75] (*Figure 1.1*).

The rates of mitosis, cell turnover, and migration have been studied only in a single anencephalic human newborn[38]. The rate of cell migration from crypt to villus was 1/3 and 1/2 that found in mature human intestine[49,59].

As early as eight weeks, lymphocytes have been observed as isolated cells in the mucosal mesenchyme and were found in increasing numbers in the epithelium of

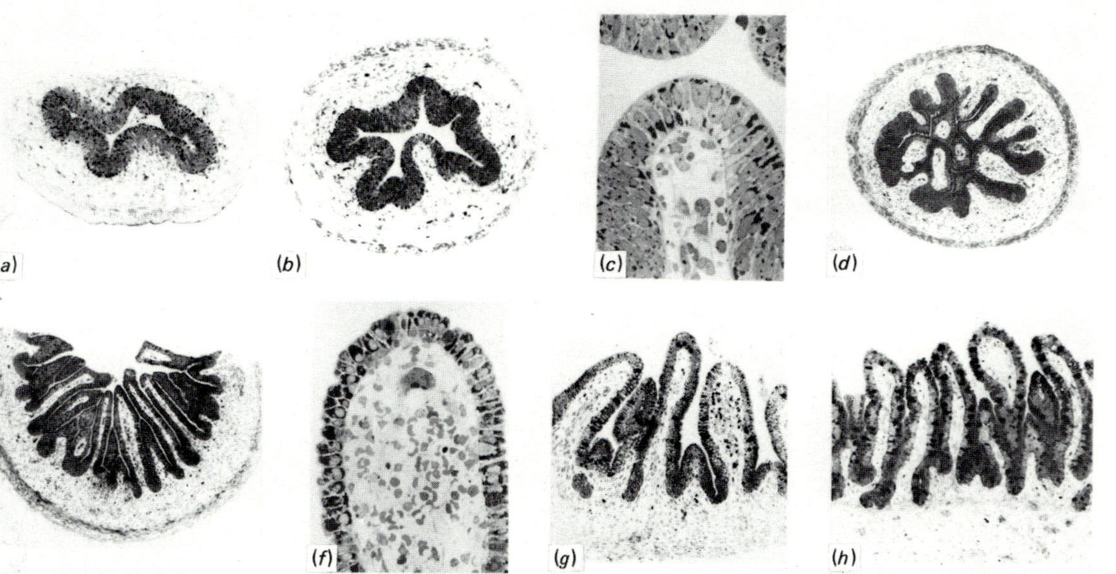

Figure 1.1 Morphological maturation of the human small intestine. (*a*) small intestine, 7–8 weeks, showing multilayered epithelium; (*b*) duodenum, 8 weeks, with rounded projections of epithelium to form primitive villus; (*c*) high power view of villus in (*b*) showing lack of nuclear polarity; (*d*) duodenum, 9 weeks, demonstrating 'occlusion' of lumen by actively proliferating villi; (*e*) duodenum, 11–12 weeks, showing well developed villi and early crypt formation; (*f*) high power view of (*e*) demonstrating more nuclear polarity than in (*c*); (*g*) ileum, 12–13 weeks, with well developed villi and immature crypts; (*h*) duodenum, 20 weeks – note more uniform villi, deep crypts, and numerous goblet cells. All tissues were embedded in Epon; sections are 1.0 μm, stained with Richardson's stain. Original magnifications (*a*), (*b*) × 130; (*c*), (*f*) × 400; (*d*) × 75; (*e*), (*g*), (*h*) × 80. Graciously provided by Dr Jerry S. Trier and Dr Pamela Colony. (From Grand *et al.*[30], courtesy of the Editor and Publishers, *Gastroenterology*)

11- to 20-week fetuses. The ultrastructure of the intraepithelial lymphocytes suggested that the cells were capable of pinocytotic activity[64]. In addition, M cells which have been implicated in antigen absorption[65,88] have tentatively been identified in fetal small intestine[61].

DEVELOPMENT OF TRANSPORT PROCESSES

Sugars

Glucose uptake has been studied using everted gut sacs obtained from human fetuses 11–19 weeks of gestation[49]. In the youngest fetuses studied, uptake against a concentration gradient was just detectable and rose 4-fold by 19 weeks. In the younger fetuses, jejunal uptake exceeded that in the ileum, but in older fetuses no such differential was found. By measuring transmural potential difference Jirsova *et al.*[44] and Levin *et al.*[55] confirmed these findings, although active transport could not truly be studied as no short circuit current was applied. At 11–12 weeks, the glucose-stimulated potential difference increased markedly and was 5-fold higher by 16 weeks[44], although at 21 weeks the potential difference had reached only 3/5 of the adult value[55]. In the ileum, no change in the potential difference was found in response to glucose until 14.5–16 weeks when the value equalled that in the jejunum[55]. Lactose generated no increase in potential difference up to 15 weeks; sucrose did produce a small increase. The absence of intestinal lactase, but presence of sucrase, at this fetal age will be discussed below.

Assuming that these changes in potential difference directly reflect true increases in sugar transport, and using data derived from a variety of perfusion studies, Younoszai has calculated that sugar transport (*Figure 1.2*) continues to develop

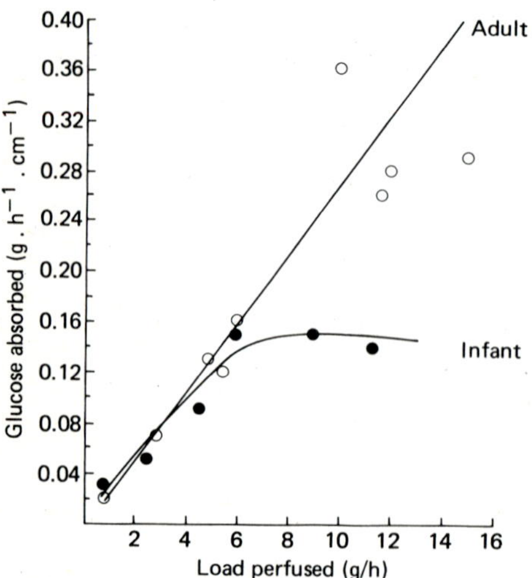

Figure 1.2 Glucose absorption during jejunal perfusion in humans. 'Infant' refers to subjects younger than 1 year of age. Data adapted from Younoszai[90]. (From CIBA Foundation Symposium 70, courtesy of the Publishers, *Development of Mammalian Absorptive Processes*)

postnatally[90]. In infants up to 12 months old, jejunal glucose absorption does not increase at perfusion rates greater than 4.5 g/h, whereas in the adult, jejunal glucose absorption is linear up to a perfusion rate of 30 g/h. Similarly, the apparent Km for glucose absorption is 5.8 mmol in infants[57] and 20 mmol or more for adults[25]. Thus, the capacity for glucose absorption rises markedly after the infancy period, either because of an increase in the number of sites of transport or because of an increased capacity of already developed sites[90].

Amino acids

Data for the absorption of amino acids in the developing human fetus derive solely from experiments using everted gut sacs[55]. Transport of L-alanine has been demonstrated, and, in this system, as with glucose, increases in transmural potential difference may occur. The potential difference generated does not change with gestational age and is similar to that reported for mature intestine[55]. Further studies of the development of amino acid absorption are needed, especially since different classes of amino acids are absorbed by separate mechanisms[27].

Protein

Considerable information is available regarding the ability of fetal and neonatal intestine to absorb intact proteins, although little is known about the digestion and utilization of such protein *in utero*. Details of this process have been reviewed recently[81].

The normal human fetus derives IgG antibody transplacentally but the newborn fails to demonstrate IgA in secretions or serum. At 3–4 weeks of life, salivary IgA appears, and reaches normal adult levels by 6 weeks. IgA is absent from newborn intestinal epithelium, but it rises rapidly after birth[73]. Measurable quantities of serum IgA appear in most babies by 3 weeks of life. Human colostrum is particularly rich in IgA, and this antibody contains both antibacterial and antiviral activity[2]. Colostral antibody appears to resist degradation in the gastrointestinal tract of the neonate[72].

IgG is known to be absorbed intact from the gastrointestinal tract of the newborn,[52] as are bovine serum albumin, α-lactalbumin and other antigens[79]. Breast-fed babies appear to have greater protection from enteric infection[15,41] and septicemia[87] than formula-fed infants. The mechanism for the enhanced uptake of intact proteins is unknown, but its possible dependence upon pinocytotic activity has been suggested. In support of this hypothesis is the presence of pinocytotic vesicles ('meconium corpuscles') in the ileum of monkey and human fetuses and newborns[3,10,69]. Lev and Orlic have also demonstrated the ileal uptake of intact horseradish peroxidase after its instillation into the amniotic sac of term fetal monkeys[53]. The fate of such proteins absorbed intact has not been fully elucidated, but they presumably undergo lysosomal digestion[79].

Lipids

The functional demands for lipid absorption *in utero* are not known, yet there is increasing evidence that an enterohepatic circulation for biliary lipids exists, and that the fetal intestine is functionally active before birth. In electron microscopic studies, Kelley has demonstrated that the 10-week, human small intestine absorbs corn oil[46]. Lipid is absorbed from the lumen and is present in cytoplasmic vesicles after 2 hours of incubation; it then appears in the intercellular spaces and lamina propria. Several investigators have noted that biliary lipid secretion occurs as early as 22 weeks[14, 66]. The human fetal gall bladder contains cholesterol, lecithin and bile salts, principally the taurine conjugates of cholic and chenodeoxycholic acid. Fetal bile salt synthesis from cholesterol, and conjugation with both taurine and glycine, have been demonstrated to occur in an *in vitro* liver organ culture model by 15 weeks of gestation[22, 31]. In the human, ileal uptake of bile acids matures postnatally[23].

The meconium, but not the bile or serum, of newborn infants contains the secondary, bacterially produced bile acids, lithocholic and deoxycholic acid. As these are not normally present following birth, nor found again until a few days of age, they are most likely of maternal origin, providing further evidence for active secretion of bile acid *in utero*[71].

The function of pancreatic enzymes and bile acids in the processing of the considerable quantities of lipid present in the amniotic fluid before birth is unexplored.

Following birth, the pre-term infant, and to a lesser extent, the full-term infant, absorb lipid inefficiently. Indeed, in the neonate, the intraluminal phase of lipid absorption is incomplete. Bile salt concentrations are often below the critical micellar concentrations required for the formation of mixed micelles[83], and fecal lipid of newborn infants contains unhydrolyzed glycerides, principally monoglycerides, which suggests either incomplete solubilization of intraluminal lipid or possibly a mucosal defect in lipid intake[83]. Lipid absorption improves during the first 4–6 weeks of life from a low of 65–70 percent of intake for many small premature infants, to nearly 80–85 percent of intake in the full-term newborn.

This improvement is closely correlated with an increase in intraluminal and serum[74] bile salt concentrations. Using stable isotope techniques it has been shown that bile acid synthesis is diminished in the full-term infant when compared to the adult[82]. In the premature infant, this is further reduced[84]. However, when prematures are studied after delivery from mothers treated with corticosteroids or phenobarbital during pregnancy, the infants' bile salt pool size and intraluminal bile salt concentrations are nearly twice those of infants of untreated mothers and equal to values found in the full-term infants[84]. These findings suggest that normally the intestinal absorption of bile salts is reduced in premature infants, and that multiple factors, including medication administered to the mother during pregnancy, influence the functional maturity of the liver and the gastrointestinal tract in the developing infant.

The mucosal phase of lipid absorption is relatively unexplored in either developing animal or human models. There is little information concerning the synthetic pathway for triglyceride synthesis from absorbed monoglycerides or fatty acid, or data concerning the protein synthesis necessary for chylomicron formation. In rats, fatty acid uptake and esterification have been shown to be inversely related to age from suckling to adult[42], but a recent study in groups of children 0–19 months and 20–38 months found little difference between these age groups[40]. Much more information concerning the critical steps in lipid absorption is needed before the mechanisms responsible for the improvement in lipid absorption during development are fully understood.

Vitamin B_{12}

The metabolism of this vitamin during human development has been extensively reviewed by others[32, 50]. Vitamin B_{12} is readily transferred across the human placenta by a mechanism which does not require transcobalamin II[32]. The fetal plasma contains both transcobalamin I and II, plus a third B_{12} binding protein termed fetal transcobalamin (FTC) whose function is unknown; it does not act as a transfer protein from tissue to tissue (e.g. liver to bone marrow), and is not present in adult plasma[50]. The human fetus actively takes up the vitamin, and its pattern of distribution is somewhat different from that in the adult[68]. In fetuses studied in mid-gestation, the liver contained the greatest concentration of the vitamin by comparison to the other organs, but it was 1/3 the values for mature liver. Luhby and colleagues have demonstrated that the term human newborn can absorb 75–95 per cent of a tracer dose of ^{59}Co-cyanocobalamin, a value higher than that for control adults (27–70 per cent)[58]. Luhby's data also suggest that the enhanced absorption of the vitamin in the first few days of life may be intrinsic factor-independent. Indeed, low intrinsic factor secretion at this age is known to occur[1]. Intrinsic factor-independent absorption of vitamin B_{12} has not been verified in the human, but does occur in the newborn rat[11, 28] and is apparently related to the pinocytotic absorption of intact proteins. Considerable data are needed regarding not only possible intrinsic factor-independent B_{12} absorption in the human, but also the developmental biochemistry of the ileal receptor mechanism.

DEVELOPMENT OF ENZYMES

The most extensively studied area of human intestinal development is that of enzyme ontogenesis, and the data available show considerable differences in the patterns obtained in the human when compared to studies of the most commonly used experimental animals[37] (*Figure 1.3*).

Sucrase, maltase, isomaltase (α-glucosidases)

Sucrase, maltase and palatinase (isomaltase) are all at levels comparable to those in mature intestine even in the youngest fetuses studied. Except for an increase at

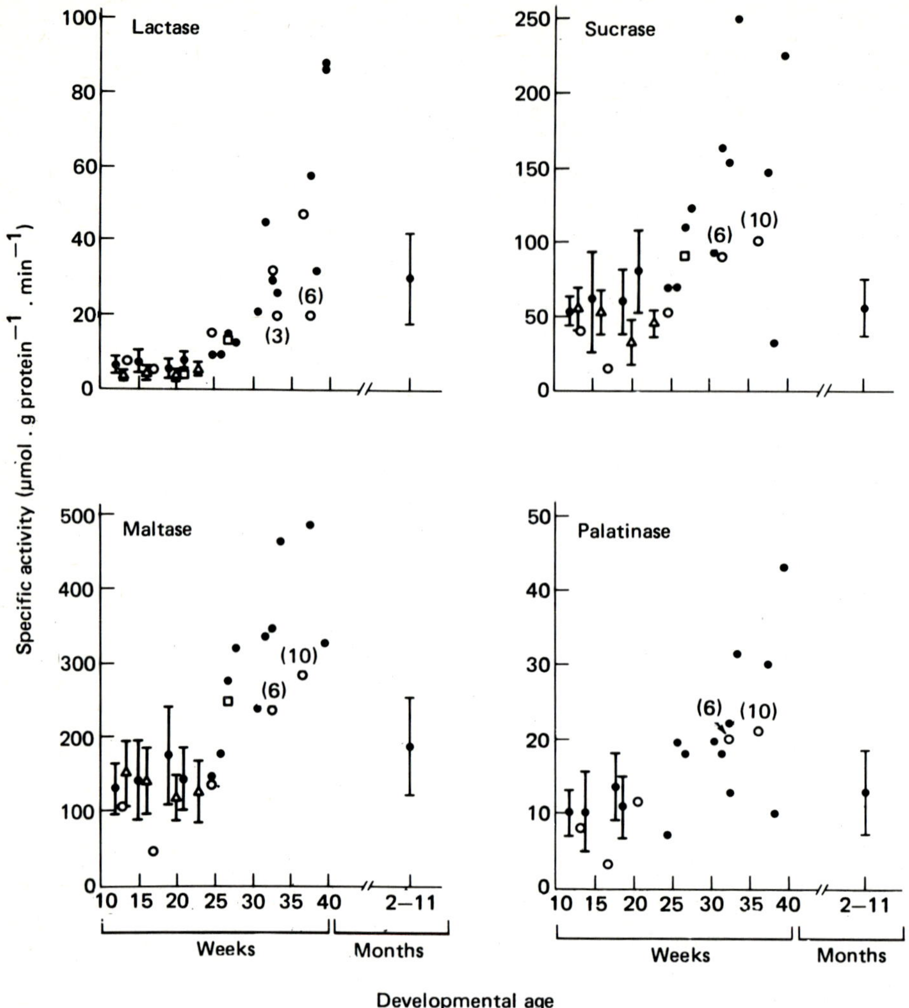

Figure 1.3 Development of disaccharidase activities in human fetal jejunum. Data adapted from references 20,21 (○), 43 (△), (4) (●). Normal gestation is 40 weeks in the human. Numbers in parentheses refer to number of observations. (From Grand *et al.*[30], courtesy of the Editor and Publishers, *Gastroenterology*)

term, the activities remain unchanged throughout development[5,6]. The α-glucosidases show maximal specific activity in the proximal jejunum in 17–24 week old fetuses, a distribution comparable to that found in adults[63]. These patterns are considerably different from those seen in experimental animals, where α-glucosidase activities begin to rise only in the suckling period, paralleling the fall in lactase activity[37]. Precocious induction of α-glucosidase activity can be achieved in animals after corticosteroid treatment, but no data are available regarding control by hormones during human development.

Lactase

Lactase activity is detectable, but at very low levels from 12 to 24 weeks of gestation when it begins to increase[5,8]. Toward the end of gestation a marked enhancement in activity occurs, bringing the levels at term to 2–4 times the values later found in normal infants 2–11 months of age[6]. Some time after birth, lactase levels apparently fall, but available data are insufficient to permit an estimation of the exact timing of this postnatal decline. Similarly, the mechanism by which the late gestational rise occurs has not been studied. As in adults, the highest specific activity of lactase in fetuses of 17–24 weeks' gestation is obtained in the proximal jejunum, and the overall pattern is comparable to that seen in adults[5,63].

The similarity of this pattern of lactase development to that seen in experimental animals is intriguing. In the rat, rabbit, cat, and guinea pig, lactase levels increase markedly in the last few days of gestation, remain high during the nursing period, and undergo a post-weaning decline to adult levels[37,45]. In most studies, lactase levels cannot be increased once the adult values are reached, although occasional data to the contrary have appeared[13,86]. Hypophysectomy or thyroidectomy will prevent the post-weaning decline in the rat if performed early in the suckling period, and thyroxine will establish precocious maturation if given during nursing[89].

In the human, the possibility of a relationship between intestinal lactase levels and endocrine status has not been investigated. While the overall pattern of lactase development in the human appears to be similar to that in experimental animals, the timing is quite different. The late gestational rise in the human occupies the entire third trimester, whereas in experimental animals it occurs late in the third trimester. The subsequent decline in activity in experimental animals occurs as nursing is completed, while the decline in the human is prolonged and is probably independent of nursing. The lactase levels found in normal infants 2–11 months old are comparable to those in the 34-week fetus; however, they are lower than those in full-term intestine ($29.9 \pm 11.2\,\mu\text{moles}\cdot\text{g protein}^{-1}\cdot\text{min}^{-1}$) with a range which overlaps that found in normal adults[54,63].

Interestingly, there is a marked late gestational rise in human fetal cortisol production[30] which correlates well with the increase in disaccharidase activities in fetal intestine. However, the sensitivity of the developing human intestine to changes in the levels of cortiocosteroids has not been investigated.

In view of the late gestational rise in lactase activity, it is of interest that so few premature newborns demonstrate clinical intolerance to lactose. Indeed, in a recent study, premature infants fed a lactose-containing formula showed comparable numbers of stools, weight gain and serum albumin levels when compared to an age-matched control group fed a formula in which lactose was replaced by glucose[30]. Although in some studies, lactose absorption, as measured by blood glucose levels, appears to be impaired in the premature infant, diarrhea does not necessarily accompany the performance of lactose tolerance tests[12]. Thus, despite the potential for lactose intolerance in premature infants, it appears relatively uncommonly.

An extensive discussion of the genetic control of adult lactose intolerance is beyond the scope of this review and is discussed elsewhere[45]. Nevertheless, it is of interest that lactose intolerance occurs in approximately 20 percent of Caucasians and 80–90 percent of non-Caucasians by or before age 5 years[18, 45]. Recent studies have also shown that at and after 5 years, lactase levels in intestinal biopsies become more variable than those in younger subjects, that a group with low lactase levels is identifiable, and that milk intolerance occurs in some of these patients[51, 85]. Lactose is not necessary to maintain normal lactase levels, as galactosemic children fed lactose-free diets from birth have normal lactose tolerance later in life[47].

Alkaline phosphatase

Alkaline phosphatase activity is detectable in the jejunum in 11-week old fetuses, and rises 4-fold by 23 weeks of gestation, but at this time is still considerably lower than the levels reported for mature jejunum[20]. These biochemical data correlate well with the histochemical findings reported by Lev *et al.*[54] A recent study reports an electrophoretically distinguishable fetal form of alkaline phosphatase, which was replaced by the adult form of intestinal alkaline phosphatase at about 38–42 weeks gestation[62].

Peptidases

Studying a variety of dipeptidases in homogenates of human fetal intestine, Lindberg has found that, at all ages, the highest specific activities occur in the proximal small intestine, but that there is no significant increase in specific activities with age from 11 to 23 weeks of gestation[56]. In contrast, Auricchio *et al.*[9] found the highest peptidase activities between 16 and 22 weeks gestation in the distal third of the intestine, although the difference among intestinal segments was not statistically significant. The γ-glutamyl peptidase was higher in fetuses than adults or children, while aminopeptidase A was significantly lower than in adults or children. Dipeptidylaminopeptidase IV and carboxypeptidase were at adult levels in the youngest fetuses. Oligoaminopeptidase increased over the period studied to achieve adult levels. At comparable fetal ages, the hydrolysis of glycyl-tripeptide is equally active in jejunum and ileum and is unchanged by gestational age[44]. By contrast, leucine aminopeptidase activity rises with gestational age, and by 16 weeks acquires a significant proximal to distal difference, the distal values being twofold greater than the proximal[44]. The significance of the early differentiation of these enzyme systems is unclear at present.

The development of enteropeptidase (enterokinase) has been studied in human fetuses[4, 5]. The data demonstrate that the enzyme appears late in gestation and increases 2-5-fold by the first year of life.

Lysosomal enzymes

An extensive investigation of the development of intestinal lysosomal enzymes has been published[5]. There was no significant difference between the mean values of α-glucosidase, β-galactosidase, and arylsulfatase in the youngest and oldest fetuses studied. However, the activities of β-glucuronidase, N-acetyl-β-glucosaminidase and acid phosphatase showed a significant tendency to increase with gestational age, while β-glucosidase activity fell significantly. These data demonstrate the early maturation of the lysosomal enzyme system in the human intestine (*Figure 1.4*). They also point out that biochemical identification of lysosomal hydrolases is possible at a time in gestation when organized lysosomal structures cannot be seen

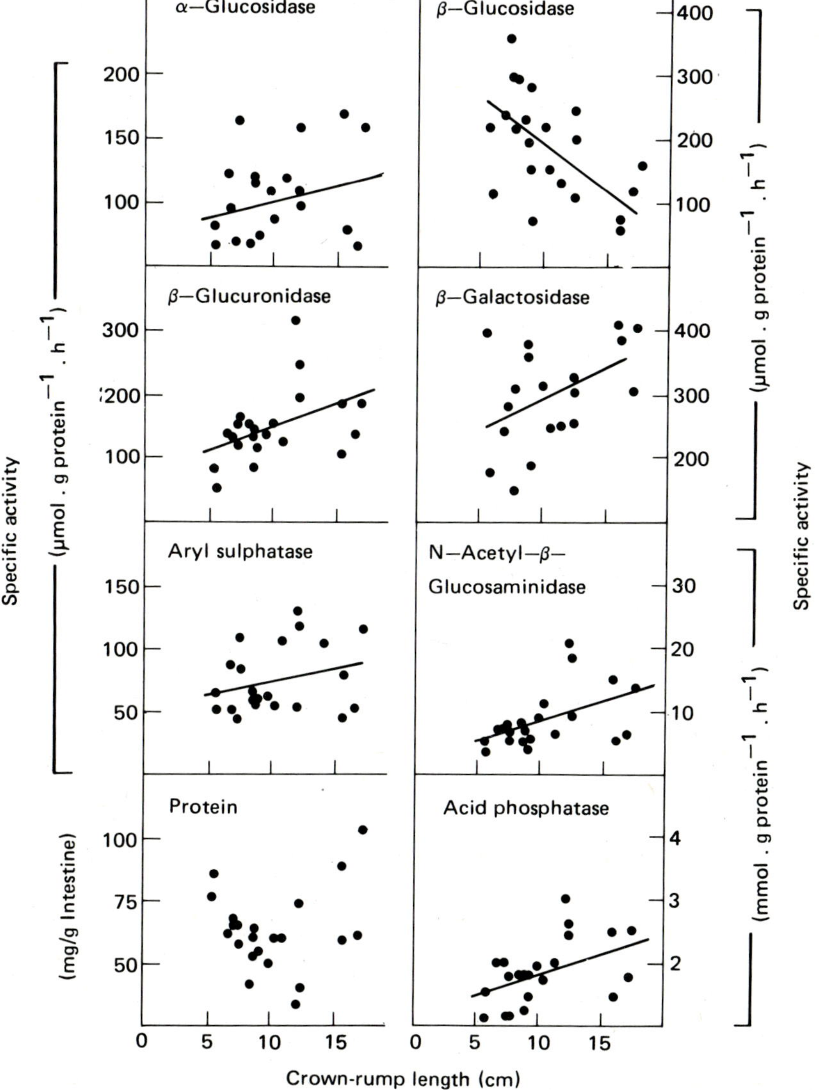

Figure 1.4 Development of lysosomal hydrolases in human fetal jejunum. Calculated linear regression is shown for each enzyme. For further details *see*[5]. (From Grand *et al*[30] courtesy of the Editor and Publishers, *Gastroenterology*)

with the electron microscope. Thus, until 13–14 weeks, the time when lysosomes can be seen ultrastructurally, the lysosomal hydrolases are either free in the cytosol or are packaged in a manner which is not identifiable morphologically. Considerable further work is needed to elucidate the significance of these findings.

POSTNATAL DEVELOPMENT

As discussed above, the human small intestine is morphologically mature at the time of birth, but some of its functions are not yet fully developed. Three areas of current activity are the investigation of the incompleteness of the intestinal permeability barrier, the role of lingual and breast milk lipases in lipid digestion in newborns, and the appearance of intestinal flora.

Ultrastructural examination of fetal intestine has revealed the presence of surface invaginations and endocytic vesicles in the distal intestinal cells, similar to the structures observed in rat intestine prior to closure, when uptake of intact macromolecules ceases at weaning[17]. These structures may permit uptake of intact macromolecules and if this capability persists into the neonatal period may allow passage of antigens as well as making the infant more susceptible to infection. There is evidence that the newborn intestine does have increased permeability to macromolecules compared to older infants[80]. Udall *et al.*[76] demonstrated decreased antigen penetration following colostrum feeding, suggesting that there may be a 'mucosal growth factor' in colostrum which accelerates intestinal maturation. In addition, recent studies in neonatal and more mature rabbits have documented a decreased level of immunoreactive BSA in serum with increasing age showing that this antigen is transported intact in newborns, but that permeability is lost with maturation[77,78].

In newborns the overall process of lipid absorption is less efficient than in adults, although, for their size, infants consume more lipid, which may constitute 40–50 percent of their total calories[34]. At least part of the reduced lipid absorption is due to immaturity of pancreatic function and low levels of pancreatic lipase[91] and immaturity of synthesis and secretion of bile salts[82–84]. It has recently been demonstrated that human breast milk contains a bile salt stimulated lipase which is active in infants' intestine[26,39]. This lipase is found only in milk from primates and Fredrikzon *et al.*[26] suggest that it may function in enhancing utilization of vitamin A. In contrast to the low activity at birth of pancreatic lipase, Hamosh and Hand[35] demonstrated that lingual lipase increased dramatically in rats after birth. In the newborn infant, lingual lipase initiates lipid hydrolysis in the stomach and probably compensates for low pancreatic lipase activity, as well as helping to overcome the temporary bile salt deficiency[34].

The postnatal acquisition of intestinal flora has also begun to receive increased attention. The fetal intestine is sterile. Subsequent bacterial colonization depends upon the type of feeding and gastric acidity. In the first few hours after birth, small quantities of enterococci and coliforms may be found. If breast feeding ensues, from day 1–4 *Lactobacillus bifidus* is the predominant organism found in the intestine. Human milk contains several growth promoting factors for this organism, thereby preventing undue growth of enteric pathogens. Human milk also contains bacteriostatic proteins, lactoferrin and lysozyme; the former preferentially binds iron and inhibits growth of *E. coli*, while the latter, in conjunction with IgA, facilitates bacterial wall digestion[43].

If formula is fed from day one, the intestinal flora rapidly include *Lactobacillus acidophilus*, coliforms, enterococci and anaerobes. *Bacteroides* species can be found in breast-fed infants late in the first month.

The reduced gastric acidity of the neonatal stomach[1] undoubtedly permits bacterial colonization of the small intestine, but the functional significance of these variations in flora are not completely understood. Several workers have noted the absence of secondary bile acids from the duodenal bile or stools of newborns for up to several days, indicating that the flora responsible for this metabolic process are absent[71]. Furthermore, Chiles *et al.*[16] have recently shown that flora responsible for hydrolysis of lactose are absent from the colon for at least seven days after birth. The accumulating data support the contention that intestinal flora participate in the adaptive responses of the neonatal intestine to the extrauterine environment.

CONCLUSION

In contrast to the most thoroughly studied laboratory animals, the small intestine of the human newborn is largely mature both structurally and functionally. Recent evidence suggests that deficiencies in pancreatic lipase and in bile salt synthesis and secretion are compensated for by availability of both breast milk lipase and lingual lipase.

The major functional deficiency appears to be the increased permeability of the newborn intestine to macromolecules which may play a significant role in some disease states, especially those involving immune responses to foreign antigens.

Acknowledgements

Supported in part by USPHS Research Grants (Nos. AM-14523 and HD-14498) from the National Institutes of Health.

References

1 AGUNOD, M., YAMAGUCHI, N., LOPEZ, R., LUHBY, A. L. and GLASS, G. B. J. Correlative study of hydrochloric acid, pepsin and intrinsic factor secretion in newborns and infants. *American Journal of Digestive Diseases*, **14,** 400–414 (1969)

2 AMMANN, A. J. and STIEHM, E. R. Immune globulin levels in colostrum and breast milk and serum from formula- and breast-fed newborns. *Proceedings of the Society for Experimental Biology and Medicine*, **122,** 1098–1099 (1966)

3 ANDERSEN, H., BIERRING, F., MATTHIESSEN, M. and EGEBERG, J. On the nature of the meconium corpuscles in human foetal intestinal epithelium. *Acta Pathologica et Microbiologica Scandanavica*, **61,** 377–393 (1964)

4 ANTONOWICZ, I. The role of enteropeptidase in the digestion of protein and its development in human small intestine. In *Development of Mammalian Absorptive Processes*, 169–187. CIBA Foundation Symposium 70, Amsterdam, Excerpta Medica. (1979)

5 ANTONOWICZ, I., CHANG, S. K. and GRAND, R. J. Development and distribution of lysosomal enzymes and disaccharidases in human fetal intestine. *Gastroenterology*, **67,** 51–58 (1974)

6 ANTONOWICZ, I. and LEBENTHAL E. Developmental pattern of small intestinal enterokinase and disaccharidase activities in the human fetus. *Gastroenterology*, **72,** 1299–1303 (1977)

7 AREY, L. B. *Development Anatomy*. Philadelphia, W. B. Saunders Company (1974)

8 AURICCHIO, S., RUBINO, A. and MURSET, G. Intestinal glycosidase activities in the human embryo, fetus and newborn. *Pediatrics*, **35,** 944–954 (1969)

9 AURICCHIO, S., STELLATO, A. and DeVIZIA, D. Development of brush border peptidases in human and rat small intestine during fetal and neonatal life. *Pediatric Research*, **15,** 991–995 (1981)

10 BIERRING, F., ANDERSEN, H., EGEBERG., J., BRO-RASMUSSEN, F. and MATTHIESSEN, M. On the nature of the meconium corpusles in human fetal intestinal epithelium. *Acta Pathologica et Microbiologica Scandanavica*, **61,** 365–376 (1964)

11 BOASS, A. and WILSON, T. H. Development of mechanisms for intestinal absorption of vitamin B 12 in growing rats. *American Journal of Physiology*, **204,** 101–104 (1963)

12 BOELLNER, S. W., BEARD, A. G. and PANOS, T. C. Impairment of intestinal hydrolysis of lactose in newborn infants. *Pediatrics*, **36,** 542–550 (1965)

13 BOLIN, T. D., PIRELA, R. C. and DAVIS, A. E. Adaptation of intestinal lactase in the rat. *Gastroenterology*, **57,** 406–409 (1969)

14 BONGIOVANNI, A. M. Bile acid content of gallbladder of infants, children and adults. *Journal of Clinical Endocrinology*, **25,** 678–685 (1965)

15 BULLEN, C. L. and WILLIS, A. T. Resistance of the breast-fed infant to gastroenteritis. *British Medical Journal*, **3,** 338–343 (1971)

16 CHILES, C., WATKINS, J. B., BARR, R., TSAI, P. Y. and GOLDMANN, D. A. Lactose utilization in the newborn: role of colonic flora. *Pediatric Research*, **13,** 365 (1979)

17 CLARK, S. L. The ingestion of proteins and colloidal materials by columnar absorptive cells of the small intestine in suckling rats and mice. *Journal of Biophysical and Biochemical Cytology*, **5,** 41–50 (1959)

18 COOK, G. C. Lactase activity in newborn and infant in Baganda. *British Medical Journal*, **1,** 527–530 (1967)

19 CORNES, J. S. Number, size and distribution of Peyer's patches in the human small intestine. *Gut*, **6,** 225–233 (1965)

20 DAHLQVIST, A. and LINDBERG, T. Fetal development of the small intestinal disaccharidase and alkaline phosphatase activities in the human. *Biology of the Neonate*, **9,** 24–32 (1965)

21 DAHLQVIST, A. and LINDBERG, T. Development of the intestinal disaccharidase and alkaline phosphatase activities in the human fetus. *Clinical Science*, **30,** 517–528 (1966)

22 DeBELLE, R., BROWN, A., BLACKLOW, N., DONALDSON, R. M. and LESTER, R. Organ culture of fetal liver. A new modal system. *Pediatric Research*, **7,** 292 (1973)

23 DeBELLE, R. C., VAUPSHAS, V., VITULLO, B. B., HABER, L. R., SHAFFER, E., MACKIE, G. G., OWEN, H., LITTLE, J. M. and LESTER, R. Intestinal absorption of bile salts: immature development in the neonate. *Journal of Pediatrics*, **94,** 472–476 (1979)

24 DEREN, J. J. Gastrointestinal development. In *Intrauterine Development*, edited by A. C. Barnes, 221–232. Philadelphia, Lea and Febiger (1968)

25 FORDTRAN, J. S. and INGELFINGER, F. J. Absorption of water, electrolytes and sugars from the human gut. In *Handbook of Physiology*, edited by C. F. Code, 1491–1512. Washington, D.C., American Physiology Society (1968)

26 FREDRIKZON, B., HERNELL, O., BLACKBERG, L. and OLIVECRONA, T. Bile salt-stimulated lipase in human milk. Evidence of activity *in vivo* and of a role in the digestion of milk retinol esters. *Pediatric Research*, **12,** 1048–1052 (1978)

27 FREEMAN, H. J. and KIM, Y. S. Digestion and absorption of protein. *Annual Review of Medicine*, **29,** 99–116 (1978)

28 GALLAGHER, N. D. and FOLEY, K. E. Corticosteroids and the development of intrinsic factor mediated vitamin B 12 absorption in the rat. *Gastroenterology*, **62,** 247–254 (1972)

29 GRAND, R. J. and MONTGOMERY, R. K. Development of the gastrointestinal tract. In *Food Intolerance*, edited by R. K. Chandra. New York, Elsevier/North Holland (in press)

30 GRAND, R. J., WATKINS, J. B. and TORTI, F. M. Development of the human gastrointestinal tract. *Gastroenterology*, **70,** 790–810 (1976)

31 HABER, L. R., VAUPSHAS, V., VITULLO, B. B., SEEMAYER, T. A. and DeBELLE, R. C. Bile acid conjugation in organ culture of human fetal liver. *Gastroenterology*, **74,** 1214–1223 (1978)

32 HALL, C. A. Congenital disorders of vitamin B 12 transport and their contribution to concepts (editorial). *Gastroenterology*, **65,** 684–686 (1973)

33 HAMILTON, W. J., BOYD, J. D. and MOSSMAN, H. W. *Human Embryology*. Baltimore, Williams and Wilkins Company (1966)

34 HAMOSH, M. A review. Fat digestion in the newborn: role of lingual lipase and preduodenal digestion. *Pediatric Research*, **13,** 615–622 (1979)

35 HAMOSH, M. and HAND, A. R. Development of secretory activity in serous cells of the rat tongue. *Development Biology*, **65,** 100–113 (1978)

36 HART, S. L. and MIR, M. S. Adrenoceptors in the human foetal small intestine. *British Journal of Pharmacology*, **41,** 567–569 (1971)

37 HENNING, S. J. Postnatal development: Coordination of feeding, digestion and metabolism. *American Journal of Physiology*, **241,** 199–214 (1981)

38 HERBST, J. J., SUNSHINE, P. and KRETCHMER, N. Intestinal malabsorption in childhood. *Advances in Pediatrics*, **16,** 11–64 (1969)

39 HERNELL, O., BLACKBERG, L. and OLIVECRONA, T. Human milk lipases. In *Textbook of Gastroenterology and Nutrition in Infancy*, edited by E. Lebenthal, 347–354. New York, Raven Press (1981)

40 HEUBI, J. E., PARTIN, J. C., SCHUBERT, W. K. and McGRAW, C. A. Small intestinal mucosal fatty acid uptake and esterification in infants and children. *Pediatric Research*, **13,** 781–782 (1979)

41 HINTON, N. A. and MacGREGOR, R. R. A study of infections due to pathogenic serogroups of *Escherichia coli. Canadian Medical Association Journal*, **79,** 359–354 (1958)

42 HOLTZAPPLE, T. G., SMITH, G. and KOLDOVSKY, O. Uptake, activation and esterification of fatty acids in the small intestine of the suckling rat. *Pediatric Research*, **9,** 786–791 (1975)

43 JELLIFFE, D. B. and JELLIFFE, E. F. P. *Human Milk in the Modern World*. Oxford, Oxford University Press (1978)

44 JIRSOVA, W., KOLDOVSKY, O., HERINGOVA, A., HOSKOVA, J., JIRASEK, J. and UHER, J. The development of the functions of the small intestine of the human fetus. *Biology of the Neonate*, **9,** 44–49 (1965)

45 JOHNSON, J. D., KRETCHMER, N. and SIMOONS, F. J. Lactose malabsorption: its biology and history. *Advances in Pediatrics*, **22,** 197–237 (1975)

46 KELLEY, R. J. An ultrastructural and cytochemical study of developing small intestine in man. *Journal of Embryology and Experimental Morphology*, **29,** 411–430 (1973)

47 KOGUT, M. D., DONNELL, G. N. and SHAW, K. N. F. Studies of lactose absorption in patients with galactosemia. *Journal of Pediatrics*, **71,** 75–81 (1967)

48 KOLDOVSKY, O. Hormonal and dietary factors in the development of digestion and absorption. *Current Concepts in Nutrition*, **1,** 135–206 (1972)

49 KOLDOVSKY, O., HERINGOVA, A., JIRSOVA, V., JIRASEK, J. E. and UHER, J. Transport of glucose against a concentration gradient in everted sacs of jejunum and ileum of human fetuses. *Gastroenterology*, **48,** 185–187 (1965)

50 KUMENTO, A. Studies on the serum binding of vitamin B 12 in the newborn human infant. *Acta Paediatrica Scandinavica*, **194,** (Suppl.) 12–55 (1969)

51 LEBENTHAL, E., ANTONOWICZ, I. and SHWACHMAN, H. Correlation of lactase activity, lactose tolerance and milk consumption in different age groups. *American Journal of Clinical Nutrition*, **28,** 595–600 (1975)

52 LEISSRING, J. C., ANDERSON, J. W. and SMITH, D. W. Uptake of antibodies by the intestine of the newborn infant. *American Journal of Diseases of Children*, **103,** 160–165 (1962)

53 LEV, R. and ORLIC, D. Uptake of protein in swallowed amniotic fluid by monkey fetal intestine in utero. *Gastroenterology*, **65,** 60–68 (1973)

54 LEV, R., SIEGEL, J. I. and BARTMAN, J. Histochemical studies of developing human fetal small intestine. *Histochemie*, **29,** 103–119 (1972)

55 LEVIN, R. J., KOLDOVSKY, O., HOSKOVA, J., JIRSOVA, V. and UHER, J. Electrical activity across human foetal small intestine associated with absorption processes. *Gut*, **9,** 206–213 (1968)

56 LINDBERG, T. Intestinal dipeptidases: characterization, development and distribution of intestinal dipeptidases of the human foetus. *Clinical Science*, **30,** 505–515 (1966)

57 LUGO-DE-RIVERA, C., RODRIGUEZ, H. and TORRES-PINEDO, R. Studies in the mechanism of sugar malabsorption in infantile infectious diarrhea. *American Journal of Clinical Nutrition*, **25,** 1248–1255 (1972)

58 LUHBY, A. L., GLASS, G. B. J. and SLOBODY, L. B. Studies on gastric mucoprotein secretion in infants and children. *American Journal of Diseases of Children*, **89,** 517 (1954)

59 MacDONALD, W. C., TRIER, J. S. and EVERETT, N. B. Cell proliferation and migration in the stomach, duodenum and rectum of man: radioautographic studies. *Gastroenterology*, **46,** 405–417 (1964)

60 MOORE, K. L. *The Developing Human.* Philadelphia, W. B. Saunders Company (1974)

61 MOXEY, P. C. and TRIER, J. S. Endocrine cells in the human fetal small intestine. *Cell and Tissue Research*, **183,** 33–50 (1977)

62 MULIVOR, R. A., HANNIG, U. L. and HARRIS, H. Developmental change in human intestinal alkaline phosphatase. *Proceedings of the National Academy of Sciences, USA*, **75,** 3909–3912 (1978)

63 NEWCOMER, A. D. and McGILL, D. B. Distribution of disaccharidase activity in the small bowel of normal and lactase deficient subjects. *Gastroenterology*, **51,** 481–488 (1966)

64 ORLIC, D. and LEV, R. An electron microscopic study of intraepithelial lymphocytes in human fetal small intestine. *Laboratory Investigation*, **37,** 554–561 (1977)

65 OWEN, R. L. and JONES, A. L. Epithelial cell specialization within human Peyer's patches: an ultra-structural study of intestinal lymphoid follicles. *Gastroenterology*, **66,** 189–203 (1974)

66 POLEY, J. R., DOWER, J. C., OWEN, C. A. Jr. and STICKLER, G. B. Bile acids in infants and children. *Journal of Laboratory and Clinical Medicine*, **63,** 838–846 (1964)

67 POSTISILOVA, V., TERSTIANSKA, G. and VRANAKOVA, V. Contribution to early development of the small intestine in the human embryo. *Folia Morphologica* (*Prague*), **25,** 333–337 (1977)

68 RAPPAZZO, M. E., SALMI, H. A. and HALL, C. A. The content of vitamin B 12 in adult and foetal tissue: a comparative study. *British Journal of Haematology*, **18,** 425–433 (1970)

69 RUEBNER, B. H., KANAYAMA, R., BRONSON, R. T. and BLUMENTHAL, S. Meconium corpuscles in intestinal epithelium of fetal and newborn primates. *Archives of Pathology*, **98,** 396–399 (1974)

70 SCAMMON, R. E. and KITTELSON, J. A. The growth of the gastrointestinal tract of the human fetus. *Proceedings of the Society for Experimental Biology and Medicine*, **24,** 303–307 (1962)

71 SHARP, H. L., PELLER, J., CAREY, J. B. and KRIVIT, W. Primary and secondary bile acids in meconium. *Pediatric Research*, **5,** 274–279 (1971)

72 SHEARMAN, D. J. C., PARKIN, D. M. and McCLELLAND, D. B. L. Demonstration and function of antibodies in the gastrointestinal tract. *Gut*, **13,** 483–499 (1972)

73 SOUTH, M. S. IgA in neonatal immunity. *Annals of the New York Academy of Science*, **176,** 40–48 (1971)

74 SUCHY, F. J., BALISTRERI, W. F., HEUBI, J. E., SEARCY, J. E. and LEVIN, R. S. Physiologic cholestasis: elevation of the primary serum bile acid concentration in normal infants. *Gastroenterology*, **80,** 1037–1041 (1981)

75 TRIER, J. S. and MADARA, J. L. Functional morphology of the mucosa of the small intestine. In *Physiology of the Digestive Tract*, edited by L. R. Johnson, 925–961. New York, Raven Press (1981)

76 UDALL, J. N., PANG, K., SCRIMSHAW, N. S. and WALKER, W. A. The effect of early nutrition on intestinal maturation. *Pediatric Research*, **13,** 409 (1979)

77 UDALL, J. N., PANG, K., FRITZE, L., KLEINMAN, R. and WALKER, W. A. Development of gastrointestinal mucosal barrier. I. The effect of age on intestinal permeability to macromolecules. *Pediatric Research*, **15,** 241–244 (1981)

78 UDALL, J. N., COLONY, P., FRITZE, L., PANG, K., TRIER, J. S. and WALKER, W. A. Development of gastrointestinal mucosal barrier II: the effect of natural versus artificial feeding on intestinal permeability to macromolecules. *Pediatric Research*, **15,** 245–249 (1981)

79 WALKER, W. A. and ISSELBACHER, K. J. Uptake and transport of macromolecules by the intestine: possible role in clinical disorders. *Gastroenterology*, **67,** 531–550 (1974)

80 WALKER, W. A. Gastrointestinal host defense: importance of gut closure in control of macromolecular transport. In *Development of Mammalian Absorptive Processes*, 201–205. CIBA Foundation Symposium 70, Amsterdam, Excerpta Medica (1979)

81 WALKER, W. A. Intestinal transport of macromolecules. In *Physiology of the Gastrointestinal Tract*, edited by L. R. Johnson, 1271–1289. New York, Raven Press (1981)

82 WATKINS, J. B. Bile salt metabolism in the newborn. *New England Journal of Medicine*, **288,** 431–434 (1973)

83 WATKINS, J. B. Bile acid metabolism and fat absorption in newborn infants. *Pediatric Clinics of North America*, **21,** 501–510 (1974)

84 WATKINS, J. B., SZCZEPANIK, P., GOULD, J. B., KLEIN, P. D. and LESTER, R. Bile salt metabolism in the human premature infant. *Gastroenterology*, **69,** 706–713 (1975)

85 WELSH, J. D., POLEY, J.R., BHATIA, M. and STEVENSON, D. E. Intestinal disaccharidase activities in relation to age, race and mucosal damage. *Gastroenterology*, **75,** 847–855 (1978)

86 WEN, C. P., ANTONOWICZ, I. and TOVAR, E. Lactose feeding in lactose intolerant monkeys. *American Journal of Clinical Nutrition*, **26,** 1221–1228 (1973)

87 WINBERG, J. and WESSNER, G. Does breast milk protect against septicemia in the newborn? *Lancet*, **1,** 1091–1094 (1971)

88 WOLF, J. L., RUBIN, D. H., FINBERG, R., KAUFFMAN, R. S., SHARPE, A. H., TRIER, J. S. and FIELDS, B. N. Intestinal M cells: a pathway for entry of reovirus into the host. *Science*, **212,** 471–472 (1981)

89 YEH, K. and MOOG, F. Intestinal lactase activity in the suckling rat. *Science*, **182,** 77–79 (1974)

90 YOUNOSZAI, M. K. Jejúnal absorption of hexose in infants and children. *Journal of Pediatrics*, **85,** 446–448 (1974)

91 ZOPPI, G., ANDREOTTI, G., PAJNO-FERRARA, F., NJAI, D. M. and GABURRO, D. Exocrine pancreas function in premature and full term neonates. *Pediatric Research*, **6,** 880–886 (1972)

2
Ultrastructure of the small intestine

Kristin Henry

With the advent of the fibre-optic instruments[5, 11, 55] the small intestine throughout its length became accessible to biopsy by the peroral route, and thus available for electron microscopical study. Until then only surgical and autopsy material had been studied[33], tissues fraught with artefactual problems and difficulties in interpretation. Now there are many excellent texts, chapters and books devoted to small intestinal ultrastructure at both scanning, and transmission electron microscopical (TEM) levels in health and disease[15, 22, 35, 62, 63, 64]. As far as TEM is concerned it has been stated that there is no place for it in the routine diagnosis of diseases of the small intestine[10]. This rather defeatist attitude fortunately has not been universally accepted and there are now many conditions in which TEM provides a definitive diagnosis.

Two of the most important applications in which TEM is routinely used are in the field of gastrointestinal tumour pathology; and in the diagnosis of infectious gastroenteritis. One further contribution made by TEM is of enormous importance, and that is that by providing insight and knowledge of ultrastructure there has been improved interpretation at light microscopical level. However it cannot be sufficiently stressed that in order to extract the best results from TEM the investigator must not only be conversant with its normal appearance at EM level but should also be experienced in the diagnostic problems and aetiological considerations relating to intestinal disease; and always TEM should be carried out alongside the light microscopical findings.

The scanning electron microscope (SEM) has also been applied with much enthusiasm to the investigation of small intestinal mucosa and for pure aesthetic quality it would be difficult to improve on the beauty of the ghostly images and 'lunar landscapes' provided by some of these studies. Aestheticism apart, it has been claimed that SEM has provided no information which was either new or which could not have resulted from TEM. After all, scanning electron microscopy reveals only surface specialization and can contribute little information to the internal milieu of cells or to the cellular components and organisation of the tissue underlying surface epithelium, unless digestive techniques have been employed. This reviewer does not hold quite such a negative view as to the merits of SEM, and

it cannot be denied that the provision of three-dimensional images enable easier interpretation of structure. Recently defined cells have been further clarified and certain characteristics of intestinal surface epithelium previously thought to be fixation artefacts have been shown to be due to genuine structural differences[59]. Also where the surface is damaged in disease processes, scanning electron microscopy has provided useful information. Nevertheless, while accepting the value of scanning electron microscopy, albeit rather limited, the author will concentrate on, and illustrate only, the transmission electron microscopic (TEM) findings of the small intestinal mucosa.
The mucosa can be conveniently sub-divided into:

(1) the villous epithelium concerned with absorption;
(2) the generative epithelial cells of the crypts;
(3) various specialised cells found within the villi and crypt epithelium;
(4) the cellular components of the connective tissue of the intestine – lamina propria.

THE ABSORPTIVE EPITHELIUM OF THE VILLI

Villi are clothed by tall columnar cells interspersed by the mucus secreting goblet cells[3,4], and their morphology differs not only according to race[10], but also to anatomic location. In the duodenum the villi are much less regular than those in the jejunum and for this reason it has become customary to biopsy the jejunal mucosa just beyond the ligament of Treitz. Ileal villi are also regular but tend to be taller than those in the jejunum and contain increasing numbers of goblet cells as the large intestine is approached; it has been far less extensively studied than the jejunum in humans. The most important and numerous cell of the villous epithelium is the columnar absorptive cell, also known as the enterocyte. Complex interdigitation and desmosomal connections exist between the lateral aspects of neighbouring enterocytes, and at their apices they are held in close contact by a specialised junctional complex (*Figure 2.1*) which thus maintains structural continuity of the mucosa. Whether viewed at light microscopical, SEM or TEM levels, a most distinctive feature of the enterocyte is the apical 'brush' or striated border (*Figure 2.1*). This structure which had long intrigued light microscopists was one of the first to be elucidated by electron microscopy[1, 6, 12, 35]. It consists of a regular arrangement of microvilli of about 1 μm in length and 0.1 μm in diameter and which in the normal mucosa is coated by a glycocalyx or 'fuzzy coat'. This glycocalyx, rich in carbohydrates elaborated by the absorptive cells is believed not only to subserve a protective (immunological) function[7] but also to play an important role in the modification and/or presentation of luminal contents to the absorptive cells[31] by virtue of its enzymatic activity.

The individual microvilli are characterised by a trilaminar plasma membrane. Filaments present within the microvillous core extend down in bundles to insert within the transversely orientated fibrillary network at the cell apex and which together form the structure known as the 'terminal web' (*Figure 2.1*). The filaments

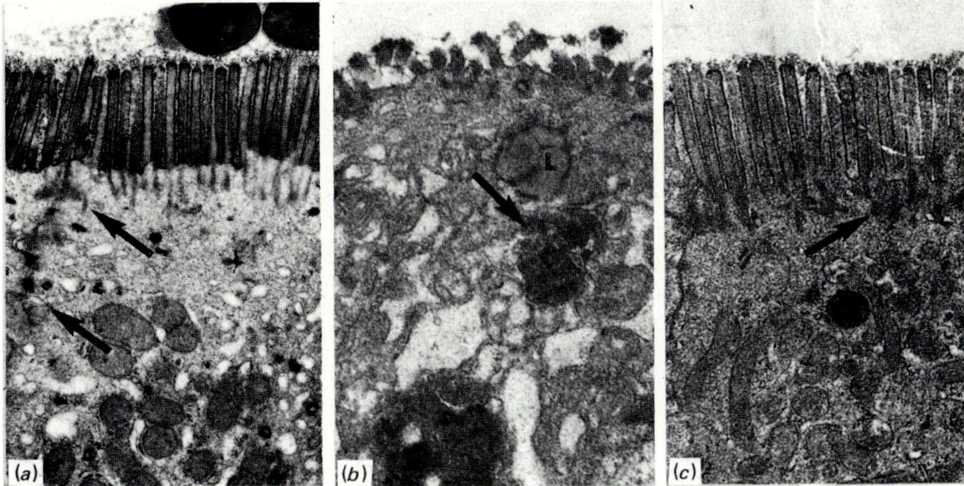

Figure 2.1 Enterocytes with striate border. (*a*) From a patient with the pre-malignant phase of alpha-chain disease showing microvilli of normal height coated by a well developed glycocalyx (arrows indicate the apical junctional complex) (*b*) From a patient with coeliac disease (gluten induced enteropathy). The microvilli are short and sparse and the glycocalyx poorly developed. Note the dilated endoplasmic reticulum, increased electron dense lysosomal structures – including a multivesicular body (arrow) – and a lipid inclusion (L). (*c*) From a patient with an enteroglucagon secreting tumour inducing mucosal hyperplasia (villi and enterocytes) with microvilli longer than normal. The arrow indicates the apical 'terminal web' composed of transversely orientated fibrils into which the fibrils from the microvillous cores insert. (× 12 000)

present in the microvillous cores have recently been shown to be actin[40]; myosin filaments present in the terminal web link the actin fibres of the individual microvilli so that the striate border subserves a contractile function. The striate border is best developed at the villous tips, which is also the zone where cell shedding occurs and thus is often referred to as the extrusion zone. Prior to cell extrusion there is individual cell death with increase in membrane permeability[49]. The striate border and apical zones of the enterocytes appear to be most vulnerable to change in certain diseases, of which the best defined are coeliac disease[37, 52] (*Figure 2.1*), tropical sprue[38], kwashiorkor[60] and other causes of malabsorption[8, 15]. Certain toxic agents of widely divergent nature, such as high acid states[25], ethanol[48, 51], and irradiation[63] also can induce cell damage and produce similar alterations; and it therefore seems that such changes in enterocyte morphology are of a non-specific nature and not necessarily the only cause of the malabsorptive state[2]. This view is supported by the fact that in two diseases which are known to be associated with profound malabsorption, namely α-chain disease and abetalipoproteinaemia the striate border reveals no abnormality (*Figure 2.1*).

Other characteristic features of enterocytes are their high content of mitochondria[64] a prominent Golgi system and the apically situated lysosomes (heterogeneous collections of acid hydrolase-containing organelles comprising the dense bodies, autophagic vesicles and multivesicular bodies, *Figures 2.1, 2.2*). There is also a well developed smooth and rough endoplasmic reticulum. A

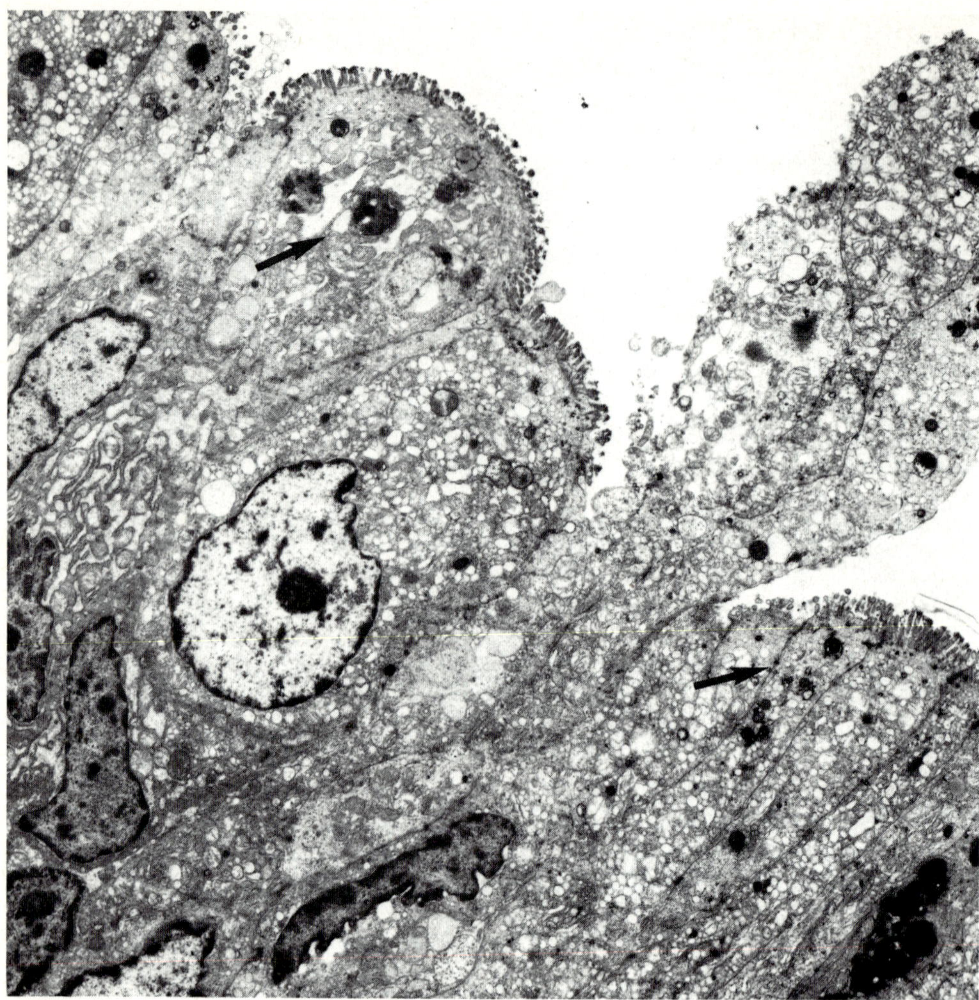

Figure 2.2 Shown here is an extrusion zone in a patient with coeliac disease and sub-total villous atrophy. Note in addition to the senescent cell, the very prominent dilatation of smooth endoplasmic reticulum, increased lysosomes (arrows) and abnormal striate border. In normal villi extrusion zones are present only at the villous tip. (× 3800)

prominent and dilated smooth endoplasmic reticulum is characteristic of senescent cells and extrusion zones[49] and a common finding in a variety of pathological states (*Figure 2.2*). The nucleus occupies the basal zone of the enterocytes, and it is in the lower half of the epithelium, which lacks junctional complexes, where there is marked variation in the degree of separation between the cell walls. Applied to the basal aspect of the enterocytes is a well formed but delicate basal lamina, which may in certain diseases, particularly coeliac disease, become thickened[56,57]. Detailed information relating to the absorptive function of enterocytes and the transfer of immunoglobulins are described in subsequent chapters and will not be considered further here.

CRYPT GENERATIVE EPITHELIUM

The crypt cells (*Figure 2.3*) are largely made up of the 'undifferentiated' precursors of the mature absorptive cells of thc villi[64]. In common with other immature cells they exhibit a high mitotic index, a high content of free ribosomes and poorly developed endoplasmic reticulum. The microvillous zone is also less well developed with fewer microvilli per cell and a less conspicuous glycocalyx. Complex interlocking with desmosomal attachments between crypt cells (including goblet and Paneth cells) is a feature and secretion granules are often observed at their luminal aspect[66]. Once the crypt cells reach the neck region and escape on to the luminal aspect maturation occurs[34]. It has been estimated that in the normal mucosa approximately three crypts serve one villus.

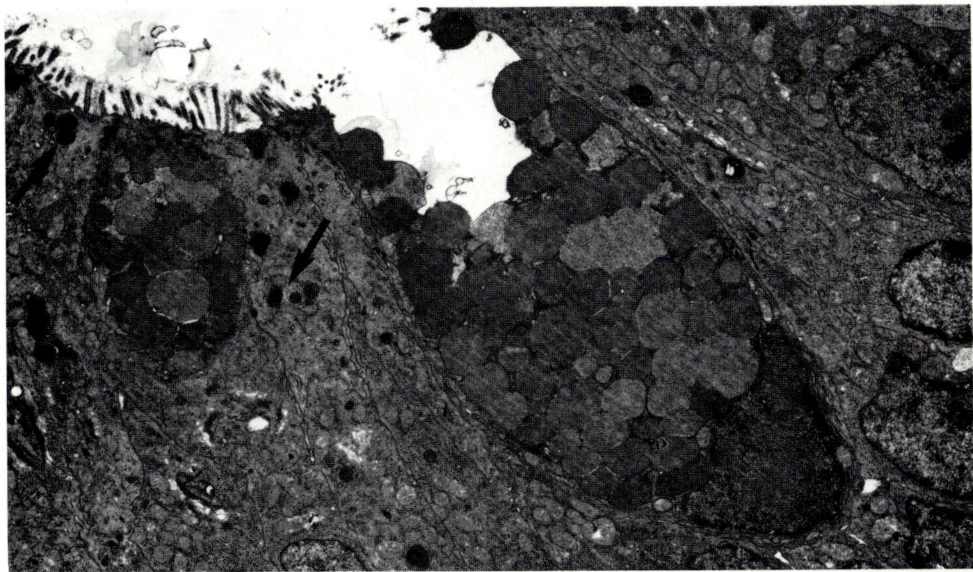

Figure 2.3 Crypt cells. Part of a normal crypt showing several generative cells rich in free fibrosomes, and a mucus secreting goblet cell which has discharged its apical content of mucus granules. Note the less well developed microvilli and the dark secretion granules (arrows) of the generative epithelium. (×3600)

SPECIALIZED MUCOSAL CELLS OTHER THAN ENTEROCYTES AND THEIR PRECURSOR CRYPT CELLS

The goblet cell

The goblet cell is a simple unicellular mucus secreting end cell incapable of division[39]. It is interspersed between the absorptive cells of the villi and the generative crypt cells with which it makes intimate contact and increases in number from the proximal to distal small intestine. Mucus is elaborated in the endoplasmic reticulum, packaged by the Golgi apparatus into mucus droplets[42] and finally discharged from the apex of the cell (*Figure 2.3*). Mucin has recently been shown to play an important role in the defence against infectious agents; and in influencing the bacterial flora of the gut. Its histochemical composition and alteration in health and disease are currently being actively explored. Filipe *et al.* have extended their studies of large intestinal mucin to the small intestine, having a particular interest in alterations in mucin secretion as a marker of potential neoplastic change[14, 23].

In the duodenum there are specialised submucosal mucous glands which connect with the crypts via ducts. These Brunner's glands have been proposed as the precursor cells of metaplastic gastric type epithelium found in the duodenum in conditions associated with a high acid environment[45].

Endocrine glands

A large group of specialised neurosecretory cells, the enteroendocrine cells, have now been defined in the gastrointestinal tract. Formerly such cells were described as argentaffin, argyrophil or enterochromaffin cells, either because of their affinity for silver or through their chromaffin reaction.

Until recently the most characteristic and numerous example was cited as the argentaffin-positive Kulchitscky cell, occurring at the base of the small intestinal crypts of Lieberkuhn. This complex family of cells has been the subject of much recent research and the number of definitive subtypes is still growing. The general term APUD cells has been proposed for this specialised system of cells based upon their functional role in secreting short chain polypeptide hormones and their uptake of and decarboxylation of the precursor substances of biological amines[16]. The APUD cell concept became linked with cells of neural crest origin; more recently the origin of APUD cells was extended to embrace cells originating from either neuroectodermal or specialised ectoderm[46]. One of the most extensively studied members of the group found in small intestine is the EC cell producing 5-hydroxytryptamine (serotonin), and which on the basis of its ultrastructural features and variation in content of different peptides has been subdivided into several subpopulations[24, 63]. Whether these enterochromaffin cells contain motilin[28] or not[29] it is of interest that duodenum in coeliac disease has been found to contain increased numbers of enterochromaffin cells[58]. At electron microscopical level the presence of specific membrane bound secretory granules is common to all APUD cell types; though depending upon the substance elaborated the secretory granules vary in size from 100 to 500 nm. There is also variability in the contour of the specific granules, with the most pleomorphic granules being those found in the various subtypes of EC (argentaffin or enterochromaffin) cells (*Figure 2.4*) and some of the most uniform, and also the largest granules (250–500 nm) being those found in the enteroglucagon producing EG or L cells, and which in addition to their uniform spherical shape lack the 'halo' separating the secretory products from the surrounding membrane. Other features shown by enteroendocrine cells are that the specific secretory granules are located in a subnuclear position, and that the cells extend to the luminal surface of the crypts and bear microvilli at their apical surface (*Figure 2.4a*). However, due to frequent tangential

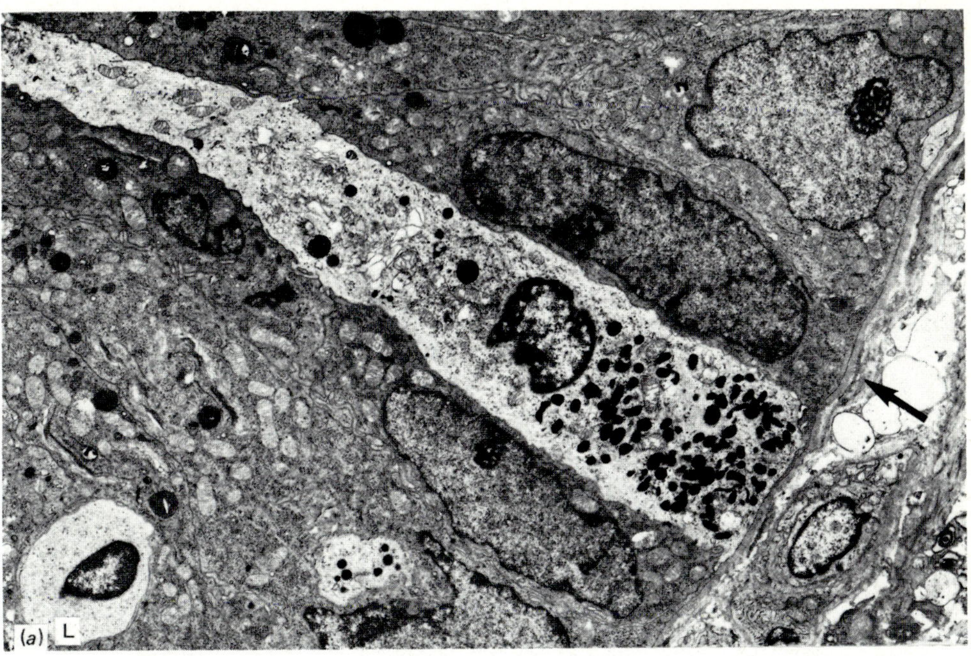

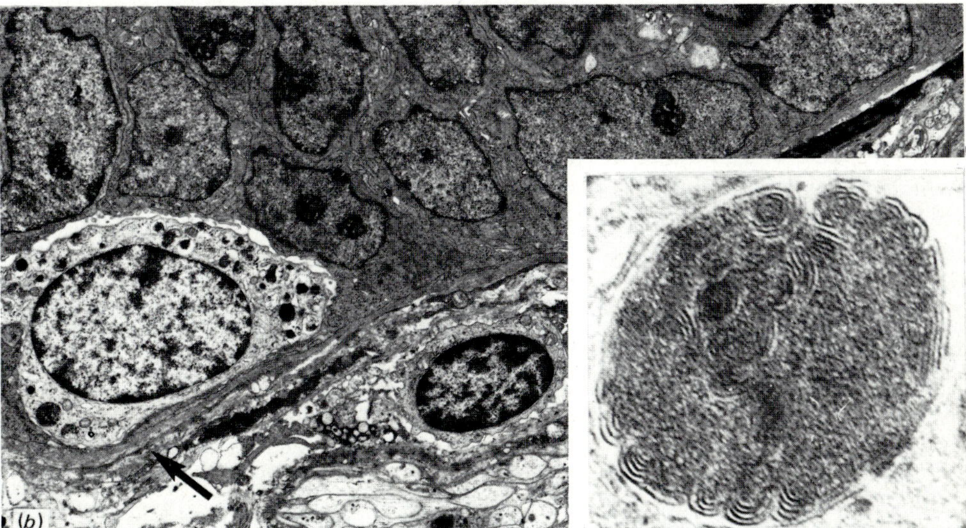

Figure 2.4 Crypt cells. (*a*) Low power view of an enterochromaffin (EC) cell. In this favourable section it can be seen that the apex of the cell extends to the crypt lumen and bears microvilli. Note the basal position of the specific granules and the intraepithelial lymphocyte (L). (*b*) A mast cell has infiltrated above the basal lamina of a crypt and superficially resembles an enteroendocrine cell. The inset reveals the classical scroll-like pattern of its granules. Arrows indicate the basal laminae. (*a*) ×3900; (*b*) ×3680; (*inset*) ×71 800

sectioning many of these cells appear to be located just above the basal lamina. It is then important not to mistake infiltrating mast cells for enteroendocrine cells (*Figure 2.4b*) which at low magnification they can mimic. It is not proposed to discuss these cells further since they are covered in a later section of this monograph.

The M cell

Owen and Jones[44] observed a specialised cell in the epithelium covering Peyer's patches. The cell was termed the M cell because of its membranous surface, which not only lacked a terminal web, microvilli and a glycocalyx, but was characterised by surface microfolds due to irregular surface projections and convolutions. These surface folds are shown to greatest advantage with the scanning electron microscope[44]. The M cell has an intimate relationship to intraepithelial lymphocytes which accumulate within the complex membranous folds or pockets and also closely interdigitate with neighbouring columnar cells. Using horseradish peroxidase as a tracer substance Owen[43] showed that M cells selectively take up protein and thus function as specialised cells in antigen absorption. Whether the M cell is a highly specialised or unique absorptive cell or whether it is entirely unrelated to the enterocyte still remains to be elucidated. The possibility that the M cell represents a particular kinetic phase of enterocyte activity relating to the presence of migrating lymphocytes should also be considered.

Paneth cell

The Paneth cell has long been recognised as a constant member of the normal crypt cell population, but, despite its distinctive and easily visualised appearance both at light and electron microscopical levels, its function has until recently been cloaked in mystery. Its characteristic ultrastructural features of large electron dense membrane bound granules extruding from the apex of the cells (*Figure 2.5*) together with a highly developed rough endoplasmic reticulum and Golgi apparatus had always suggested a specialised secretory function. One such possible function has been linked with zinc metabolism since this metal is present in higher concentration in Paneth cell granules than in any other tissue in the body; and abnormalities in the fine structure of Paneth cell granules corrected by zinc administration[4] have been observed in the rare familial disease acrodermatitis enteropathica in which there is a low plasma zinc level. Only comparatively recently, since the demonstration by Erlandsen *et al.* that Paneth cells contain lysozyme[20] – indeed in jejunum they are the main source of lysozyme[47] – and immunoglobulin[21,50], has this cell become recognised as of supreme importance in the phagocytosis of microorganisms[18,19]. Indeed evidence has emerged that the Paneth cell, albeit a fixed cell of the crypts, is not only a member of the mononuclear phagocytic cell system but also influences the intestinal bacterial flora by phagocytosis and/or secretion of lysozyme. Thus the observations by Ward, Ferguson and Eastwood[67] that Paneth cells and lysozyme activity are reduced in

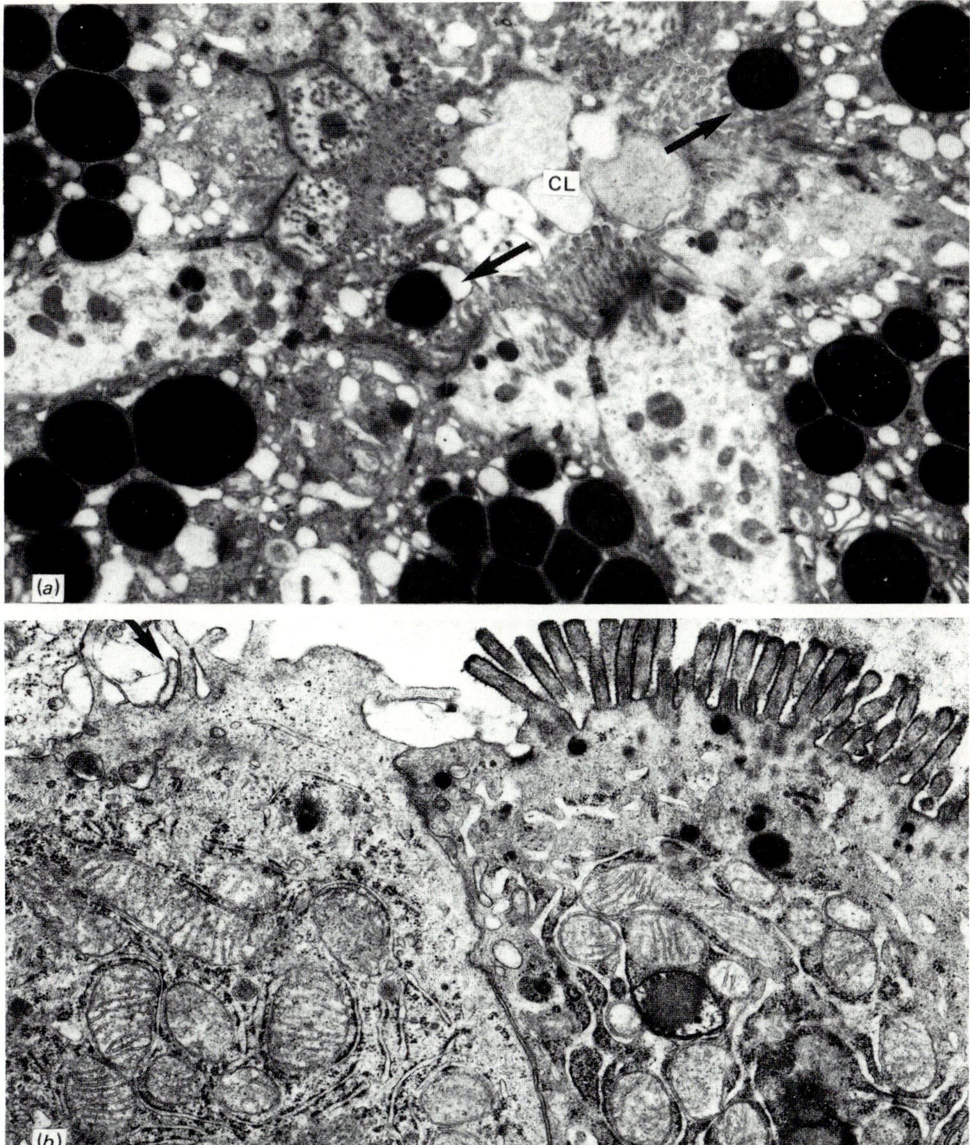

Figure 2.5 Crypt cells. (*a*) Transverse section of a crypt showing Paneth cells with granules (arrows) extruding into the crypt lumen (CL); Note the apical microvilli. (*b*) Part of a 'tuft' cell with narrow apex bearing few microvilli (arrow) adjacent to a normal crypt cell. Note the numerous mitochondria. (*a*) ×9700; (*b*) ×16 500

coeliac disease is of considerable interest. However, others[53] were unable to confirm a reduction in the Paneth cells. Nevertheless the Paneth cell is emerging as a cell of immense importance in intestinal homeostasis and EM studies of qualitative as well as quantitative alterations in its granule content are likely to prove rewarding.

The tuft cell

This cell, recognised throughout the alimentary tract as well as in respiratory tissue[30, 41] has been called a variety of names since first observed in mice and later in human intestine[63]. Its incidence varies considerably from less than 1 per cent of the colonic crypt cell population to much higher levels as, for example, in rat stomach. The term 'tuft' derives from its long and well developed microvilli which project into the lumen and are often seen to best advantage in scanning electron microscopy[30]. The apex of the cell is narrow compared to neighbouring crypt cells (*Figure 2.5*) and although it bears only approximately 90 microvilli, these are extremely well developed with filamentums extending into the cytoplasm and interdigitating with the cytoplasmic organelles. No secretory activity has been demonstrated and no features to suggest these cells belong to the APUD cell series. Other cytological features which distinguish the 'tuft' cell from other crypt cells are the high mitochondrial content[30] and an often prominent apical vesiculation of smooth endoplasmic reticulum. Their function is still debated and range from that of a specialised sensory receptor cell to a specialised absorptive cell.

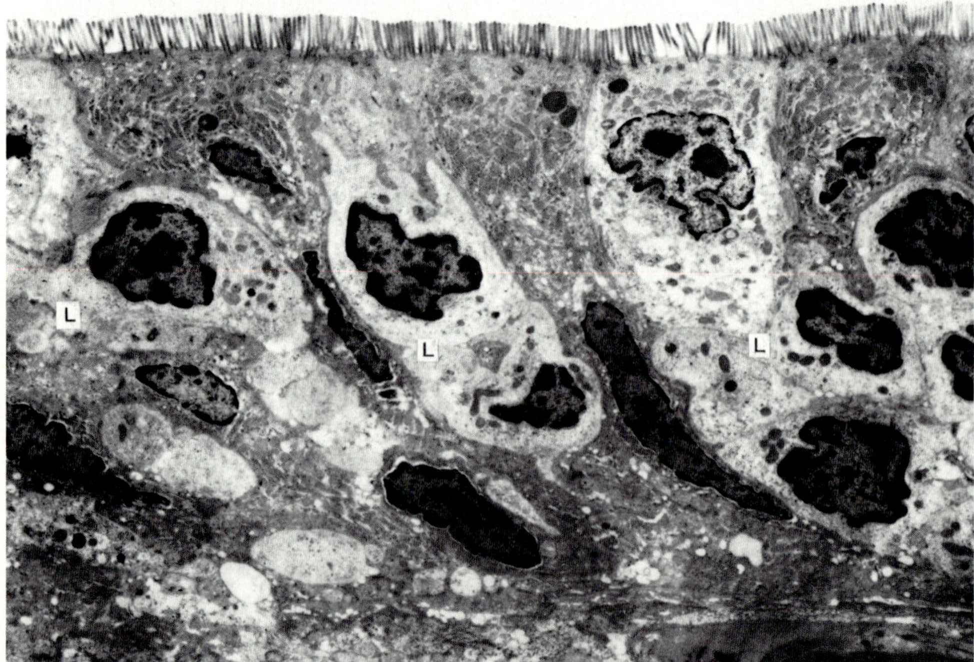

Figure 2.6 **Intraepithelial lymphocytes (theliolymphocytes) are a constant finding in normal mucosa, and are increased in many intestinal disorders. Illustrated here are increased numbers (L) in a patient with the premalignant phase of α-chain disease. Note the 'mature' appearance of the lymphocytes and absence of any plasmacytoid differentiation. (×3600)**

Intraepithelial lymphocytes

Lymphocytes are a constant finding in the crypts and villous epithelium[22, 65] in both normal individuals and those with intestinal disease. The majority of such intraepithelial lymphocytes or theliolymphocytes are, in the author's experience, mature cells (*Figure 2.6*), but less well differentiated or blast forms[36] are also encountered; intraepithelial lymphocytes showing plasma cell differentiation have not been observed. They are derived from the indiginous lymphoid population of the lamina propria (*see below*) and can often be seen crossing the basal lamina. Close contact exists between the lymphocyte and epithelial cell cytoplasm. Conditions in which their numbers are significantly increased include coeliac disease[57] and tropical sprue[38], diseases known to be related to immunological mechanisms[56] and more specifically to cell mediated mechanisms. Recent studies have tended to confirm their T-cell nature[54] and in this context it is of interest that lymphocytes present in the relatively normal epithelium overlying the plasma cell/lymphoplasmacytoid infiltrate in premalignant α-chain disease show no plasma cell differentiation (*Figure 2.6*). On the other hand, other than a sometimes prominent lysosomal content, there are no ultrastructural features present as described in some T cells: the nuclei lack a convoluted appearance, there is no cytoplasmic glycogen and there are no cytoplasmic microfibrils. Nevertheless evidence is accumulating that intraepithelial lymphocytes are distinct from lamina propria lymphocytes; and on the basis of one recent study on the preparation and purification of mouse small intestine, lymphocytes formed two quite distinct populations[13].

LAMINA PROPRIA

Lamina propria is the name given to the connective tissue of the intestinal mucosa. The term is somewhat inappropriate for not only is the lamina propria important in providing structural integrity to the absorptive epithelium by means of its connective tissue and smooth muscle cells, but it also forms a major component of the peripheral or secondary lymphoreticular system.

Lymphoreticular tissue

Lymphocytes and plasma cells are scattered throughout the connective tissue of the intestinal mucosa and are also found as aggregates of non-encapsulated lymphoid tissue with formation of germinal centres lying beneath the mucosal epithelium. Such lymphoid aggregates increase in number and size towards the terminal ileum, where they are known as Peyer's patches, and appendix. As mentioned above and shown in *Figure 2.6* lymphocytes are also found in the epithelium and there is still controversy as to the origin of these intraepithelial lymphocytes[3]. Part of the problem appears to lie in the failure to separate the lamina propria lymphocytes from the intraepithelial lymphocytes. Where such separation has been achieved[13] then, at least in mice, the intraepithelial lymphocytes appear to belong to a different subtype of lymphocyte. The immunological function of gut associated lymphoid tissue or GALT will be discussed elsewhere in this monograph. Suffice it to say that in human lamina propria the majority of lymphoid cells which consist of plasma cells, plasma cell precursors (plasmablasts) and small mature lymphocytes appear on morphological grounds to be of B lymphocytic origin. So also are the

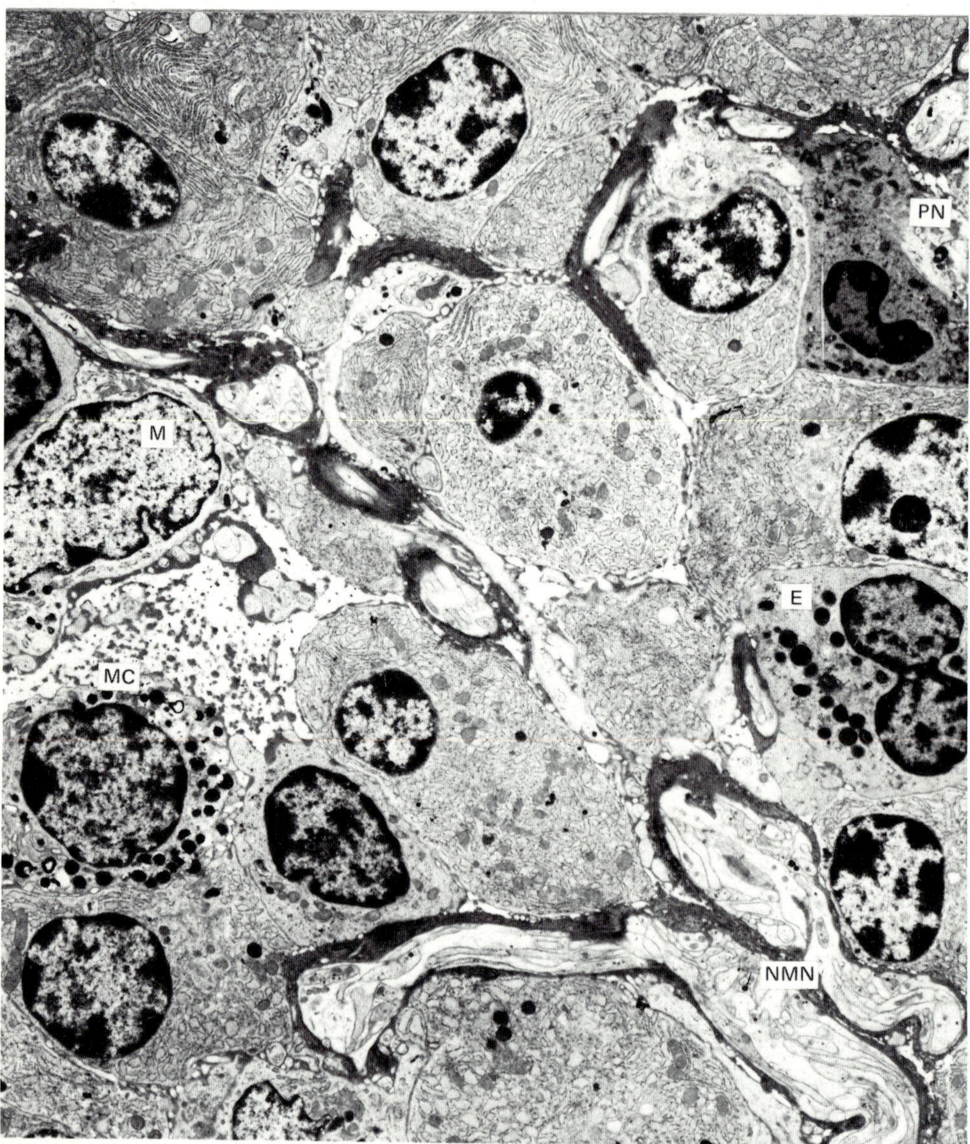

Figure 2.7 Lamina propria containing in addition to numerous plasma cells, a polymorph neutrophil (PN), an eosinophil (E), a mast cell (MC) and a macrophage (M). The tubular profiles (NMN) are non-myelinated nerve fibres. Gluten challenge in a patient with treated coeliac disease. (×3800)

lymphoid follicles and germinal centres, which are comparable to similar B cell structures occurring throughout the body. There is however one important difference and that is that even the larger lymphoid aggregations are unencapsulated. And as described earlier there is a very distinctive cell, the M cell, found in the epithelium overlying the lymphoid aggregates which appears to provide a very special environment for lymphoid cells migrating upwards into the epithelium.

Plasma cells are increased in a non-specific manner in a wide variety of small intestinal disorders[17, 38, 52, 57] of which the three most striking examples are untreated coeliac disease (*Figure.2.7*), some cases of tropical sprue and in the premalignant phase of α-chain disease (*Figure 2.8b*). However, on ultrastructural grounds alone it is not always possible to distinguish between the reactive plasma cells in coeliac disease or sprue on the one hand, and the monoclonal/neoplastic but premalignant plasma cells on the other[17, 27]. Interestingly, where there is migration of lymphocytes into the overlying epithelium in α-chain disease these lymphocytes never show plasma cell differentiation (*Figure 2.6*); and it is probable that here too they represent a non-B and possible T cell population of lymphocytes. Plasma cells are characterised by an eccentric nucleus with a peripherally condensed nuclear chromatin pattern, a cytoplasm with an abundance of rough endoplasmic reticulum often filled with electron-dense secretory products, and a prominent Golgi apparatus, the structure responsible for the perinuclear 'halo' or hof observed at light microscopical level. The cytoplasm may also contain globular secretory products (Russell bodies), crystals of immunoglobulin and spherical electron-dense lysosomal structures. Plasmablasts contain a more centrally placed nucleus with a large and generally central nucleolus, and a much less well developed rough endoplasmic reticulum and Golgi apparatus. They can and must be distinguished from immunoblasts, which may also be found in the lamina propria as well as within the germinal centres of lymphoid follicles, by the more abundant and coarser chromatin pattern of their nuclei and their content of rough endoplasmic reticulum[27]. In the author's view the majority of primary lymphomas of the gastrointestinal tract (including those complicating coeliac disease and α-chain disease) are not only of a B lymphocytic nature but are also in a significant proportion composed of plasma cells or a mixture of plasmablastic or plasmacytoid cells[26]. Reports of gastrointestinal involvement by a T cell malignancy appear to be exceptionally rare and thus the paper on intestinal involvement in a patient with Sézary syndrome is of considerable interest[9].

Macrophages (mononuclear phagocytic cells)

Macrophages are a constant component of the lamina propria though their numbers vary considerably. They are increased in 'non-specific' inflammation, in many infections, e.g. Whipple's disease[32], and are usually present in impressive numbers in coeliac disease. In most conditions there is nothing specific about their ultrastructural findings in that they all exhibit increased numbers of primary and secondary lysosomes lacking any special features. There are however two exceptions which will permit a definitive diagnosis to be made on the basis of the

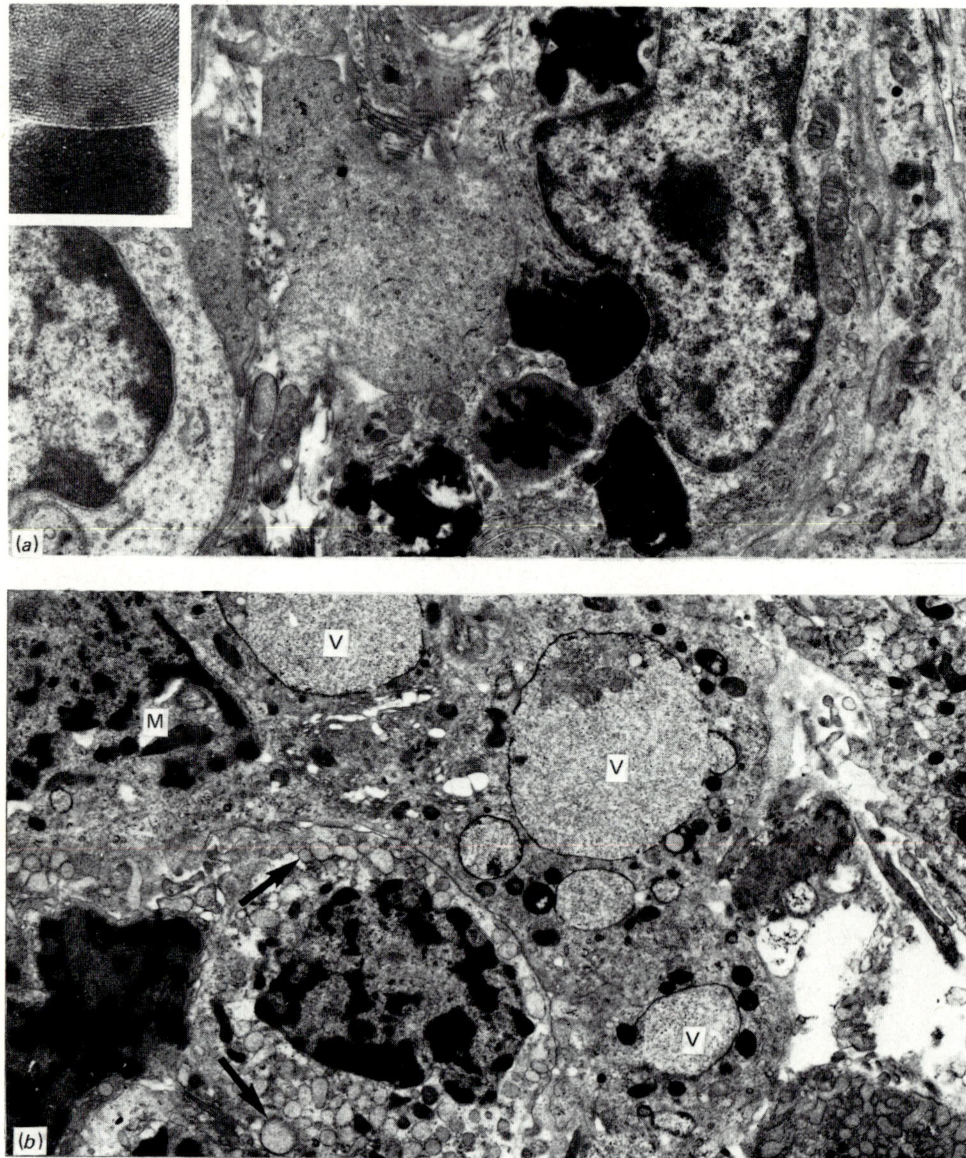

Figure 2.8 Macrophages. (*a*) Shows a macrophage from a pathogen-free piglet which is filled with abundant dense polymorphous secondary lysosomes, characteristic of the effects of neomycin ingestion; and which in the inset reveal a crystalline structure. (*b*) An example of a macrophage from a patient with the premalignant phase of α-chain disease in which there are large vesicular lysosomes (V) containing finely granular material similar to that present in the cisternae of the rough endoplasmic reticulum of the plasma cells (arrows). M, nucleus of macrophage. (*a*) ×10 500; (*inset*) ×113 000; (*b*) ×5900

macrophage inclusions. One is in Whipple's disease[15] where the degraded bacteria can be identified within the phagolysosomes and the other is following therapy with, or experimentally fed, neomycin which induces large amorphous and exceedingly dense macrophage inclusions (*Figure 2.8a*) showing at high magnification a characteristic paracrystalline structure (*Figure 2.8a*, inset)[61]. In a third disease, namely premalignant α-chain disease, the condition may be suspected by the presence of macrophages containing very large, relatively lucent lysosomes, which at high magnification can be seen to contain granular electron-dense material similar to that present in the adjacent plasma cells (*Figure 2.8b*).

Other cellular components

Varying in number in the so-called normal state, and in inflammatory conditions are mast cells, polymorph neutrophils and eosinophils. Mast cells are often

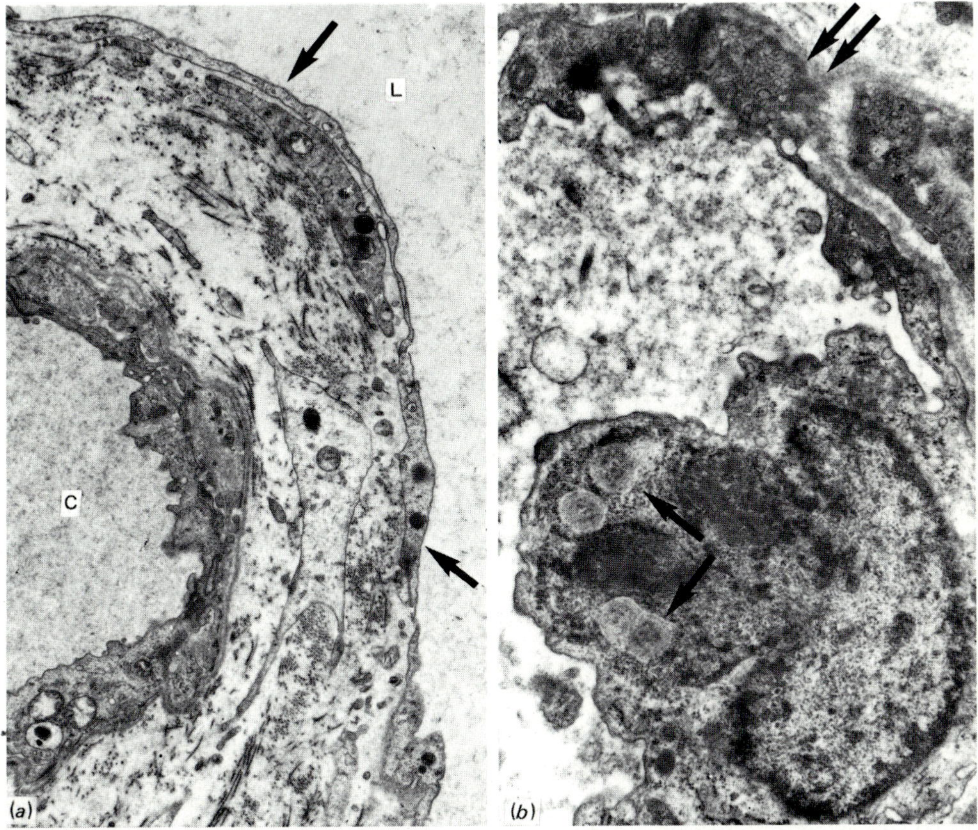

Figure 2.9 Vessels. (*a*) In this field is part of a capillary (C) and a lacteal (L). Note the attenuated lining (arrow) of the lacteal in comparison to the capillary. (*b*) Part of a capillary with markedly hyperplastic nucleus. Note nuclear bodies (arrows) and the basal lamina (double arrow). Gluten challenge in coeliac disease. (*a*) ×6700 (*b*) ×2500

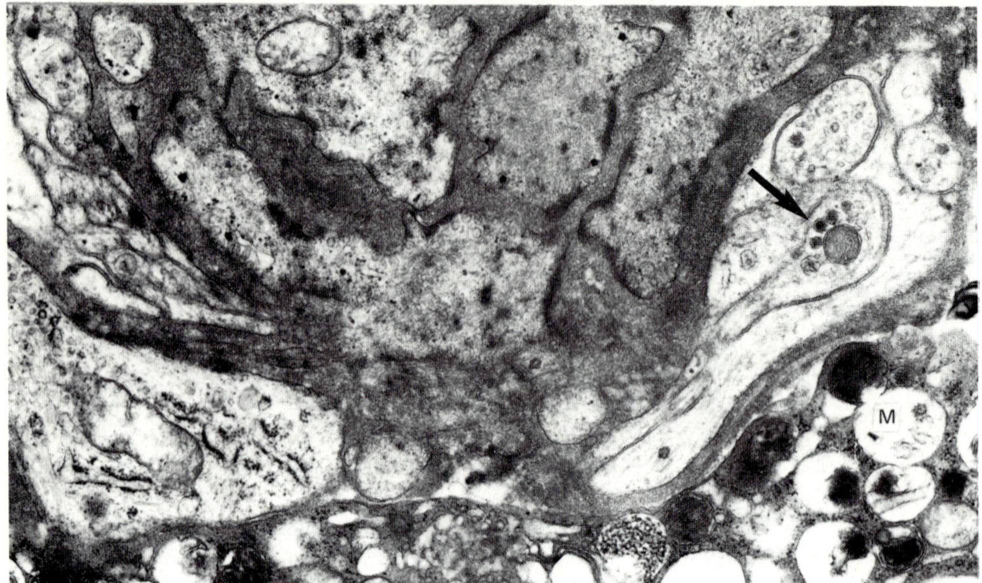

Figure 2.10 Transversely sectioned smooth muscle bundle, adjacent to which is a non-myelinated nerve fibre containing dense core granules (arrow) and part of the cytoplasm of a mast cell (M) (× 18 000)

extremely numerous in gluten-induced enteropathy and other non-specific inflammatory infiltrations, where they are often seen infiltrating the epithelium of crypts (*Figure 2.4b*) and where they may be mistaken for enterochromaffin cells. However, their specific secretory granules, rich in heparin and histamine but in man *not* 5-hydroxytryptamine (serotonin), have a very specific scroll-like and laminar pattern allowing them at high magnification to be distinguished with ease from the enterochromaffin cells. In an experiment involving gluten challenge to coeliac patients in remission one of the earliest responses to occur was the influx of polymorph neutrophils and eosinophils, migrating out from the small vessels in the lamina propria, together with increased numbers of mast cells and macrophages (*Figure 2.7*)[16]. The capillary endothelial cells on gluten challenge assume a more bulky configuration with hyperplastic nuclei containing nuclear bodies; small clumps of platelets are seen in the capillary lumen.

Under normal circumstances the capillary endothelial cytoplasm forms a thin fenestrated layer (*Figure 2.9*) surrounded by a well developed basal lamina. The lymphatics or lacteals unlike capillaries lack a well defined basal lamina and fenestrations are absent. Junctional complexes are however a frequent finding between the complex interdigitations of the lymphatic endothelial cytoplasm. Smooth muscle, other than that associated with blood vessels is a normal constituent of lamina propria extending in from the muscularis mucosae between the crypts and up into the villi along the lacteals. In patients with villous atrophy of various causes, the muscle bundles often appear prominent due to increase in width, and at ultrastructural level appear contracted. One of the most striking findings on gluten challenge was the contracted muscle fibres seen in the shortened villi (*Figure 2.10*)[16]. Non-myelinated nerve fibres are associated with the smooth muscle fibres and are frequently seen in very close association (*Figure 2.10*).

References

1 ANDERSEN, K. J., VON DER LIPPE, G., MORKRID, L. and SCHJONSBY, H. Purification and characterisation of guinea pig intestinal brush borders. *Biochemical Journal*, **152,** 157–159 (1975)

2 ARAYA, M. and WALKER-SMITH, J. A. Specificity of ultrastructural changes of small intestinal epithelium in early childhood. *Archives of Disease in Childhood*, **50,** 844–855 (1975)

3 BOCKMAN, D. E. and COOPER, M. D. Early lymphoepithelial relationships in human appendix. A combined light and electron microscopic study. *Gastroenterology*, **68,** 1160–1168 (1975)

4 BOHANE, T. D., GETZ, E., HAMILTON, J. R. and GALL, D. G. Acrodermatitis enteropathica. Zinc and the Paneth cell. A case report with family studies. *Gastroenterology*, **73,** 587–592 (1977)

5 BRANDBORG, L. L., RUBIN, C. E. and QUINTON, W. E. A multipurpose instrument for suction biopsy of the oesophagus, stomach, small bowel and colon. *Gastroenterology*, **33,** 1–16 (1959)

6 BROWN, A. J. Microvilli of the human jejunal epithelial cell. *Journal of Cell Biology*, **12,** 623–627 (1972)

7 BROWN, W. R., ISOBE, Y. and NAKANE, P. Studies on translocation of immunoglobulins across intestinal epithelium. II. Immunoelectron microscopic localisation of immunoglobulins and secretory component in human intestinal mucosa. *Gastroenterology*, **71,** 985–995 (1976)

8 CHEN, H. C., REYES, V. and FRESH, J. W. An electron microscopic study of the small intestine in human cholera. *Virchows Archiv Abteilung B*, **7,** 236–259 (1971)

9 COHEN, M. I., WIDERLITE, L. W., SCHECHTER, G. P., JAFFE, E., FISHMANN, A. B., SCHEIN, P. G. and MACDONALD, J. S. Gastrointestinal involvement in the Sezary syndrome. *Gastroenterology*, **73,** 143–149 (1977)

10 CREAMER, B. *The Small Intestine*. London, Heinemann (1974)

11 CROSBY, W. H. and KUGLER, H. W. Intraluminal biopsy of the small intestine. *American Journal of Digestive Diseases*, **2,** 236–241 (1957)

12 DALTON, A. J. Electron micrography of epithelial cells of the gastrointestinal tract and pancreas. *American Journal of Anatomy*, **89,** 109–134 (1951)

13 DAVIES, M. D. J. and PARROTT, D. M. Preparation and purification of lymphocytes from epithelium and lamina propria of mouse small intestine. *Gut*, **22,** 481–488 (1981)

14 DAWSON, P. A. and FILIPE, M. I. An ultrastructural and histochemical study of the mucus membrane adjacent to and remote from carcinoma of the colon. *Cancer*, **37,** 2388–2398 (1976)

15 DOBBINS, W. O. Diagnostic pathology of the intestine and colon. In *Diagnostic Electronmicroscopy*, Volume 1, edited by B. F. Trump and R. T. Jones, 253–346. New York, John Wiley & Son (1978)

16 DOE, W. F., HENRY, K. and BOOTH, C. C. Complement in coeliac disease. In *Coeliac Disease*, edited by W. Th. J. M. Hekkens and A. S. Pena. Leiden, H. E. Stenfert Kroese B. V. (1975)

17 DOE, W. F., HENRY, K., HOBBS, J. R., AVERY-JONES, F., DENT, C. E. and BOOTH, C. C. Five cases of alpha chain disease. *Gut*, **13,** 947–957 (1972)

18 ERLANDSEN, S. L. and CHASE, D. G. Paneth cell function: phagocytosis and intracellular digestion of intestinal micro-organisms. I. *Hexamita muris. Journal of Ultrastructure Research*, **41,** 296–318 (1972)

19 ERLANDSEN, S. L. and CHASE, D. G. Paneth cell function: phagocytosis and intracellular digestion of intestinal micro-organisms. II. Spiral micro-organisms. *Journal of Ultrastructure Research*, **41,** 319–333 (1972)

20 ERLANDSEN, S. L., PARSONS, J. A. and TAYLOR, T. D. Ultrastructural immunocytochemical localisation of lysozyme in the Paneth cells of man. *Journal of Histochemistry and Cytochemistry*, **22,** 401–413 (1974)

21 ERLANDSEN, S. L., RODNING, C. B., MONTERO, C., PARSONS, J. A., LEWIS, E. A. and WILSON, I. D. Immunocytochemical identification and localization of immunoglobulin A within Paneth cells of the rat small intestine. *Journal of Histochemistry and Cytochemistry*, **24,** 1085–1092 (1976)

22 FERGUSON, A. and MURRAY, D. Quantitation of small intraepithelial lymphocytes in human jejunum. *Gut*, **12,** 988–994 (1971)

23 FILIPE, M. I. and FENGER, C. Histochemical characteristics of mucins in the small intestine. A comparative study of normal mucosa, benign epithelial tumours and carcinoma. *Histochemical Journal*, **11,** 277–287 (1979)

24 FORSSMANN, W. G. The ultrastructure of the endocrine cells in the normal and pathological gastrointestinal mucosa. In *Chromaffin, Enterochromaffin and Related Cells*, edited by R. E. Coupland and T. Fujita. Amsterdam, Elsevier (1976)

25 GIAMPOLO, C., FELDMAN, D., REYNOLDS, E. S., DZAV, V. J. and SZABO, S. Ultrastructural characterisation of proprionitrile-induced duodenal ulcer in the rat. *Federal Proceedings of Federation of the American Societies of Experimental Biology*, **34,** 227 (1975)

26 HENRY, K. and FARRER-BROWN, G. Primary lymphomas of the gastrointestinal tract. I. Plasma cell tumours. *Histopathology*, **1,** 53–76 (1977)

27 HENRY, K. and FARRER-BROWN, G. *A Colour Atlas of Thymus and Lymph Node Histopathology – with Ultrastructure*, London, Wolfe Medical Publications (1981)

28 HEITZ, P., KASPER, M., KRAY, G., POLAK, J. M. and PEARSE, A. G. H. Immunoelectrocytochemical localisation of motilin in human duodenal enterochromaffin cells. *Gastroenterology*, **74,** 713–717 (1978)

29 HELMSTAEDTER, V., KREPPEIN, W., DOMSCHKE, W., MITZREGG, P., YAMAHARA, N., WUNSCHE, E. and FORSSMANN, W. G. Immunohistochemical localisation of motilin in endocrine non-enterochromaffin cells of the small intestine of humans and monkeys. *Gastroenterology*, **76,** 897–902 (1979)

30 ISOMAKE, A. M. A new cell type (tuft cell) in the gastrointestinal mucosa of the rat. *Acta Pathologica et Microbiologica Scandinavica, Series A* (Suppl.) 240 (1973)

31 ITO, S. Form and function of the glycocalyx on free cell surfaces. *Philosophical Transactions of the Royal Society, London*, **268,** 55–66 (1974)

32 LAMBERTY, J., VARELA, P. Y., FONT, R. G., JARVIS, B. W. and COOVER, J. Whipple's disease: light and electron microscopy study. *Archives of Pathology*, **98,** 325–330 (1974)

33 LOEHRY, C. A. and CREAMER, B. Post-mortem study of small intestinal mucosa. *British Medical Journal*, **1,** 827–829 (1966)

34 LOJDA, Z. Cytochemistry of enterocytes and of other cells in the mucous membrane of the small intestine. *Biomembranes*, **4A,** 43–122 (1974)

35 MARSH, M. N. The scanning electron microscope and its application to the investigation of intestinal structure. In *Recent Advances in Gastroenterology*, edited by J. Badenoch and B. M. Brooke. Edinburgh, Churchill-Livingstone (1972)

36 MARSH, M. N. Studies of intestinal lymphoid tissue. I. Electron microscopic evidence of 'blast transformation' in epithelial lymphocytes of mouse small intestinal mucosa. *Gut*, **16,** 665–674 (1975)

37 MARSH, M. N., BROWN, A. C. and SWIFT, J. A. The surface ultrastruture of the small intestinal mucosa of normal control subjects and of patients with untreated and treated coeliac disease using the scanning electron microscope. In *Coeliac Disease*, edited by C. C. Booth and R. H. Dowling. Edinburgh, Churchill-Livingstone (1970)

38 MATHAN, M., MATHAN, V. I. and BAKER, S. J. An electron microscopic study of jejunal mucosal morphology in control subjects and in patients with tropical sprue in Southern India. *Gastroenterology*, **68,** 17–32 (1975)

39 MERZEL, J. and LEBLOND, C. P. Origin and renewal of goblet cells in the epithelium of the mouse small intestine. *American Journal of Anatomy*, **124,** 281–299 (1966)

40 MOOSEKER, M. K. and TILNEY, L. G. Organisation of an action filament-membrane complex. Filament polarity and membrane attachment in the microvilli of intestinal epithelial cells. *Journal of Cell Biology*, **67,** 725–743 (1975)

41 NABEYAMA, A. and LEBLOND, C. P. 'Caveolated cells' characterised by deep surface invaginations and abundant filaments in mouse gastrointestinal epithelia. *American Journal of Anatomy*, **140,** 147–166 (1974)

42 NEUTRA, M. and LEBLOND, C. P. Synthesis of the carbohydrate of mucus in the Golgi complex as shown by electron microscope radio-autography of goblet cells from rats injected with glucose H. *Journal of Cell Biology*, **30,** 119–136 (1966)

43 OWEN, R. L. Sequential uptake of horseradish peroxidase by lymphoid follicle epithelium of Peyer's patches in the normal unobstructed mouse intestine: an ultrastructural study. *Gastroenterology*, **72,** 440–451 (1977)

44 OWEN, R. L. and JONES, A. L. Epithelial cell specialisation within human Peyer's patches: an ultrastructural study of intestinal lymphoid follicles. *Gastroenterology*, **66,** 189–203 (1974)

45 PATRICK, W. J., DENHAM, D. and FORREST, A. P. Mucous change in the human duodenum: a light and electron microscopic study and correlation with disease and gastric acid secretion. *Gut*, **15,** 767–776 (1974)

46 PEARSE, A. G. E. The APUD cell concept and its implications in pathology. *Pathology Annual*, **9,** 27–41 (1974)

47 PEETERS, T. and VAN TRAPPEN, G. The Paneth cell: a source of intestinal lysozyme. *Gut*, **16,** 553–558 (1975)

48 PORTELA-GOMES, G., MARTINS, M. M. and CORREIA, J. P. Ultrastructural changes in jejunal epithelial cells in liver cirrhosis. *Scandinavian Journal of Gastroenterology*, **9,** 657–663 (1974)

49 POTTEN, C. S. and ALLEN, T. D. Ultrastructure of cell loss in the intestinal mucosa. *Journal of Ultrastructural Research*, **60,** 272–277 (1977)

50 RODNING, C. B., WILSON, I. D. and ERLANDSEN, S. L. Immunoglobulins within human small intestinal Paneth cells. *Lancet*, **1,** 984–987 (1976)

51 RUBIN, E., RYBAK, B. J., LINDENBAUM, J., GERSON, C. D., WALKER, G. and LIEBER, C. S. Ultrastructural changes in the small intestine induced by ethanol. *Gastroenterology*, **63,** 801–814 (1972)

52 RUBIN, W. Coeliac disease. *American Journal of Clinical Nutrition*, **24,** 91–111 (1971)

53 SCOTT, H. and BRANDTZAEG, P. Enumeration of Paneth cells in coeliac disease: comparison of conventional light microscopy and immunofluorescent staining for lysozyme. *Gut*, **22,** 812–816 (1981)

54 SELBY, W. S., JANOSSY, G. and JEWELL, D. P. Immunohistological characteristics of intraepithelial lymphocytes of the human gastrointestinal tract. *Gut*, **22,** 169–176 (1981)

55 SHINER, M. Jejunal biopsy tube. *Lancet*, **1,** 17–19 (1965)

56 SHINER, M. Ultrastructural changes suggestive of immune reactions in the jejunal mucosa of coeliac children following gluten challenge. *Gut*, **14,** 1–12 (1973)

57 SHINER, M. Cell distribution in the jejunal mucosa in coeliac disease. In *Coeliac Disease*, edited by W. Th. J. M. Hekkens and A. S. Pena. Leiden, Stenfert Kroese B. V. (1975)

58 SJÖLUND, K., ALUMENTS, J., BERG, N. O., HAKANSON, R. and SUNDLER, F. Enteropathy of coeliac disease in adults: increased number of enterochromaffin cells in the duodenal mucosa. *Gut*, **23,** 42–48 (1982)

59 SPERRY, D. G. and WASSERSUG, R. J. A proposed function for microridges on epithelial cells. *Anatomical Record*, **185,** 253–258 (1976)

60 THERON, J. J., WITTMAN, W. and PRINSLOO, J. G. The fine structure of the jejunum in kwashiorkor. *Experimental Molecular Pathology*, **14,** 184–192 (1971)

61 THOMPSON, G. R., HENRY, K., EDINGTON, N. and TREXLER, P. C. Effect of neomycin on cholesterol metabolism in the germ-free pig. *European Journal of Clinical Investigations*, **2,** 365–371 (1972)

62 TONER, P. G. and CARR, K. E. The digestive system. In *Biomedical Research Applications of Scanning Electron Microscopy*, edited by G. M. Hodges and R. C. Hallowes. London, Academic Press (1979)

63 TONER, P. G., CARR, K. E. and AL YASSIN. The small intestine. In *Electron Microscopy in Human Medicine*, Volume 7, edited by J. Vincents Johannessen, 132–168. New York, McGraw Hill (1980)

64 TONER, P. G., CARR, K. E., FERGUSON, A. and MACKAY, C. Scanning and transmission electron microscopic studies of human intestinal mucosa. *Gut*, **11,** 471–481 (1970)

65 TONER, P. G. and FERGUSON, A. Intraepithelial cells in human intestinal mucosa. *Journal of Ultrastructural Research*, **24,** 329–344 (1971)

66 TRIER, J. S. Studies on small intestinal crypt epithelium. II. Evidence for and mechanisms of secretory activity by undifferentiated crypt cells of the human small intestine. *Gastroenterology*, **47,** 480–495 (1964)

67 WARD, M., FERGUSON, A. and EASTWOOD, M. A. Jejunal lysozyme activity and the Paneth cell in disease. *Gut*, **20,** 55–58 (1979)

3
Biochemical anatomy of the enterocyte

T. J. Peters

The aim of this chapter is to discuss a biochemical approach to the study of the subcellular organelles of the enterocyte. The principal properties of these structures will be considered and examples of disordered function will be described. The article will concentrate principally on human tissue but where relevant, animal studies will be discussed. Thus the approach will be a quantitative discussion of the cell biology and pathology of the enterocyte.

METHODOLOGY

Although morphological and ultrastructural studies are being increasingly provided with a quantitative foundation, at present they are essentially descriptive and subjective. It is therefore often difficult to determine whether the ultrastructural alterations found in certain cells truly reflect a generalized consequence of the disease or are simply a chance, patchy alteration. In addition, ultrastructural studies do not indicate the functional integrity of the organelles. There is a tendency to assume that ultrastructural abnormalities must reflect functional impairment. This is not necessarily so. For example the mitochondrial enlargement found in alcoholic fatty liver is associated with favourable functional adaptation to the increased ethanol load and does not reflect organelle damage[22].

The techniques of subcellular fractionation permit the isolation of the various tissue organelles. In the analytical, rather than preparative approach[38,39], all the organelles in a particular tissue sample can be studied in a single experiment. This will avoid the criticism of selectivity in evaluating the pathological changes. Subcellular fractionation is usually performed by centrifugation techniques in which organelles are separated on the basis of differences in density and size or combinations thereof[14]. Alternative techniques which are being used with increasing frequency include, free flow electrophoresis, two phase partition, affinity chromatography with organelle specific ligands and gel filtration. Two phase counter-current partition is of particular potential value. It is a gentle, rapid separation procedure in which excellent organelle integrity is preserved[30]. Cells, organelles and macromolecules are separated on the basis of differences in surface charge and membrane composition[16].

Separation of organelles on the basis of density differences

In the study of human tissue it has been necessary to perform subcellular fractionation on milligram quantities of tissue as obtained by biopsy techniques, compared with conventional centrifugation methods which require gram quantities of tissue. Two developments have been essential in performing these studies. The small volume (35 ml) automatic zonal rotor of Henri Beaufay[8] allows rapid (approximately 30 min) separation of the organelles from biopsy tissue samples, although a recent report[51] has reported similar results using surgically resected specimens and a commercially available zonal rotor. The use of highly sensitive enzyme assays, generally employing radiolabelled or fluorimetric substrates is the second requirement.

Figure 3.1 is a diagram of the fractionation procedure. In this technique[37] portions of a jejunal biopsy specimen (approximately 10 mg) are homogenized in isotonic sucrose and the undisrupted cells (crypt cells, lymphocytes, etc.), nuclei and large brush border fragments are removed by low speed centrifugation. The

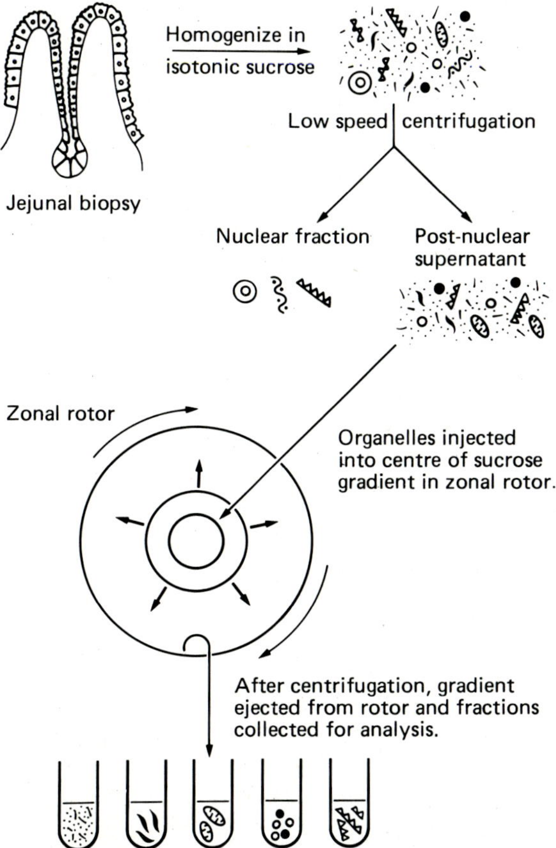

Figure 3.1 Flow diagram of homogenization and analytical subcellular fractionation of human jejunal biopsy sample

post-nuclear supernatant is injected into the centre of the zonal rotor which contains a sucrose gradient. Under high speed sedimentation the various organelles gravitate out to their equilibrium densities. After centrifugation, the gradient is ejected from the rotor and a series of fractions are collected. Although this is the

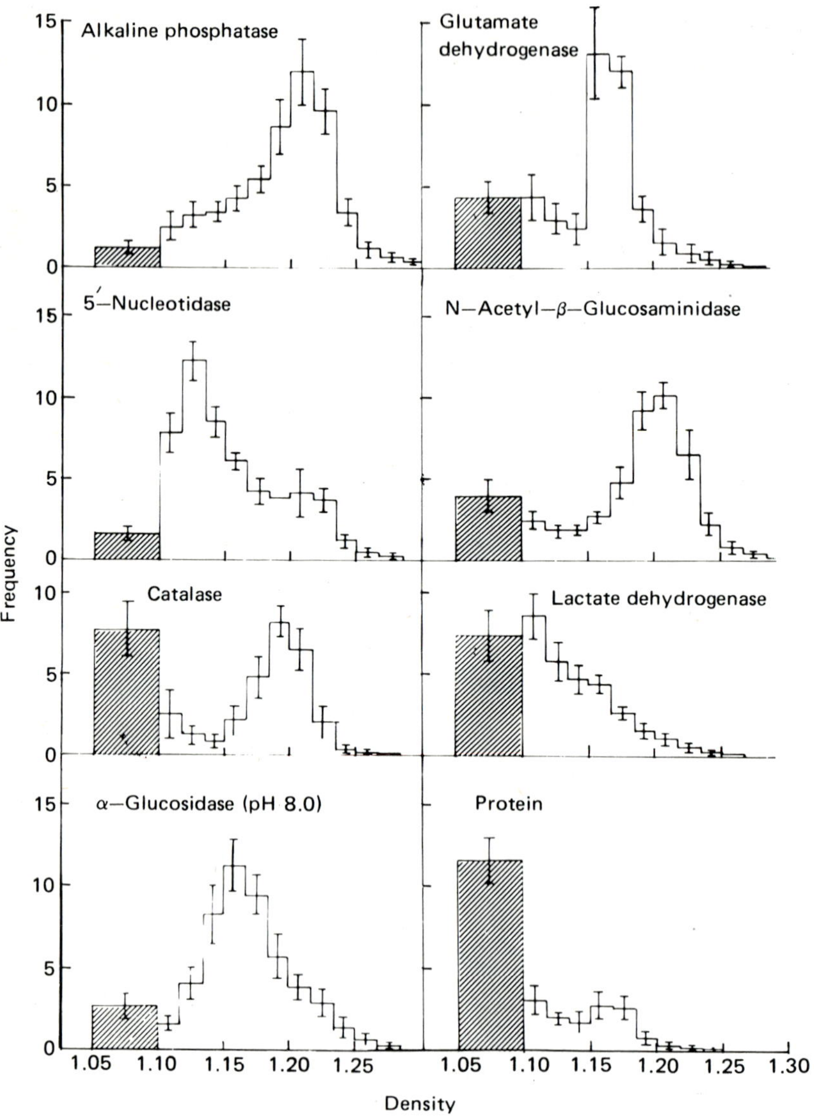

Figure 3.2 Density gradient centrifugation of post-nuclear supernatant from control jejunal biopsy homogenates. (Mean (± SD) enzyme distributions are shown.) The cross-hatched area represents activity remaining with the original sample layer and is assumed to represent soluble enzymes. (From Peters[37], courtesy of the Editor and Publishers, *Clinical Science and Molecular Medicine*)

general principle of the analytical approach to subcellular fractionation, there are clearly many possible variations.

Studies with human intestine have used post-nuclear supernatant fractions routinely as a starting material for the gradient centrifugation. In this manner organelle contributions from crypt and interstitial cells are minimized. However, the large organelles, nuclei and intact brush borders are sedimented with the undisrupted cells and are therefore not subjected to the gradient centrifugation step. *Figure 3.2* shows the distribution of the principal organelles from a series of control jejunal biopsies. Distinct distributions are present, for basal–lateral membrane (5′-nucleotidase), endoplasmic reticulum (α-glucosidase, pH 8.0), mitochondria (glutamate dehydrogenase), peroxisomes (catalase), lysosomes (N-acetyl-β-glucosaminidase) and brush border (alkaline phosphatase). Note that lactate dehydrogenase, a cytosolic marker, is largely recovered in the sample layer but some activity is particle-bound, probably to the endoplasmic reticulum.

Having characterized the distribution of organelles in the sucrose gradients with these marker enzymes, it becomes possible to determine the localization of hitherto unassigned enzymes. *Figure 3.3* compares the subcellular distribution of a series of dipeptidases and tripeptidases in normal human jejunum. Clearly the dipeptidase activity is almost exclusively cytosolic whereas tripeptidase is equally divided between the cytosolic and a particulate (brush border) fraction. Further studies[32, 34] have shown that higher oligopeptidases are almost exclusively located to the brush border fraction.

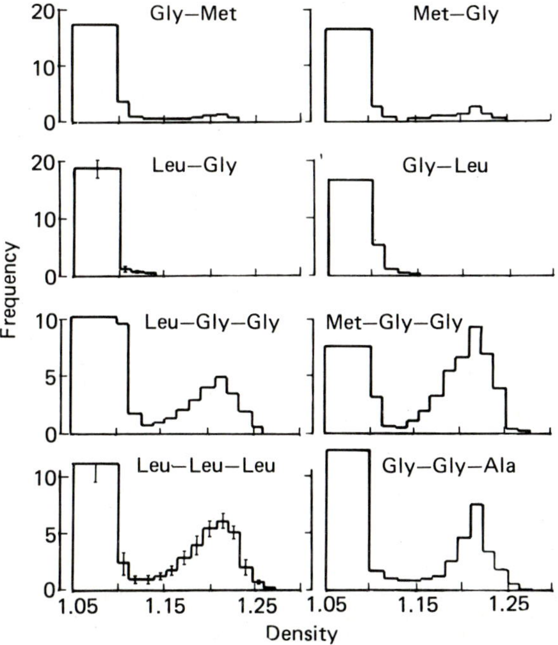

Figure 3.3 Distribution of peptidase activities following density gradient centrifugation of post-nuclear supernatant from control jejunal biopsy homogenates. (From Nicholson and Peters[34], courtesy of the Editor and Publishers, *European Journal of Clinical Investigation*)

Use of fluorescent enzyme substrates

In these experiments highly sensitive enzyme assays have to be used because the tissue sample size is small. The fractionation procedure involves a dilution (approximately one-tenth) of the tissue activity and further dilution of the gradient fractions may be necessary to overcome any inhibition due to the high sucrose concentrations. For this reason we have used several novel or modified fluorescent assay procedures[31, 33, 40, 42]. Of particular value has been the use of 4-methyl umbelliferyl substrates. Studies on the distribution of α-glucosidase activity are illustrated in *Figure 3.4*. This activity has a complex distribution. These results and

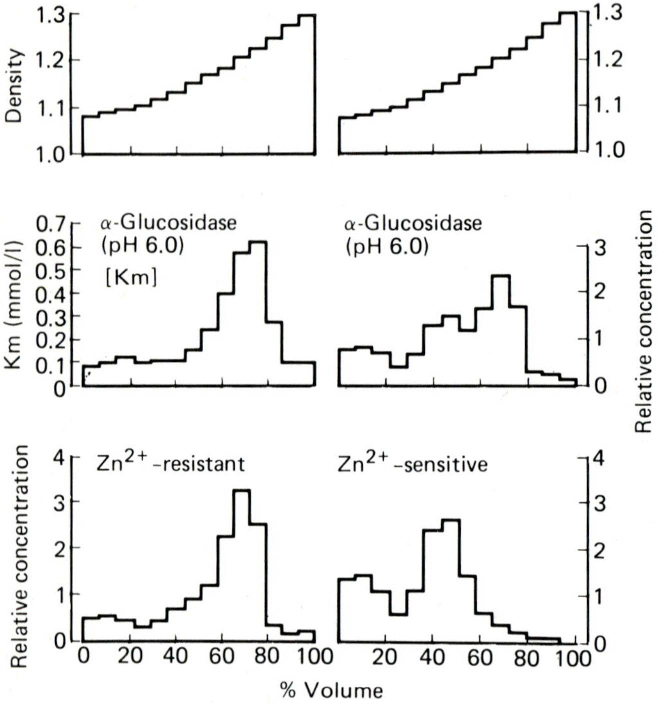

Figure 3.4 Distribution of α-glucosidase activities following density gradient centrifugation of post-nuclear supernatants from control jejunal biopsy homogenates. Activities are plotted against volume distribution along the gradient. Densities of individual fractions are shown in top panels. Fractionation experiments performed as in[37]. Kinetic constants calculated by direct linear plot method[15]

other findings may be summarized as follows. The brush border contains a neutral α-glucosidase of relatively high Km (approximately 0.5 mmol/l) which is strongly inhibited by TRIS but not by Zn^{2+}. This activity probably corresponds to maltase activity when assayed with natural substrates[11]. The endoplasmic reticulum contains an α-glucosidase with a more alkaline pH optimum and a lower apparent Km (approximately 0.1 mmol/l) for its substrate. This activity is strongly inhibited by Zn^{2+} but is relatively resistant to TRIS. The cytosolic fraction contains an α-glucosidase with similar properties to the endoplasmic reticulum marker. These markers have proved to be particularly useful in the recent demonstration of a tocopherol acetate esterase in mucosal cell endoplasmic reticulum[27].

Further examples of the heterogeneity of marker enzymes along the density gradient are illustrated in *Figures 3.5 and 3.6. Figure 3.5* compares the distribution of alkaline phosphatase, a brush border marker enzyme, assayed in the presence of D- (control) and L-phenylalanine. In control experiments, this enzyme has a major brush border component ($\rho = 1.22$) and minor basal–lateral ($\rho = 1.12$) and cytosolic components. L-Phenylalanine inhibits the total activity by approximately 90 per cent. The residual activity is found largely in the cytosolic fraction with a small brush border component. This result clearly shows similarities between the brush border and basal–lateral alkaline phosphatase activities, a finding confirming preparative fractionation procedures[18]. It also indicates that the cytosolic activity is probably due to a distinct enzyme form.

Figure 3.6 compares the total fluoride inhibitable and fluoride-resistant acid phosphatase in the gradient fractions. The bulk of the acid phosphatase is inhibited by fluoride ions showing a broad peak, modal density 1.20 $g \cdot cm^{-3}$, with a small soluble component. This distribution is similar to other lysosomal marker enzymes. The fluoride-resistant activity, approximately one-third of the total, is localized to the cytosol and endoplasmic reticulum. This multiple location of acid phosphatase, when assayed with fluorigenic and chromatogenic substrates, has been previously reported in other tissues particularly liver[47].

One of the disadvantages of analytical subcellular fractionation by single-step sucrose density gradient centrifugation is the overlap in distribution of several organelles. Many subcellular fractionation studies, either by differential pelleting or discontinuous gradient centrifugation, yield discrete fractions which have been labelled nuclear, mitochondria, microsomes, etc. This approach frequently gives a false impression of organelle purity. Continuous gradient centrifugation, although

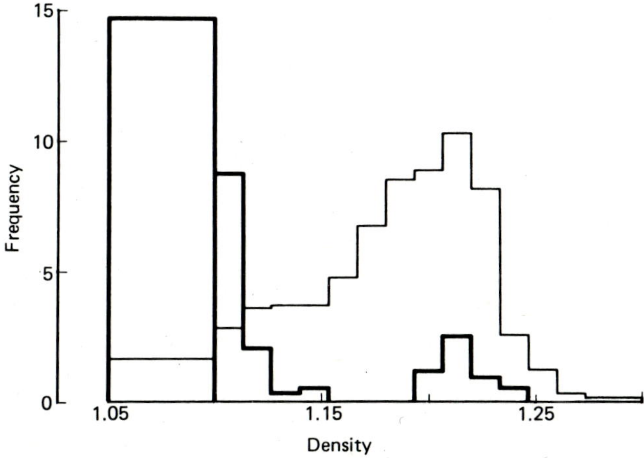

Figure 3.5 Distribution of alkaline phosphatase, assayed in the presence of either D-phenylalanine (thin line) or L-phenylalanine (thick line). A post-nuclear supernatant of control jejunal biopsy homogenate was fractionated by the standard technique[37]

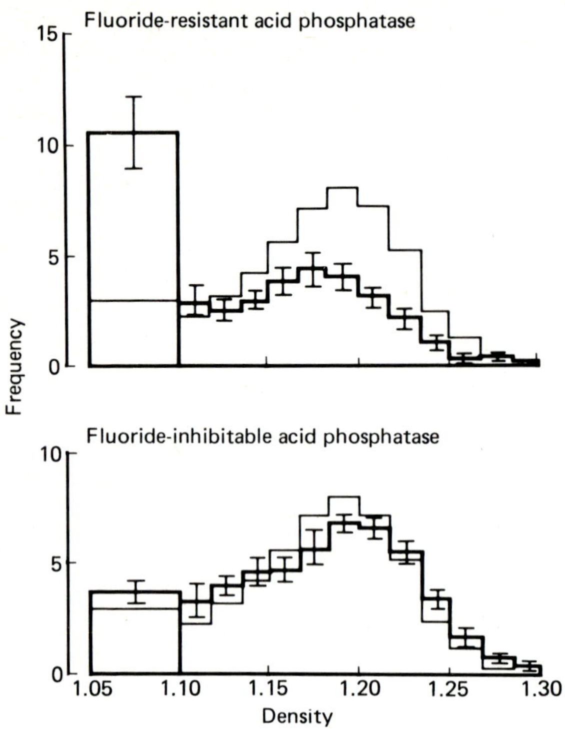

Figure 3.6 Distribution of acid phosphatase following density gradient centrifugation of post-nuclear supernatant from normal jejunal biopsy (thick line). Total acid phosphatase (thin line) distribution taken from[37]. Fluoride (2 mmol/l) resistant and inhibitable activity determined with 4-methyl umbelliferyl phosphate.

superficially less appealing, gives a more representative picture of organelle distributions. Nevertheless this approach may yield equivocal localizations of certain cell components. Examination of the enzyme distributions in *Figure 3.2* shows considerable overlap between alkaline phosphatase (brush border) and N-acetyl-β-glucosaminidase (lysosomes) and between glutamate dehydrogenase (mitochondria) and alkaline α-glucosidase (endoplasmic reticulum). These and other examples of equivocal distribution data can be resolved by the use of selective organelle perturbants. These are illustrated in *Figure 3.7–3.9*.

Figure 3.7 compares the distribution of the principal organelle marker enzymes when either fresh or digitonin-treated jejunal biopsy homogenates are subjected to analytical subcellular fractionation. Digitonin has highly specific and selective effects on the various subcellular organelles. These differential effects vary markedly with the concentration of digitonin used in the homogenization medium. More accurately, the digitonin-tissue cholesterol ratio probably determines the effect of this agent. Digitonin, a dense ($\rho = 1.35\,g{\cdot}cm^{-3}$) cardiac glycoside, binds to accessible cholesterol residues in the various cell membranes[1]. Up to a certain concentration, digitonin progressively increases the density of the membranes containing cholesterol. At higher concentrations, which differ markedly for each organelle, digitonin exerts its more traditional detergent action. This may lead to the release of certain membrane components[52,54] or to complete membrane disruption with recovery of its enzymic components in the cytosol[37,47]. Thus the contents of vesicular organelles e.g. lysosomes will be released into the soluble fraction. A further, recently recognised[36], effect of digitonin is to render the organelle membrane permeable to sucrose and thereby increase the equilibrium density of the organelle in the sucrose gradient.

These differential effects are well-illustrated in subcellular fractionation studies of the human jejunum (*Figure 3.7*). Mitochondria, peroxisomes and endoplasmic reticulum are unaffected by low concentrations of digitonin but plasma membrane components viz. brush border and basal lateral membranes, show a significant increase in equilibrium density. In contrast, lysosomes, as reflected by N-acetyl-β-glucosaminidase, are disrupted and their enzymes released into the soluble fraction. Note the effect of digitonin on the distribution of γ-glutamyl transferase. Both brush border and basal–lateral components of this activity show a density shift from 1.13 and 1.21 to 1.17 and 1.24 $g \cdot cm^{-3}$, respectively. This approach of isolating a membrane fraction before and after digitonin treatment offers a

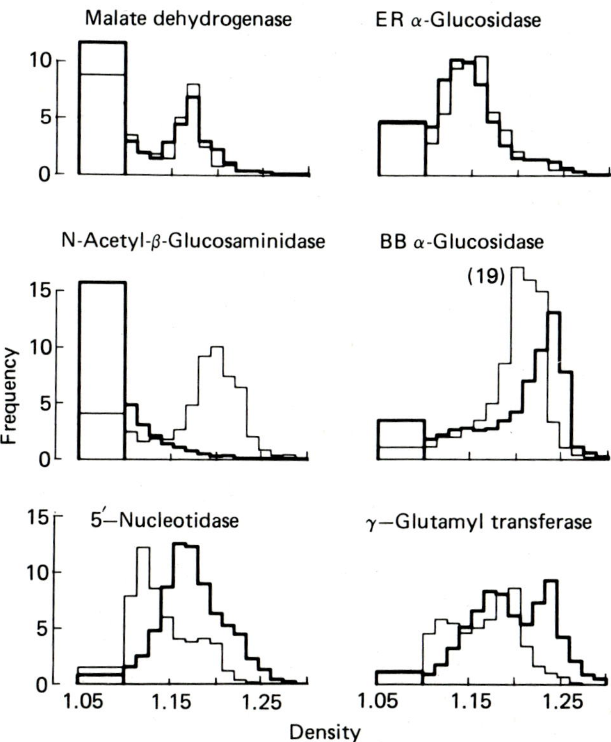

Figure 3.7 Effect of digitonin on the distribution of organelles in sucrose density gradients. Control data (thin line). Biopsies homogenized in isotonic sucrose containing 0.2 mg/ml digitonin shown in thick line. (From Peters[37], courtesy of the Editor and Publishers, *Clinical Science and Molecular Medicine*)

relatively simple and rapid approach to the isolation of plasma membranes to a high state of purity[36].

This selective effect of digitonin on the various membranes of the enterocyte can be used to confirm the localization of unassigned components whose distribution is otherwise equivocal. An example is illustrated in *Figure 3.8*. The distribution of the two tripeptidase activities shows a particulate component in the density region 1.18 – 1.23 g·cm^{-3} and it is uncertain from control experiments (see *Figure 3.3*) whether this represents a lysosomal or brush border distribution. Fractionation experiments performed in the presence of digitonin clearly show that the peptidase activity shifts, like the brush border enzymes, to a higher density and unequivocally assigns the activities to this organelle. Similar results have been obtained with isolated enterocytes from guinea pig and rat[25, 54].

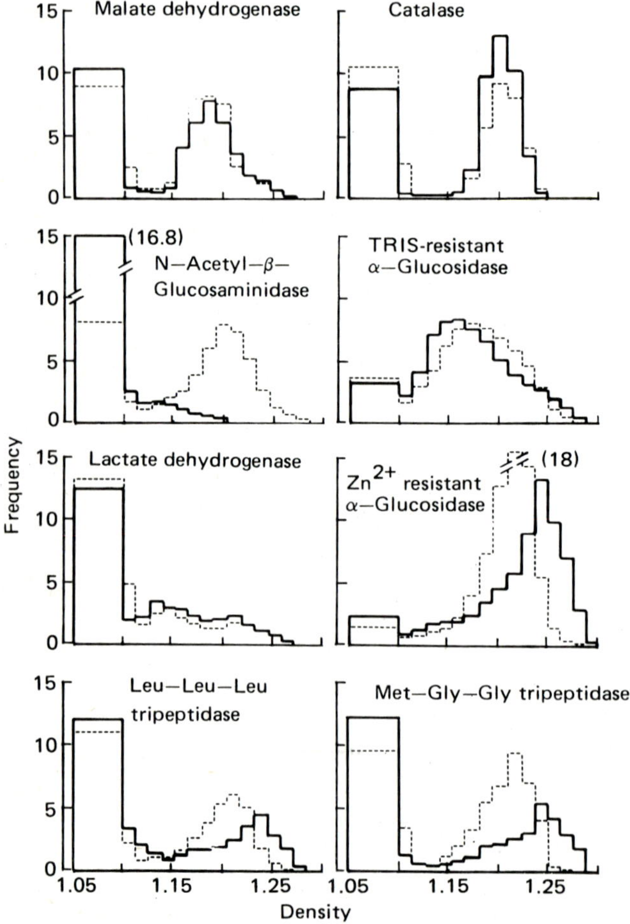

Figure 3.8 Effect of digitonin on the distribution of peptidase activities. Jejunal biopsies from normal subjects homogenized in the absence (interrupted line) or presence (continuous line) of digitonin. (From Nicholson and Peters[34], courtesy of the Editor and Publishers, *European Journal of Clinical Investigation*)

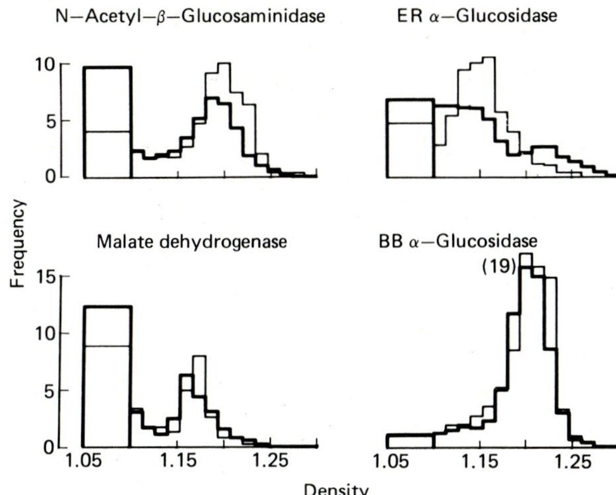

Figure 3.9 Effect of pyrophosphate on the distribution of organelles in sucrose density gradients. Control data (thin line) taken from[37]. Biopsies homogenized in the presence of isotonic sucrose containing 15 mmol/l sodium pyrophosphate shown in thick line

Figure 3.9 illustrates the use of pyrophosphate, a selective perturbant of the endoplasmic reticulum. This reagent releases bound ribosomes from the membranes of the endoplasmic reticulum[1, 3, 29, 52] and, as these components are major determinants of the density distribution of these membranes[55], stripping off the ribosomes would be expected to cause a selective decrease in the density of these membranes. There is clearly a marked decrease in the median density of the endoplasmic reticulum α-glucosidase but no significant alteration in the brush border α-glucosidase. Pyrophosphate appears to cause some damage to other organelles as more N-acetyl-β-glucosaminidase and malate dehydrogenase is recovered in the soluble fraction.

Other specific organelle perturbants can be employed. Thus lysosomes can be loaded with exogenous reagents which either increase, (e.g. ferritin[2], colloidal gold[19], dextran[28]) or decrease, (e.g. Triton WR1339[53], cholesterol[41]) their equilibrium density. An ingenious approach has been used to selectively increase the density of mitochondria by exploiting the unique localization of succinate dehydrogenase to this organelle. Mitochondrial fractions[12] or whole homogenates[10, 21] are pre-incubated with succinate and nitro-blue tetrazolium. The mitochondria accumulate large amounts of dense insoluble formazan and, on subsequent density gradient centrifugation, show a marked increase in density. Loading mitochondria with Mn^{2+} and PO_3^- has also been used to enhance mitochondrial separation from enterocyte plasma membranes[17]. A similar approach utilizing the glucose-6-phosphatase activity of endoplasmic reticulum has been used to isolate these membranes[26]. Recently attempts are being made with some success to selectively increase the density of specific membrane components by incubating tissue homogenates with ferritin-labelled antibodies specifically directed against constituents of these membranes[9].

Subcellular fractionation of whole homogenates

The studies described so far have used density gradient centrifugation of post-nuclear supernatants prepared from tissue extracts. More recently[49] we have adopted the approach of subjecting the whole homogenate to single-step gradient centrifugation. This considerably shortens the procedure allowing isolation of organelles with greater integrity and is particularly useful for studies on plasma membranes as significant amounts of this organelle are lost with the nuclear fraction. Disadvantages of the whole homogenate fractionation technique are that more vigorous homogenisation, with possible damage to the more fragile organelles, is necessary to ensure complete disruption of the cells. Undisrupted cells including contaminating erythrocytes, sediment deep into the gradient forming a distinct band which may overlap with specific organelle peaks. This is a particular problem with nuclear studies as these organelles have similar sedimentation characteristics to intact cells.

Figure 3.10 shows the distribution of certain marker enzymes following single-step fractionation of a jejunal biopsy homogenate. Comparing the distribution to those found with fractionated post-nuclear supernatants (*Figure 3.2*), similar patterns are obtained. The brush border components, as might be expected, are more distinct. Certain organelles e.g. mitochondria and basal–lateral membranes have higher equilibrium densities and there is a greater degree of lysosomal disruption. For many purposes whole homogenate centrifugation offers a significant improvement over conventional studies.

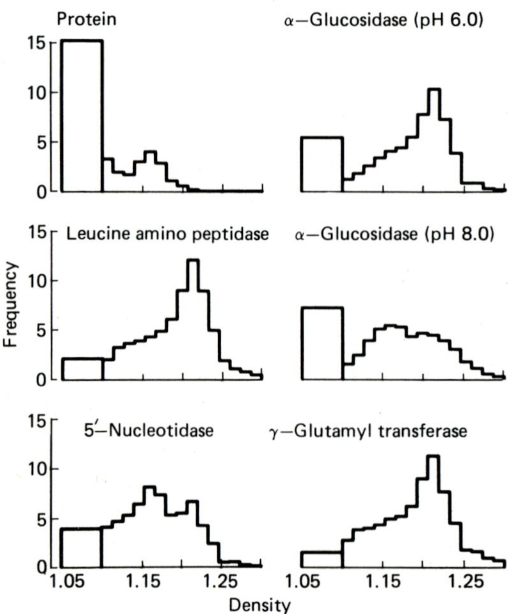

Figure 3.10 Density gradient centrifugation of homogenate of control jejunal biopsy. Fractionation procedure performed as in[37]

Separation of organelles on the basis of size differences

Centrifugation procedures can also separate organelles on the basis of differences in sedimentation coefficient. This parameter, under isotonic conditions, usually relates to organelle diameter. This type of separation is the basis of organelle fractionation by differential pelleting when tissue homogenates are subjected to sequential centrifugation for increasing g min integrals. This is a lengthy procedure and is not readily applicable to tissue biopsy fragments. The use of shallow sucrose gradients to separate organelles due to size differences is, however, applicable to biopsy-sized amounts of tissue. Although organelles show a far greater size distribution than density distribution, it is likely that, under altered physiological or pathological situations, changes in organelle size are more likely to occur than variations in organelle density. In addition, less organelle damage resulting from hypertonic centrifugation media or from hydrostatic effects of prolonged high speed centrifugation occurs. Separation of organelles on the basis of differences in sedimentation coefficients correlates better with ultrastructural observations on the organelles within intact tissue. This is particularly useful when organelles, e.g. hormone granules, intracellular vesicles, which have not been fully characterized with respected to marker constituents, are studied. This approach, illustrated in

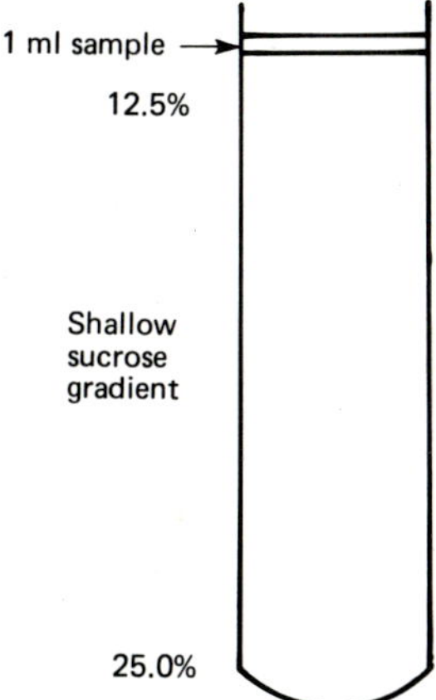

Figure 3.11 Diagram of use of swinging bucket rotor for the determination of sedimentation coefficients of subcellular organelles. Experimental details in[13]

Figure 3.11, has mainly been applied to a study of the regulatory peptide granules in human biopsy specimens but reference data for mitochondria also have been obtained[13]. Results are illustrated in *Table 3.1*. There is a rough correlation between sedimentation coefficient and particle size as determined by electron microscopy but no relationship between organelle density and sedimentation coefficient. Clearly this approach should prove of particular value in characterizing organelles which have been little studied and for exploring specific organelle alterations in disease.

Table 3.1 Rate zonal centrifugation of human jejunal biopsies (From Dawson *et al.*[13], courtesy of the Editor and Publishers, *Clinica Chimica Acta*)

Component	*Sedimentation coefficient* ($S_{20w} \times 10^{-13}$)	*Equilibrium density in sucrose* ($g \cdot cm^{-3}$)	*Diameter (nm)*
Motilin	3020	1.20	160
Gastrin	3240	1.22	190
Enteroglucagon	4920	1.25	210
Gastric inhibitory peptide	7050	1.22	350
Somatostatin	7540	1.23	310
Mitochondria	12800	1.16	500 × 2500

FUTURE CONSIDERATION FOR ANALYTICAL SUBCELLULAR FRACTIONATION

In this review the importance of the analytical approach to subcellular fractionation has been stressed. With this approach the major organelles have been characterized and it should be on the basis of this information that preparative methods for the isolation of a particular organelle are made. This is particularly important if an organelle is to be isolated from both normal and pathological tissue especially if the properties of the organelle differs in the two situations. Using this approach, especially with the aid of selective membrane perturbants, it is possible to design isolation procedures which are capable of rapidly isolating particular organelles to a high degree of purity[36]. Further application of this approach should prove highly profitable.

This review has considered the principal organelles of the enterocyte but others of equal importance, e.g. Golgi, endocytic vacuoles, shuttle vesicles, intercellular junctional complexes, endoskeleton, can be studied by similar techniques. In particular, the importance of Golgi in the biosynthesis of the brush border glycocalyx should encourage the study of this organelle in both normal and diseased enterocytes. Galactosyl transferase has proved a useful marker for this organelle in rat jejunum[24, 48] and suitable isolation procedures should prove relatively easy to devise.

APPLICATION OF THE ANALYTICAL APPROACH TO THE STUDY OF ORGANELLE PATHOLOGY

Although not the prime aim of this article, an example of how the techniques of analytical subcellular fractionation can be used to study the organelle pathology of damaged enterocytes is shown in *Figure 3.12*. The gradient distribution of the brush border marker enzyme, alkaline phosphatase, from homogenates of biopsies from patients with coeliac disease is compared to those from control subjects. Biopsies from untreated patients with subtotal villus atrophy show approximately a quarter of the specific activity of alkaline phosphatase of control tissue. Density gradient

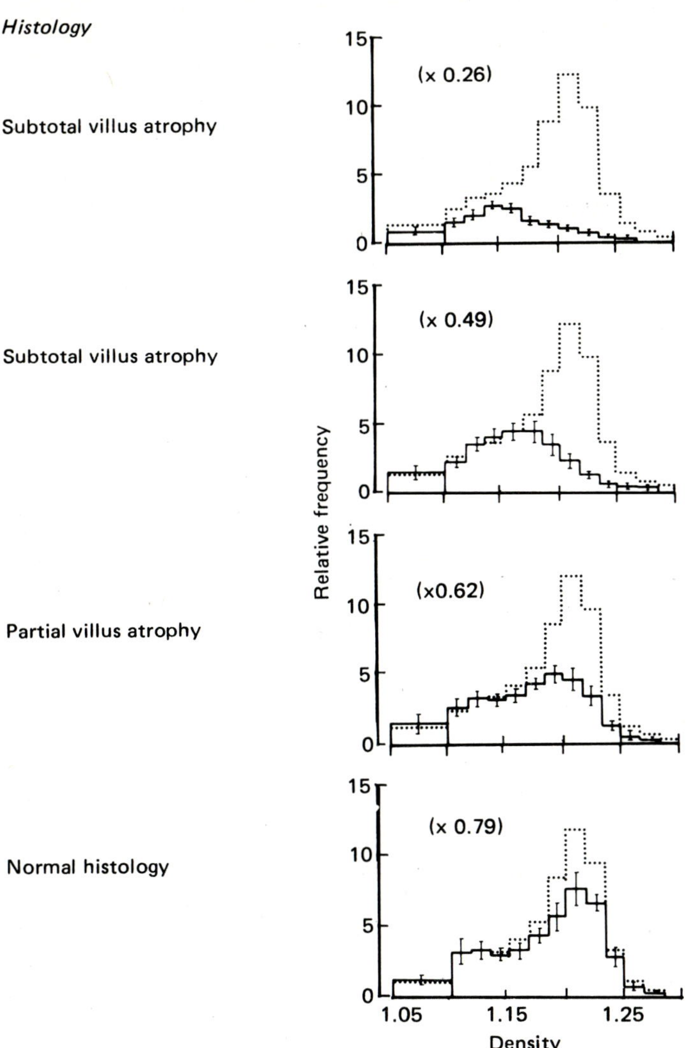

Figure 3.12 Distribution of alkaline phosphatase activity in sucrose density gradients from control subjects (interrupted line) and patients with coeliac disease (continuous line). (From Peters *et al.*[43], courtesy of the Publishers, *Perspectives in Coeliac Disease*)

centrifugation reveals striking differences in the distribution of the enzyme activity in the two patient groups. Most of the activity is associated with the endoplasmic reticulum with only small amounts of enzyme in brush border membranes of lower than normal density. As is well known, treatment of these patients by gluten withdrawal leads to almost complete restoration to normality of the enterocyte damage. Sequential enzymic assays and subcellular fractionation studies can be used to quantitate the organelle improvements. Treatment by gluten-withdrawal for 2–4 weeks usually leads to no detectable histological improvement but clearly the enzyme specific activity has doubled and the density distribution of the brush border membrane is increased. Prolonged, strict gluten withdrawal may lead to histologically normal mucosa but the brush border alkaline phosphatase activity clearly remains persistently subnormal. This figure illustrates the alterations in a single organelle in a particular syndrome. Similar information can be obtained for other organelles[45]. In addition this approach can be used to distinguish at a biochemical level, subcategories of disease classes, e.g. responsive and non-responsive coeliac disease[44], and to investigate other conditions where morphological changes in the gut are present[20, 35, 46] or suspected[11, 23, 50] both in man and animals[4–7].

Acknowledgements

I am grateful to the succession of research fellows and technicians who have contributed to this work and to Ms Rosamund Greensted for secretarial assistance.

References

1 AMAR-COSTESEC, A., WIBO, M., THINES-SEMPOUX, D., BEAUFAY, H. and BERTHET, J. Analytical study of microsomes and isolated subcellular membranes from rat liver. 4 Biochemical, physical and morphological modifications of microsomal components induced by digitonin, EDTA and pyrophosphate. *Journal of Cell Biology*, **62,** 717–745 (1974)

2 ARBORGH, B., ERICSSON, J. L. E. and GLAUMANN, H. Method for the isolation of iron-loaded lysosomes from rat liver. *FEBS Letters*, **32,** 190–194 (1973)

3 BALASUBRAMANIAN, S., VENKATESAN, S., MITROPOULOS, K. A. and PETERS, T. J. The submicrosomal localisation of acyl coenzyme A-cholesterol acyltransferase and its substrate and of cholesterol esters in rat liver. *Biochemical Journal*, **174,** 863–872 (1978)

4 BATT, R. M., BUSH, B. M. and PETERS, T. J. Morphological and biochemical studies of a naturally-occurring enteropathy in the dog resembling chronic tropical sprue in man. *Gastroenterology*, **76,** 1096 (1979)

5 BATT, R. M., BUSH, B. M. and PETERS, T. J. Biochemical changes in the jejunal mucosa of dogs with naturally occurring exocrine pancreatic insufficiency. *Gut*, **20,** 709–715 (1979)

6 BATT, R. M. and PETERS, T. J. Subcellular fractionation studies on peroral jejunal biopsies from the dog. *Research in Veterinary Science*, **26,** 94–100 (1978)

7 BATT, R. M., WELLS, G. P. and PETERS, T. J. Studies on the effects of prednisolone on the enterocyte at a subcellular level. *Clinical Science and Molecular Medicine*, **55,** 435–443 (1978)

8 BEAUFAY, H. La centrifugation en gradient de densitee. These d'Agregation de l'Enseignement Superieur Universite Catholique de Louvain Ceuterick SA, Louvain, Belgium (1966)

9 BROWN, A. E. and ELOVSON, J. Subfractionation of liver membrane preparations by specific ligand-induced density perturbation. *Biochimica Biophysica Acta*, **597,** 247–262 (1980)

10 COLAS, B. and MAROUX, S. Simultaneous isolation of brush border and basolateral membrane from rabbit enterocytes. Presence of brush border hydrolases in the

basolateral membrane of rabbit enterocytes. *Biochimica Biophysica Acta*, **600,** 406–420 (1980)

11 COOPER, B. T., CANDY, D. C. A., HARRIES, J. T. and PETERS, T. J. Subcellular fractionation studies of the intestinal mucosa in congential sucrase–isomaltase deficiency. *Clinical Science*, **57,** 181–185 (1979)

12 DAVIES, G. A. and BLOOM, F. E. Subcellular particles separated through a histochemical reaction. *Analytical Biochemistry*, **51,** 429–435 (1973)

13 DAWSON, J., BRYANT, M. G., BLOOM, S. R. AND PETERS, T. J. The sedimentation coefficients of human jejunal gut hormone storage granules. *Clinica Chimica Acta* (in press)

14 De DUVE, C., BERTHET, J. and BEAUFAY, H. Gradient centrifugation of cell particles: theory and application. *Progress in Biophysics and Biophysical Chemistry*, **9,** 325–369 (1959)

15 EISENTHAL, R. and CORNISH-BOWDEN, A. The direct linear plot. A new graphical procedure for estimating enzyme kinetic parameters. *Biochemical Journal*, **139,** 715–720 (1974)

16 FISHER, D. The separation of cells and organelles by partitioning in two polymer aqueous phases. *Biochemical Journal*, **196,** 1–10 (1981)

17 GRATECOS, D., KNIBIEHLER, M., BENOIT, V. and SEMERIVA, M. Plasma membranes from rat intestinal epithelial cells at different stages of maturation. I Preparation and characterization of plasma membrane subfractions originating from crypt cells and from villous cells. *Biochimica Biophysica Acta*, **512,** 508–524 (1978)

18 HANNA, S. D., MIRCHEFF, A. K. and WRIGHT E. M. Alkaline phosphatase of basal lateral and brush border plasma membrane. *Journal of Supramolecular Structure*, **11,** 451–466 (1979)

19 HENNING, R. and PLATTNER, H. Isolation of rat liver lysosomes by loading with colloidal gold. *Biochimica Biophysica Acta*, **354,** 114–120 (1974)

20 HEUMAN, R., BOERYD, B., BOLIN, T., MAGNUSSON, K.-E., SJODAHL, R. and TAGESSON, C. Subcellular fractionation of human intestinal mucosa by large scale zonal centrifugation. *Acta Chirugica Scandinavica*, **146,** 195–201 (1980)

21 HOLLOWAY, B. R., THORP, J. M., SMITH, G. D. and PETERS, T. J. Analytical subcellular fractionation and enzyme analysis of liver homogenates from control and clofibrate-treated rats, mice and monkeys with reference to the fatty acid oxidizing enzymes. *Annals of the New York Academy of Sciences*, (in press)

22 JENKINS, W. J. and PETERS, T. J. Mitochondrial enzyme activities in liver biopsies from patients with alcoholic liver disease. *Gut*, **19,** 341–344 (1978)

23 JONES, P. E., PALLIS, C. and PETERS, T. J. Morphological and biochemical findings in jejunal biopsies from patients with multiple sclerosis. *Journal of Neurology Neurosurgery and Psychiatry*, **42,** 402–406 (1979)

24 KIM, Y. S., PERDOMO, J., OCHOA, P. and ISAACS, R. A. Regional and cellular localization of glycosyl transferase in rat small intestine. Changes in enzymes with differentiation of intestinal epithelial cells. *Biochimica Biophysica Acta*, **391,** 39–50 (1975)

25 LEWIS, B. A., ELKIN, A., MICHELL, R. H. and COLEMAN, R. Basolateral plasma membrane of intestinal epithelial cells. Identification by lactoperoxidase-catalysed iodination and isolation after density perturbation with digitonin. *Biochemical Journal*, **152,** 71–84 (1975)

26 LEWIS, J. A. and TATA, J. R. Heterogeneous distribution of glucose-6-phosphatase in rat liver microsomal fractions as shown by adaptation of a cytochemical technique. *Biochemical Journal*, **134,** 69–78 (1973)

27 MATHIAS, P. M., HARRIES, J. T., PETERS, T. J. and MULLER, D. P. R. Studies on the *in vivo* absorption of micellar solution of tocopherol and tocopherol acetate in the rat: demonstration and partial characterization of a mucosal esterase localized to the endoplasmic reticulum of the enterocyte. *Journal of Lipid Research*, **22,** 829–837 (1981)

28 MEYER, A. E. and WILLIGHAGEN, R. G. The activity of glucose-6-phosphatase, adenosine triphosphatase, succinic dehydrogenase after dextran and polyvinylpyrrolidone uptake by liver *in vitro*. *Biochemical Pharmacology*, **12,** 973–980 (1963)

29 MITROPOULOS, K. A., VENKATESAN, S., BALASUBRAMANIAN, S. and PETERS, T. J. The submicrosomal localization of 3 hydroxy-3-methyl glutaryl coenzyme A reductase, cholesterol 7a hydroxylase and cholesterol in rat liver. *European Journal of Biochemistry*, **82,** 419–429 (1978)

30 MORRIS, W. B. and PETERS, T. J. Microanalytical partition of rat liver homogenates by poly(ethylene glycol)-dextran counter-current distribution. *European Journal of Biochemistry*, **121,** 421–426 (1982)

31 NICHOLSON, J. A. and PETERS, T. J. Fluorimetric assay for intestinal peptidases. *Analytical Biochemistry*, **87,** 418–424 (1978)

32 NICHOLSON, J. A. and PETERS, T. J. Subcellular distribution of hydrolase activities for glycine and leucine homopeptides in human jejunum. *Clinical Science and Molecular Medicine*, **54,** 205–207 (1978)

33 NICHOLSON, J. A. and PETERS, T. J. Fluorimetric assay for human intestinal glycine peptidases. *Clinica Chimica Acta*, **91,** 153–158 (1979)

34 NICHOLSON, J. A. and PETERS, T. J. The subcellular localization of peptide hydrolase activity in the human jejunum. *European Journal of Clinical Investigation*, **9,** 349–354 (1979)

35 O'MORAIN, C., SMETHURST, P., LEVI, A. J. and PETERS, T. J. Mucosal enzyme abnormalities in rectal biopsies in inflammatory bowel disease. *Clinical Science*, **61,** 20P (1981)

36 PEASE, R. J., BASSET, M., SMITH, G. D. and PETERS, T. J. Studies on the integrity of prolactin-containing vesicles in rat liver. *Biochemical Society Transactions*, (in press)

37 PETERS, T. J. The analytical subcellular fractionation of jejunal biopsy specimens. Methodology and characterisation of the organelles in normal tissue. *Clinical Science and Molecular Medicine*, **51,** 557–574 (1976)

38 PETERS, T. J. Application of analytical subcellular fractionation techniques and tissue enzymic analysis to the study of human pathology. *Clinical Science and Molecular Medicine*, **53,** 505–511 (1977)

39 PETERS, T. J. Investigation of tissue organelles by a combination of analytical subcellular fractionation and enzymic microanalysis: a new approach to pathology. *Journal of Clinical Pathology*, **34,** 1–12 (1981)

40 PETERS, T. J., BATT, R. M., HEATH, J. R. and TILLERAY, J. The microassay of intestinal disaccharidases. *Biochemical Medicine*, **15,** 145–148 (1976)

41 PETERS, T. J. and De DUVE, C. Lysosomes of the arterial wall. II Subcellular

fractionation of aortic cells from rabbits with experimental atheroma. *Experimental and Molecular Pathology*, **20,** 228–256 (1974)

42 PETERS, T. J., HEATH, J. R., WANSBROUGH-JONES, M. and DOE, W. F. Enzyme activities and properties of lysosomes and brush borders in jejunal biopsies from control subjects and patients with coeliac disease. *Clinical Science and Molecular Medicine*, **48,** 259–267 (1975)

43 PETERS, T. J., JONES, P. E., JENKINS, W. J. and NICHOLSON, J. A. Analytical subcellular fractionation of jejunal biopsy specimens from control subjects and patients with coeliac disease. In *Perspectives in Coeliac Disease*, edited by B. McNicholl, C. F. McCarthy and P. F. Fottrell, 423–443. Lancaster, MTP Press (1978)

44 PETERS, T. J., JONES, P. E., JENKINS, W. J. and WELLS, G. Analytical subcellular fractionation of jejunal biopsy specimens: enzyme activities, organelle pathology and response to corticosteroids in patients with nonresponsive coeliac disease. *Clinical Science and Molecular Medicine*, **55,** 293–300 (1978)

45 PETERS, T. J., JONES, P. E. and WELLS, G. Analytical subcellular fractionation of jejunal biopsy specimens: enzyme activities, organelle pathology and response to gluten withdrawal in patients with coeliac disease. *Clinical Science and Molecular Medicine*, **55,** 285–292 (1978)

46 PETERS, T. J., JONES, P. E., WELLS, G. and COOK, G. C. Sequential enzyme and subcellular fractionation studies on jejunal biopsy specimens from patients with postinfective tropical malabsorption. *Clinical Science*, **56,** 479–486 (1979)

47 PETERS, T. J. and SEYMOUR, C. A. Analytical subcellular fractionation of needle –biopsy specimens from human liver. *Biochemical Journal*, **174,** 435–446 (1978)

48 PETERS, T. J. and SHIO, H. Subcellular fractionation studies on isolated rat jejunal enterocytes with special reference to the separation of lysosomes, peroxisomes and mitochondria. *Clinical Science and Molecular Medicine*, **50,** 355–366 (1976)

49 SMITH, G. D. and PETERS, T. J. Analytical subcellular fractionation of rat liver with special reference to the localisation of putative plasma membrane marker enzymes. *European Journal of Biochemistry*, **104,** 305–311 (1980)

50 STIEL, D. and PETERS, T. J. Enzymic alterations in duodenal mucosa of rats with cysteamine-induced peptic ulceration. *Clinical Science*, **61,** 15–16P (1981)

51 TAGESSON, C., BOLIN, T., HEUMAN, R., MAGNUSSON, K.-E., NORRBY, K. and SJODAHL, R. Subcellular fractionation of human intestinal mucosa by large-scale zonal centrifugation. I Characterization of subcellular organelles in the distal part of the ileum. *Scandinavian Journal of Gastroenterology*, **15,** 353–362 (1980)

52 TILLERAY, J. and PETERS, T. J. Analytical subfractionation of microsomes from the liver of control and Gunn strain rats. *Biochemical Society Transactions*, **4,** 248–250 (1976)

53 TROUET, A. Immunisation de lapins par des lysosomes hepatiques de rats traites au Triton WR 1339. *Archives International Physiologie et Biochimie*, **72,** 698–700 (1964)

54 WELLS, G. P., NICHOLSON, J. A. and PETERS, T. J. Subcellular localisation of di- and tri-peptidases in guinea pig and rat enterocytes. *Biochimica Biophysica Acta*, **569,** 82–88 (1979)

55 WIBO, M., AMAR-COSTESEC, A., BERTHET, J. and BERTHET, H. Electron microscope examination of subcellular fractions. III Quantitative analysis of the microsomal fraction isolated from rat liver. *Journal of Cell Biology*, **51,** 52–71 (1971)

4
In vitro methods and their applications

J. S. Hugon, R. Calvert and D. Menard

INTRODUCTION

Intestinal mucosa is the most recent tissue to be studied by *in vitro* methods. Its high degree of differentiation and the rapid turnover of many of its components are thought to be the main factors in the rapid deterioration of morphological and physiological aspects of the mucosa. Three methods have nevertheless been used to study intestinal metabolism *in vitro*: the everted sac technique, the culture of isolated intestinal cells and organ culture.

The everted sac method is used for physiological studies of very short duration. Morphological preservation of the mucosa does not extend for more than 45 minutes under the best conditions. No attempts have been made to maintain normal growth with this technique, so we shall not discuss this point any further. An interesting surgical technique has been developed by Eloy *et al.*[25,26] allowing *ex vivo* vascular perfusion of isolated canine or rat small bowel under which a steady state can be maintained for 2 to 3 hours.

An important amount of work has dealt with the isolation and culture of separated intestinal cells. Although some interesting results have been obtained, these cells, generally, remain viable for a very short time.

Organ culture of gut mucosa has been made possible by the pioneering work of Browning and Trier[13]. Since this date, numerous studies have been reported on the human intestine *in vitro* and have been reviewed by several authors. Organ culture of the small intestine of adult laboratory animals has been studied less and the purpose of this review is to focus on this contribution and to underline the course of future research. Indeed, recent observations have been extended to the fetal and neonatal mammalian intestine with promising results.

Preceding chapters have shown that intestinal epithelial cells present a rather undifferentiated aspect in the crypt but as they migrate onto the villi they become highly polarized, mature enterocytes with many enzymes and absorptive or secretory pathways. The stimuli triggering this crucial differentiation are unknown and appear to be very difficult to analyze *in vivo* where luminal, humoral and neurogenic factors interact with the mucosa. Culture systems in which the cell or tissue environment can be controlled precisely should therefore bring important information about the specific roles of these factors.

EPITHELIAL CELL CULTURE

A reproducible method of culturing isolated intestinal cells while preserving growth and differentiation has not yet been obtained[43]. However, several techniques allow the isolation of intact epithelial cells from adult animals[37]. The methods used are mechanical agitation, enzymic dissociation or chelating agents, and are frequently combined. These procedures and their effects on cell viability have been reviewed[24]. The highest yields of viable cells appear after the use of chelating agents combined with some type of mechanical agitation. Bjerknes and Cheng[8] have recently described a simple technique for obtaining non-contaminated epithelial cells. The method is very rapid and provides the opportunity of studying kinetic parameters and turnover time of the whole epithelium using flow cytometric procedures. On the other hand, Quaroni *et al.*[66] have been able to maintain in culture an intestinal cell line exhibiting many physiological characteristics of crypt cells and several transport systems[46].

The sequential isolation of villus and crypt cells has revealed differential profiles of enzymic activities along the crypt–villus axis, illustrating the maturation of enterocytes[65]. Numerous metabolic studies have been done on the isolated cells of the intestine, including investigations of the synthesis and transport of triglycerides, localization of hormonal receptors, and RNA synthesis[64], but the limited survival has restricted the study to only two or three hours duration. Ziomek *et al.*[85] have shown that in isolated intestinal epithelial cells, membrane proteins, specifically alkaline phosphatase and leucine amino peptidase are progressively distributed over the entire cell surface migrating from the brush border zone. These observations may explain why numerous attempts to maintain these isolated cells in culture have generally failed: the epithelial cells lose their polarity and are unable to differentiate into mature enterocytes.

ORGAN CULTURE

Adult small intestine

Methods

In humans, intestinal explants are generally obtained by suction biopsies or during major intestinal surgery. In animals, biopsies have been used from monkeys, dogs and rabbits. These biopsies are immediately divided into small pieces no more than 1 mm^3. In small animals like mice or guinea pigs, a segment of intestine is taken after sacrifice. The gut is opened and fixed on a waxed dish and thoroughly washed with oxygenated Hanks' solution. The serosa is stripped away and small explants are excised. This method makes it possible to obtain a large number of explants from the same intestinal region. The explants are placed, with villi upwards, on a stainless screen placed on the central well of a sterile Falcon dish. Medium is added to the level of the base of the explants. The dishes are maintained in a high humidity environment by a circular filter pad saturated with distilled water. The covered dishes are placed in special containers in a 37°C incubator and gassed for 15 minutes with a mixture of 95 per cent O_2, 5 per cent CO_2.

The ideal medium for intestinal organ culture has not yet been established and seems to depend on the metabolic requirements of the animals. Browning and Trier[13] have successfully used Trowell T8 medium for human biopsies. This medium has been and remains the most frequently used for human intestine culture. However, RPMI-1640, NCTC-135 or a mixture of Trowell and NCTC have been tried with apparent success by several authors. For intestinal cultures from adult animals, the same media have been used, except for mice where there is insufficient preservation. In this case, a medium composed of nine parts DMEM-Hepes and one part NCTC-135 enriched with 10 per cent fetal bovine serum, gave the best morphological and kinetic results compared with seven other media[30, 31].

All the authors added antibiotics to the media in the form of penicillin, streptomycin or gentamycin. The addition of fetal bovine serum seems a pre-requisite for adequate preservation of structure and function. The temperature of incubation should be maintained at 36–37°C to allow for normal metabolism. The particular requirements for the culture of the fetal and neonatal intestine will be discussed later.

Adult animal intestine

VIABILITY AND METABOLISM DURING CULTURE

There is only a limited number of studies analyzing the *in vitro* behaviour of adult mammalian intestine. Kagnoff *et al.*[48, 49] maintained rabbit jejunal mucosa for 24 hours *in vitro* and recorded active protein, glycoprotein and IgA synthesis. Moreover, radiolabelled proteins increased steadily in the culture medium after 3 hours.

Haffen *et al.*[36] using two different methods of organ culture and three different media, have demonstrated on a morphological basis that canine duodenal and jejunal mucosa could not be preserved more than 24 hours, and rat mucosa, no more than a few hours, but that guinea pig intestine survived for more than 24 hours. This last observation was confirmed by our study of guinea pig duodenum in organ culture for up to 48 hours[51, 52]. However, the mitotic and thymidine labelling indexes and several enzyme activities decreased after 24 hours of culture[51–53].

Mouse duodenal and jejunal explants have been cultured for 48 hours. Near normal morphology of the mucosa was preserved and mitotic activity and DNA synthesis remained at a high level[30, 31]. The protein content was not modified. Brush border enzymes increased in the tissues and were secreted into the medium giving a total increase of 250 per cent of the activity present in the fragments at the start of the culture[4]. Protein synthesis was maintained at a steady rate during 48 hours[7]. Gel electrophoresis showed that the same proteins were present on the brush border membrane at the start and end of culture and had been renewed[5, 6, 7]. An increasing fraction of the enzyme secreted during culture was in a particulate form probably bound to microvesicles coming from the microvilli[5, 6, 7]. This

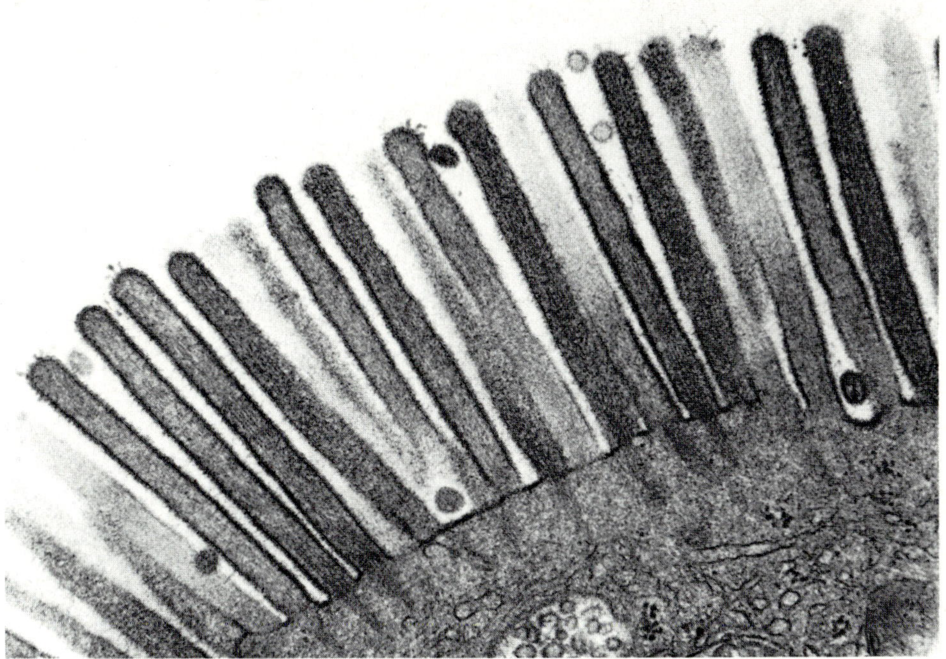

Figure 4.1 Brush border region from an absorbing cell of the adult mouse jejunum cultured for 24 h. Numerous microvesicles are being shed from the microvillus membrane. (× 57 600)

shedding process most likely indicates enhancement of a normal turnover mechanism of membrane-bound enzymes already described *in vivo*[61] (*Figure 4.1*).

The regulation of cholesterol and lipoprotein synthesis has been studied in organ culture of canine[33] and rabbit ileum[79, 80]. It was shown that the regulation of cholesterol synthesis was maintained *in vitro* and that endogenous cholesterol synthesis was a prerequisite for intestinal cell renewal and differentiation. It was also demonstrated that lipoproteins, insulin and glucagon were regulators of cholesterol synthesis[55]. Moreover, cholesterol synthesis increased during lipoprotein deprivation, and was suppressed by low density lipoprotein but stimulated by very low density and high density lipoproteins[79, 80].

IN VITRO RESPONSE TO NUTRIENTS, HORMONES AND DRUGS

Several studies have analyzed the action of drugs or hormones on the intestine in organ culture. Deoxycholate, indole and bacterial endotoxin destroyed the villous architecture of rabbit jejunal mucosa[3]. Protein synthesis was impaired but the brush border enzyme activities were not modified. Mak *et al.*[59] have shown in rabbit intestinal mucosa cultured for 24 hours, that cytochalasin-B, at different doses, does not alter glycoprotein, protein and secretory IgA synthesis. Some morphological alterations have nevertheless been observed in mouse duodenum after the addition of 50 μg/ml of cytochalasin-B[45]. Shields *et al.*[76] have been unable to detect an increase in protein synthesis of duodenal, jejunal or ileal explants of rabbits after 24 hours of culture in the presence of pentagastrin. In our laboratory, pentagastrin added at different doses to an organ culture of adult mouse jejunum or duodenum did not modify DNA or protein synthesis, brush border enzyme activities, nor the DNA and protein content after different periods of culture up to 48 hours[17, 18]. EGF, a potent growth factor acting on various tissues and cells, and a powerful mitogen, was added at doses of 15–800 ng/ml to an organ culture of adult mouse jejunum. No stimulatory effect on DNA or protein synthesis and no increase in brush border enzyme activities was recorded[17, 18]. Fructose (4 mg/ml) added to the culture medium of mouse jejunal fragments provoked an important increase of glucose-6-phosphatase activity in less than 6 hours and a threefold increase in 24 hours[16].

Cholera toxin added to explants of rabbit jejunum cultured for 12 hours provoked an increase in mucosal cAMP and fructose phosphatase activities[73]. Theophylline had the same action in 15 minutes proving that the increase of cAMP is sufficient to induce modification of gluconeogenesis and glycolysis[74]. In rabbit jejunal biopsies maintained in organ culture, Krawitt[57] was able to demonstrate in mucosal cells an accumulation of vitamin D_3, but no evidence of intestinal hydroxylation of the same vitamin. Rothenberg *et al.*[71] using organ culture of ileal segments from guinea pigs demonstrated that vitamin B_{12} became coupled with transcobalamin-2 from mucosal origin and not from the circulating blood.

Human intestine

VIABILITY AND EXPERIMENTAL RESULTS IN NORMAL INTESTINE

Several reviews summarize those works dealing with organ culture of human intestine[38, 58, 70, 81, 82]. We shall therefore only survey the more recent observations. The viability of the human intestine in organ culture has been demonstrated by several authors[39]. Protein and glycoprotein synthesis was maintained. Normal turnover of brush border enzymes has been demonstrated[54]. The protein content of the explants, however, decreased with time[62]. Explants synthesized and secreted apolipoprotein A-1, incorporated palmitic acid into lipoprotein and secreted newly synthesized lipoprotein during a 24-hour culture[67–69]. Block *et al.*[11] showed that the apical lysosomes of the absorptive cells exhibited a crinophagic role in sequestring glycoproteins delayed in their migration by colchicine treatment. They also demonstrated that horseradish peroxidase and lactoperoxidase entered the apical membrane by pinocytosis and were subsequently segregated in the lysosomes but that ferritin was not interiorized[12].

DISEASED INTESTINE

Few intestinal diseases have been investigated using organ culture technique. However, coeliac sprue has been extensively studied with *in vitro* methods and much controversy has arisen over the results obtained from these short duration cultures[47]. The literature on the subject has been reviewed by Trier[82], but several new works have in part resolved some of the discrepancies between laboratories. Trier and Browning[83] demonstrated that morphologically, intestinal biopsies from coeliac sprue patients improved during culture in gluten-free medium. Large lysosomes and abnormal lipid vacuoles disappeared and the cuboidal diseased cells were replaced by polarized absorptive cells. This improvement could be prevented by the addition of gluten or its toxic moiety to the culture medium[50]. Moreover, the labelling *in vitro* of the proliferative zone of the intestinal crypt showed an increase in DNA synthesizing cells and their migration rate in biopsies from non-treated coeliac sprue patients compared with normal volunteers[27,28]. However, Hauri *et al.*[40] have challenged these observations and found no difference between intestinal biopsies of coeliac diseased children, cultured with or without various toxic fractions of gliadin. On the other hand, the role of histocompatibility type on gluten sensitivity *in vivo* was demonstrated by Falchuk *et al.*[29]. The explants taken from the intestine of HLA-B8 negative patients frequently failed to develop gluten induced damage *in vitro* in contrast to HLA-B8 positive patients. Recently, Howdle *et al.*[44] have observed a significant increase in the height of the cells, after 24 hours of culture, from untreated patients and a significant decrease after culture in the presence of gluten. The biopsies from normal volunteers or patients with various intestinal diseases did not show this sensitivity to the presence or absence of gluten in the medium. It seems possible, therefore, to find *in vitro* tests able to help and even to decide on the diagnosis of coeliac sprue. Using organ culture and *in vitro* sensitivity to gluten, Klaeveman *et al.*[56] were able to assume that ulcerative ileojejunitis is indeed a complication of an underlying gluten-sensitive enteropathy which clinically does not respond to gluten-free diet.

Ginsel *et al.*[34] studied the transport of ^{3}H-fucose glycoprotein in intestinal biopsies from patients with a lysosome storage disease (fucosidosis). They observed more newly synthesized glycoproteins in lysosomes than were seen in normal controls. This could be explained by the lack of lysosomal hydrolases normally involved in the degradation process of glycoproteins.

ORGAN CULTURE OF NEONATAL SMALL INTESTINE

The neonatal small intestine which presents specific characteristics in terms of cellular turnover, enzyme levels and pinocytotic activity [42] changes into adult form during weaning. Few studies evaluated the ideal conditions for maintaining explants of neonatal small intestine. In 1964, Doell and Kretchmer[22] reported that jejunum from 5-day-old rats can be cultured in Eagle's medium plus 10 per cent calf serum with 95 per cent O_2 and 5 per cent CO_2 for up to seven days. Unfortunately the temperature used and the morphological appearance of the explants were not stated. Haffen *et al.*[36] showed good morphological maintenance of 15-day-old rat and guinea pig small intestine. The duodenum and jejunum were cultured in Trowell's T8 medium supplemented with 10 per cent fetal calf serum at 37°C with 95 per cent O_2 and 5 per cent CO_2. More recently, Shields *et al.*[75] reported the successful maintenance of suckling rat ileum (4–15 days old) for 24 hours using

Hanks' balanced salt solution without fetal calf serum, at 25°C and in room air. They also reported that duodenum and jejunum are difficult to maintain well, either in this system or in a variety of other systems using different media (Eagle's, 199, T8 and NCTC-DMEM supplemented with 10 per cent fetal calf serum) and culture conditions (25 or 37°C with 95 per cent O_2 and 5 per cent CO_2 or room air). During the 24-hour culture period, ileal DNA synthesis as well as protein synthesis were maintained. Kedinger *et al.*[55] studied rat jejunum at different postnatal stages (4–21 days) cultured in RPMI medium supplemented with 10 per cent heat-inactivated fetal calf serum at 37°C with 95 per cent O_2 and 5 per cent CO_2. The morphological appearance of the explants was well preserved during the first 24 hours of culture but a considerable regression of villi occurred during the following 24 hours. Brush border membrane hydrolytic activities such as maltase, lactase and alkaline phosphatase decreased in the explants during culture compared with non-cultured intestine.

The absence of fetal calf serum in a culture system could be a major advantage since its hormonal content may interfere with the factors under study[72]. We have established that 8-day-old mouse small intestine can best be maintained for 48 hours in a serum-free culture using Leibovitz L-15 medium at 22°C and room air[60]. The histological characteristics of duodenal and ileal mucosa are preserved during culture (*Figure 4.2*). The brush border membrane hydrolytic activities are

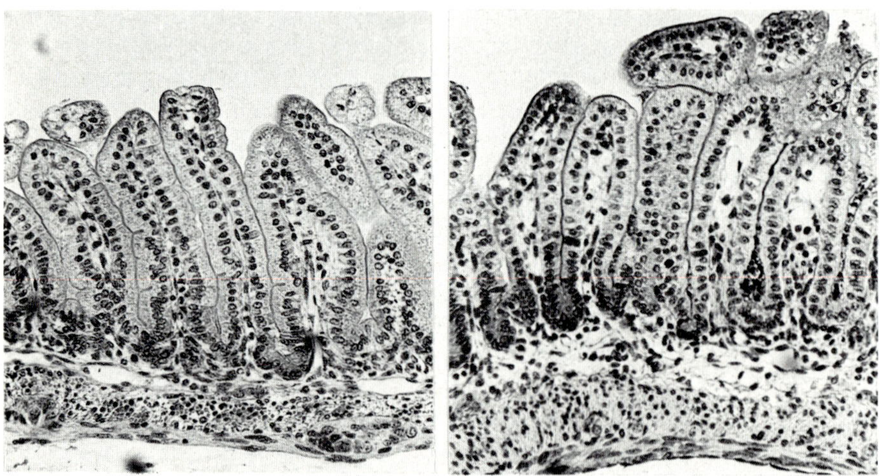

Figure 4.2 Duodenal explants of an 8-day-old suckling mouse at the beginning of the culture (*left*) and after 24 hours of culture in Liebovitz L-15 medium and room air (*right*). HPS stain. (× 42)

retained in the intestinal explants and accumulate in the culture medium. Moreover, continuous DNA and protein synthesis occurred throughout the culture.

In order to clarify the mechanism(s) by which different factors may influence either directly or indirectly the maturation of the neonatal small intestine, hormones are now being added to culture medium. Shields *et al.*[75] did not find any modifications in DNA synthesis, protein synthesis or in the proportion of soluble to membrane-bound alkaline phosphatase following addition of hydrocortisone (1μM) or thyroxine (0.01 μM) to the culture medium during 24 hours. Kedinger *et al.*[55] reported that the addition of dexamethasone (30 mg/ml) did not affect alkaline phosphatase activity but directly induced the precocious appearance of sucrase and a premature increase in maltase activity. The implications of other hormones such as EGF and insulin are under investigation[60, 77]. The maintenance of neonatal small intestine in organ culture offers a promising system for the establishment of the different factors involved either directly or indirectly in the regulatory mechanism(s) of the normal differentiation of this organ.

ORGAN CULTURE OF FETAL SMALL INTESTINE

The organ culture methodology has been applied successfully to avian small intestine for many years[63]. More recently, Black and Moog[9, 10] published milestone papers on the effect of thyroxine and hydrocortisone on duodenal explants of chick embryos cultured in defined medium. The maintenance *in vitro* of explants of fetal mammalian small intestine for the study of the different factors involved in the normal differentiation of this organ has been achieved only in the past few years.

The first trials were done with human fetal intestine, with the purpose of using the explants as substrates for the growth of viruses. Henle and Deinhardt[41] established a cell line from finely minced pieces of jejunum and ileum from a human embryo of two months gestation. After the fourth transfer fibroblasts, histocyte-like cells and small islands of poorly characterized epithelial-like cells were noted. Later, Dolin *et al.*[23] cultured small intestine from human fetuses of 9 – 16 weeks for 21 days in Leibovitz L-15 medium.

In vitro techniques have been applied to fetal intestine of rodents in an effort to study small bowel differentiation under controlled conditions. DeRitis *et al.*[20] cultured segments of jejunum from 18-day-old fetal rats for 72 hours in modified Leibovitz L-15 medium in room air at 37°C. This technique was later used to study the effect of wheat toxic proteins and peptides on *in vitro* development of rat fetal intestine[21].

The organ culture method we used for fetal mouse small intestine was adapted from the method described by Kedinger *et al.*[51, 52] for the maintenance in organ culture of adult guinea pig duodenum. The proximal third of 15-day-old fetal mouse small intestine was cultured for 72 hours at 37°C in room air with the following media: McCoy's 5A (without serum), medium 199, Swim's S-77, Trowell's T8 (without insulin) Leibovitz L-15 and RPMI- 1640[15]. We studied the effect of the addition of 17-day-old mouse amniotic fluid to Trowell's T8 medium on the formation of duodenal villi (*Figure 4.3*)[14] and also the effect of EGF on the differentiation of the endoplasmic reticulum in absorptive cells[2].

Two abstracts have reported the maintenance of fetal small intestine in organ culture for extended periods. Cho and Takeuchi[19] claim that fetal mice small intestine of 13–14 days can be grown and the mucosal structure and function maintained for up to 20 days in Tricine buffered Eagle's MEM. Recently, Truding

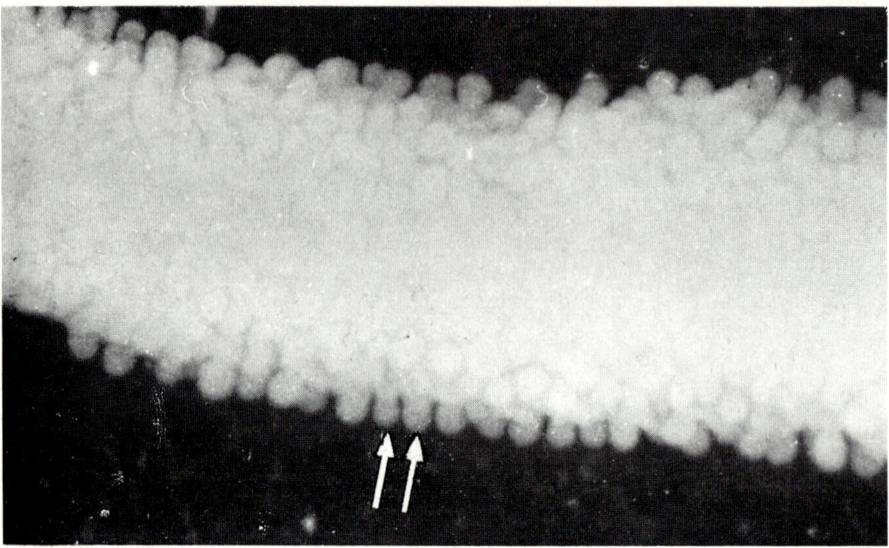

Figure 4.3 With the addition of mouse amniotic fluid (25 per cent) to Trowell T8 medium, villi are observed (arrows) over the whole surface of the explants after 24 h of culture. Without amniotic fluid villi are absent and the surface remains smooth. (×25)

et al.[84] were able to culture segments of the small intestine isolated from fetal rats of 13–22 days gestation in CMRL-1066 medium, for up to 2 months.

Epithelial–mesenchymal interactions during differentiation of the small intestine have been studied in culture. By recombination experiments Fukamachi and Takayama[32] observed that the mesenchyme of glandular stomach or forestomach was better than duodenal mesenchyme in supporting morphogenesis of rat duodenal epithelium.

The maintenance of fetal mammalian small intestine in organ culture offers a favourable system for the study of the different factors involved in the normal differentiation of this organ. The use of completely synthetic medium permits the study of the specific effect of these factors under rigidly controlled conditions.

FUTURE APPLICATIONS OF *IN VITRO* METHODS

Organ culture of intestine has been used for the study of intestinal functions and as an aid in the diagnosis of enteropathies. Many new applications could be considered.

In basic research, the method will facilitate our understanding of the regulatory mechanism for differentiation of the intestinal mucosa during the fetal and neonatal period and in adult or senescent animals. It is now possible to use the same segment of intestine from the same animal to obtain control and experimental explants and so reduce the variations between animals of the same strain. It is not compulsory, therefore, to find a universal medium which, in fact, might need to be different for each species. The main prospect will be to extend the culture period for several weeks as has already been done for the colon[1]. The goblet cells, Paneth cells and endocrine cells of the small intestine not yet studied *in vitro* could be stimulated or inhibited by various drugs allowing precise analysis of the secretory pathways. Many other intestinal functions could be investigated without interference from systemic reactions. Already lipid and glycoprotein metabolism are under study and the direct action of hormones is being investigated. The role of cells from the lamina propria and submucosa in the differentiation of the mucosa could also be evaluated.

Clinical applications are certainly numerous in the diagnosis and treatment of enteropathies. The ability to follow the synthesis of proteins and the migration of glycoproteins by incubating biopsies with an appropriate radiolabel, will give new insights into the metabolism of many intestinal disorders. The behaviour *in vitro* of intestinal explants from various intestinal diseases may allow us to discriminate between intrinsic and extrinsic factors. The addition *in vitro* of specific drugs may help in the selection of appropriate treatment. Unfortunately, the ideal conditions for successful human intestinal organ culture have not yet been established and vary from one laboratory to another. It is therefore imperative to establish, in the near future, a standard medium for the culture of human intestine.

CONCLUSION

Thirteen years after its introduction by Browning and Trier[13], organ culture of small intestine is used by many laboratories. This useful method should help in the development of different lines of intestinal research: basic studies of the factors controlling the development of fetal and neonatal intestine, fine analysis of metabolic pathways of absorption and secretion in adult intestinal mucosa and study of the alterations of the mucosal metabolism in numerous enteropathies. It is now time to apply a systematic approach to organ culture of the intestine. On the other hand, the culture of isolated epithelial cells should probably receive renewed interest. In the next five years, many new concepts in the understanding of the intestinal physiology will certainly arise from these studies.

References

1 AUTRUP, H. Explant culture of human colon. In *Methods in Cell Biology*, Volume 21, 385–401, edited by C. Harris, B. Trump and G. Stona, London, Academic Press (1980)

2 BEAULIEU, J. F. and CALVERT, R. The effect of epidermal growth factor (EGF) on the differentiation of the rough endoplasmic reticulum in fetal mouse small intestine in organ culture. *Journal of Histochemistry and Cytochemistry*, **29**, 765–770 (1981)

3 BEEKEN, W. L., ROESSNER, K. D. and KRAWITT, E. L. Effects of deoxycholate, indole, and endotoxin on organ cultures of rabbit jejunum. *Gastroenterology*, **66,** 998–1004 (1974)

4 BERTELOOT, A., CHABOT, J. G., MÉNARD, D. and JUGON, J. S. Organ culture of adult mouse intestine. III. Behavior of the proteins, DNA content and brush border membrane enzymatic activities. *In Vitro*, **15,** 294–299 (1979)

5 BERTELOOT, A., CHABOT, J. G. and HUGON, J. S. Turnover of mouse intestinal brush border membrane proteins and enzymes in organ culture. *Biochimica Biophysica Acta* **678,** 423–436, (1981)

6 BERTELOOT, A., CHABOT, J. G. and HUGON, J. S. Organ culture of adult mouse intestine. V. Vesiculation of the brush border membrane during culture. *Biology of the Cell* **42,** 109–114 (1981)

7 BERTELOOT, A. and HUGON, J. S. Proteins and enzymes of the brush border membrane of mouse intestine. Influence of organ culture on gel electrophoretic patterns. *Canadian Journal of Biochemistry* **60,** 434–443 (1982)

8 BJERKNES, M. and CHENG, H. Methods for the isolation of intact epithelium from the mouse intestine. *Anatomical Record*, **199**, 565–574, (1981)

9 BLACK, B. L. and MOOG, F. Goblet cells in embryonic intestine: accelerated differentiation in culture. *Science*, **197,** 368–370 (1977)

10 BLACK, B. L. and MOOG, F. Alkaline phosphatase and maltase activity in the embryonic chick intestine in culture. Influence of thyroxine and hydrocortisone. *Developmental Biology*, **66,** 232–249 (1978)

11 BLOCK, J., GINSEL, L. A., MULDER-STAPEL, A. A., ONDERWATER, J. J. M. and DAEMS, W. Th. The effect of colchicine on the intracellular transport of ^{3}H-fucose-labelled glycoproteins in the absorptive cells of cultured human small-intestinal tissue. *Cell and Tissue Research*, **215,** 1–12 (1981)

12 BLOCK, J., MULDER-STAPEL, A. A., GINSEL, L. A. and DAEMS, W. Th. Endocytosis in absorptive cells of cultured human small-intestinal tissue: horseradish peroxidase, lactoperoxidase, and ferritin as markers. *Cell and Tissue Research*, **216,** 1–13 (1981)

13 BROWNING, T. H. and TRIER, J. S. Organ culture of mucosal biopsies of human small intestine. *Journal of Clinical Investigation*, **48,** 1423–1432 (1969)

14 CALVERT, R. Effect of amniotic fluid and fetal bovine serum on the morphogenesis of mouse duodenal villi in organ culture. *Experientia*, **37,** 417–418 (1981)

15 CALVERT, R., MICHELETII, P. A. Selection of chemically defined medium for culturing fetal mouse small intestine. *In Vitro*, **17,** 331–344 (1981)

16 CHABOT, J.-G., MÉNARD, D. and HUGON, J. S. Organ culture of adult mouse intestine. IV. Stimulation of glucose-6-phosphatase *in vitro*. *Histochemistry*, **57,** 33–45 (1978)

17 CHABOT, J.-G. and HUGON, J. S. Lack of trophic effect of gastrin upon organ culture of adult mouse intestine. *Anatomical Record*, **196,** 30-A (1980)

18 CHABOT, J.-G. and HUGON, J. S. Stimulation of DNA synthesis in mouse intestinal mucosa by epidermal growth factor. *Journal of Cell Biology*, **87,** H-1205 (1980)

19 CHO, H. Y. and TAKEUCHI, A. Organ culture of the fetal mouse intestine. *In Vitro*, **15,** 194 (1979)

20 DeRITIS, G., FALCHUK, Z. M. and TRIER, J. S. Differentiation and maturation of cultured fetal rat jejunum. *Developmental Biology*, **45,** 304–317 (1975)

21 DeRITIS, G., OCCORSIO, P., AURICCHIO, S., GRAMENZE, F., MORISI, G. and SILANO, V. Toxicity of wheat flour proteins and protein-derived peptides for *in vitro* developing intestine from rat fetus. *Pediatric Research*, **13,** 1255–1261 (1979)

22 DOELL, R. G. and KRETCHMER, N. Intestinal invertase: precocious development of activity after injection of hydrocortisone. *Science*, **143,** 42–44 (1964)

23 DOLIN, R., BLACKLOW, N. R., MALMGREN, R. A. and CHANOCK, R. M. Establishment of human fetal intestinal organ cultures for growth of viruses. *Journal of Infectious Disease*, **122,** 227–231 (1970)

24 EADE, O. E., ST-ANDRÉ-UKENA, S., BEEKEN, W. L. Comparative viabilities of rat intestinal epithelial cells prepared by mechanical, enzymatic and chelating methods. *Digestion*, **21,** 25–32 (1981)

25 ELOY, R., RAUL, F., POUSSE, A., MIRHOM, R., ANANA, A. and GRENIER, J. F. *Ex vivo* vascular perfusion of the isolated rat small bowel. *European Journal of Surgical Research*, **9,** 96–112 (1977)

26 ELOY, R., VAULTIER, J. P., RAUL, F., MIRHOM, R., CLENDINNEN, G. and GRENIER, J. F. Hormonal stimulation of intestinal brush border enzymes release. *Research in Experimental Medicine*, **172,** 109–121 (1978)

27 FALCHUK, Z. M., GEBHARD, R. L., SESSOMS, C. and STROBER, W. An *in vitro* model of gluten-sensitive enteropathy. Effect of gliadin on intestinal epithelial cells of patients with gluten-sensitive enteropathy in organ culture. *Journal of Clinical Investigation*, **53,** 487–500 (1974)

28 FALCHUK, Z. M. and STROBER, W. Gluten-sensitive enteropathy: synthesis of antigliadin antibody *in vitro*. *Gut*, **15,** 947–952 (1974)

29 FALCHUK, Z. M., NELSON, D. L., KATZ, A. J., BERNARDIN, J. E., KASARDA, D. D., HAGUE, N. E. and STROBER, W. Gluten-sensitive enteropathy. Influence of histocompatibility type on gluten sensitivity *in vitro*. *Journal of Clinical Investigation*, **66,** 227–233 (1980)

30 FERLAND, S. and HUGON, J. S. Organ culture of adult mouse intestine. I. Morphological results after 24 and 48 hours of culture. *In Vitro*, **15,** 278–287 (1979)

31 FERLAND, S. and HUGON, J. S. Organ culture of adult mouse intestine. II. Mitotic activity, DNA synthesis and cellular migration after 24 and 48 hours of culture. *In Vitro*, **15,** 288–293 (1979)

32 FUKAMACHI, H. and TAKAYAMA, S. Epithelial-mesenchymal interaction in differentiation of duodenal epithelium of fetal rats in organ culture. *Experientia*, **36,** 335–336 (1980)

33 GEBHARD, R. L. and COOPER, A. D. Regulation of cholesterol synthesis in cultured canine intestinal mucosa. *Journal of Biological Chemistry*, **253,** 2790–2796 (1978)

34 GINSEL, L. A., ONDERWATER, J. J. M. and DAEMS, W. Th. Transport of radiolabelled glycoprotein to cell surface and lysosome-like bodies of absorptive cells in cultured small-intestinal tissue from normal subjects and patients with a lysosomal storage disease. *Virchows Archives B Cell Pathology*, **30,** 245–273 (1979)

35 GOODMAN, M. W., PRIGGE, W. F. and GEBHARD, R. L. Hormonal regulation of canine intestinal cholesterol synthesis. *American Journal of Physiology*, **240,** G274–280 (1981)

36 HAFFEN, K., KEDINGER, M. and GRENIER, J. F. Etude de la survive en culture organotypique de la muqueuse intestinale de trois espèces de mammifères. *Comptes Rendus de la Société de Biologie*, **167,** 1973–1977 (1973)

37 HAFFEN, K., LEWIN, J. M. and ROBBERECHT, P. Intérêt du modèle des cellules isolées du pancréas exocrine, de l'estomac et de l'intestin grêle pour la recherche en gastroentérologie. *Gastronetérologie Clinique et Biologique*, **3,** 267–282 (1979)

38 HAURI, H. P., KEDINGER, M., HAFFEN, K., GRENIER, J. F. and HADORN, B. Organ culture of human duodenum and jejunum. *Biological Gastroenterology*, **8,** 307–319 (1975)

39 HAURI, H. P., KEDINGER, M., HAFFEN, K., FREIBURGHAUS, A., GRENIER, J. F. and HADORN, B. Biosynthesis of brush border glycoproteins by human small intestinal mucosa in organ culture. *Biochimica Biophysica Acta*, **467,** 327–339 (1977)

40 HAURI, H. P., KEDINGER, M., HAFFEN, K., DAZE, H., HADORN, B. and HEKKENS, W. Re-evaluation of the technique of organ culture for studying gluten toxicity in coeliac disease. *Gut*, **19,** 1090–1098 (1978)

41 HENLE, G. and DEINHARDT, F. The establishment of strains of human cells in tissue culture. *Journal of Immunology*, **79,** 54–59 (1957)

42 HENNING, S. J. and KRETCHMER, N. Development of intestinal function in mammals. *Enzyme*, **15,** 3–23 (1973)

43 HOFFMAN, A. G. D. and KUKSIS, A. Culture of presumptive epithelial cells from jejunal mucosa of axenic rats. *Experientia*, **36,** 202–204 (1980)

44 HOWDLE, P. D., CORAZZA, G. D. R., BULLEN, A. W. and LOSOWSKY, M. S. Gluten sensitivity of small intestinal mucosa *in vitro*: quantitative assessment of histological change. *Gastroenterology*, **80,** 442–50 (1981)

45 HUGON, J. S. and FERLAND, S. Action de la cytochalasine B sur des explants de duodénum de souris maintenus en culture organotypique. *Journal de Microscopie*, **23,** 53a–54a (1975)

46 INUI, KEN-ICHI, QUARONI, A., TILLOTSON, L. G. and ISSELBACHER, K. J. Amino acid and hexose transport by cultured crypt cells from rat small intestine. *American Journal of Physiology*, **239,** C190–196 (1980)

47 JOS, J. and REY, L. L'apport de la culture organotypique à l'étude pathogénique de la maladie coeliaque. *Archives Françaises des Maladies de l'Appareil Digestif*, **64,** 461–464 (1975)

48 KAGNOFF, K. F., DONALDSON, R. M. and TRIER, J. S. Organ culture of rabbit small intestine: prolonged *in vitro* steady state protein synthesis and secretion and secretory IgA secretion. *Gastroenterology*, **63,** 541–551 (1972)

49 KAGNOFF, M. F., SERFILIPPI, D. and DONALDSON, R. M. *In vitro* kinetics of intestinal secretory IgA secretion. *Journal of Immunology*, **110,** 297–300 (1973)

50 KATZ, A. J. and FALCHUK, Z. M. Definitive diagnosis of gluten-sensitive enteropathy. Use of an *in vitro* organ culture model. *Gastroenterology*, **75,** 695–700 (1978)

51 KEDINGER, M., BERTELOOT, A., HAFFEN, K. and HUGON, J. S. Organ culture of adult guinea-pig intestine. II. Biochemical and ultracytochemical findings. *Histochemistry*, **40,** 311–321 (1974)

52 KEDINGER, M., HAFFEN, K. and HUGON, J. S. Organ culture of adult guinea-pig intestine. I. Ultrastructural aspect after 24 and 48 hours of culture. *Zeitschrift fur Zellforschung*, **147,** 169–181 (1974)

53 KEDINGER, M., HAFFEN, K. and HUGON, J. S. Organ culture of adult guinea-pig intestine. III. Mitotic and cellular migration. *Cell and Tissue Research*, **156,** 353–358 (1975)

54 KEDINGER, M., HAURI, H. P., HAFFEN, K., GREEN, J. R., GRENIER, J. F. and HADORN, B. Turnover studies of human intestinal brush border membrane glycoproteins in organ culture. *Enzyme*, **24,** 96–106 (1979)

55 KEDINGER, M., SIMON, P. M., RAUL, F., GRENIER, J. F., HAFFEN, K. The effect of dexamethasone on the development of rat intestinal brush border enzymes in organ culture. *Developmental Biology*, **94,** 9–21 (1980)

56 KLAEVEMAN, H. L., GEBHARD, R. L., SESSOMS, C. and STROBER, W. *In vitro* studies of ulcerative ileojejunitis. *Gastroenterology*, **68,** 572–582 (1975)

57 KRAWITT, E. L. Vitamin D uptake and hydroxylation by jejunal organ culture. *Gastroenterology*, **74,** 1051 (1978)

58 LICHTENBERGER, L. M., LECHAGO, J. and MILLER, T. A. Cell culture of human intestinal mucosa. *Gastroenterology*, **77,** 1291–1300 (1979)

59 MAK, K. M., TRIER, J. S., SERFILIPPI, D. and DONALDSON, R. M. Resistance of adult mammalian intestinal mucosa to cytochalasin B. *Experimental Cell Research*, **86,** 325–332 (1974)

60 MÉNARD, D. and MALO, C. Establishment of an *in vitro* model for studying hormonal influence on developing intestinal mucosa. *Journal of Cell Biology*, **91,** 35a (1981)

61 MISCH, D. W., GIEBEL, P. E. and FAUST, R. G. Intestinal microvilli: responses to feeding and fasting. *European Journal of Cell Biology*, **21,** 269–279 (1980)

62 MITCHELL, J. D., MITCHELL, J. and PETERS, T. J. Enzyme changes in human small bowel mucosa during culture *in vitro*. *Gut*, **15,** 805–811 (1974)

63 MOOG, F. and NEHARI, V. The influence of hydrocortisone on the epithelial phosphatase of embryonic intestine *in vitro*. *Science*, **119,** 809–810 (1954)

64 PORTEOUS, J. W., LAKE, C. M. and MORRISON, A. Transcription and translation in intestinal epithelium. *Cell Biology International Reports*, **4,** 766 (1980)

65 POTHIER, P. and HUGON, J. S. Characterization of isolated villus and crypt cells from the small intestine of the adult mouse. *Cell and Tissue Research*, **211,** 405–418 (1980)

66 QUARONI, A., WANDS, J., TRELSTAD, R. L. and ISSELBACHER, K. J. Epithelioid cell cultures from rat small intestine. Characterization by morphologic and immunologic criteria. *Journal of Cell Biology*, **80,** 248–265 (1979)

67 RACHMILEWITZ, D., FAINARU, M. and EISENBERG, S. Lipoprotein secretion and Apo-I synthesis by cultured human intestinal mucosa. *Gastroenterology*, **79,** 1081 (1978)

68 RACHMILEWITZ, D. and FAINARU, M. Apolipoprotein A-I synthesis and secretion by cultured human intestinal mucosa. *Metabolism*, **28,** 739–743 (1979)

69 RACHMILEWITZ, D., SHARON, P. and EISENBERG, S. Lipoprotein synthesis and secretion by cultured human intestinal mucosa. *European Journal of Clinical Investigation*, **10,** 125–131 (1980)

70 RAMPAL, P. and DELMONT, J. Les cultures de muqueuse d'intestin grêle. *Archives Françaises des Maladies de l'Appareil Digestif*, **64,** 159–169 (1975)

71 ROTHENBERG, S. P., WEISS, J. P. and COTTER, R. Formation of transcobalamin II-Vitamin B_{12} Complex by guinea-pig ileal mucosa in organ culture after *in vivo* incubation with intrinsic factor-vitamin B_{12}. *British Journal of Haematology*, **40,** 401–414 (1978)

72 SATO, G. H. The role of serum in cell cultures. In *Biochemical Actions of Hormones*. Volume 3, edited by G. Litwak, 391–395. New York, Academic Press (1975)

73 SCHWARTZ, C. J., KINBERG, D. V. and WARE, P. Adenylate cyclase in intestinal crypt and villus cells: stimulation by cholera enterotoxin and prostagladin E. *Gastroenterology*, **68,** 94–104 (1975)

74 SHERR, H. P., STIFEL, F. B. and HERMAN, R. H. Effect of cholera toxin on rabbit jejunal carbohydrate metabolizing enzymes. *Gastroenterology*, **75,** 711–716 (1978)

75 SHIELDS, H. M., YEDLIN, S. T., BAIR, F. A., GOODWIN, C. L. and ALPERS, D. H. Successful maintenance of suckling rat ileum in organ culture. *American Journal of Anatomy*, **155,** 375–389 (1979)

76 SHIELDS, H. M., LEVINE, G. M., YEZDIMIR, E. A., BIELUNAS, J. C. and BAIR, F. A. Effect of pentagastrin on rabbit stomach and small intestinal protein synthesis *in vitro*. *Digestive Disease and Science*, **25,** 769–775 (1980)

77 SIMON, P. M., KEDINGER, M., HAFFEN, K., RAUL, F. and GRENIER, J. F. Action of various hormones and cAMP on intestinal brush border enzymes in organ culture. *Gastroenterology*, **80,** 1286 (1981)

78 SORIANO, L. Différenciation des épithéliums du tube digestif *in vitro*. *Journal of Embryology and Experimental Morphology*, **14,** 119–128 (1965)

79 STANGE, E. F., ALAVI, M., SCHNEIDER, A., PRECLIK, G. and DITSCHUNEIT, H. Lipoprotein regulation of 3-hydroxy-3-methylglutaryl coenzyme A reductase in cultured intestinal mucosa. *Biochimica Biophysica Acta* **620,** 520–527 (1980)

80 STANGE, E. F., PRECLIK, G., SCHNEIDER, A., ALAVIN, M. and DITSCHUNETT, H. Regulation of 3-hydroxy-3-methylglutaryl-CoA reductase by endogenous sterol synthesis in cultured intestinal mucosa. *Biochimica Biophysica Acta*, **663,** 613–620 (1981)

81 TRIER, J. S. Organ culture methods in the study of gastrointestinal mucosal function and development. *New England Journal of Medicine*, **295,** 150–155 (1976)

82 TRIER, J. S. Organ culture of the mucosa of human small intestine. In *Methods in Cell Biology*, edited by C. C. Harris, B. F. Trump and G. D. Stoner, 365–384, New York, Academic Press (1980)

83 TRIER, J. S. and BROWNING, T. H. Epithelial-cell renewal in cultured duodenal biopsies in celiac sprue. *New England Journal of Medicine*, **283,** 1245–1250 (1970)

84 TRUDING, R., QUARONI, A. and WALKER, W. A. The use of fetal intestinal explants to study differentiation of the gut. *Gastroenterology*, **80,** 1305 (1981)

85 ZIOMEK, C. A., SCHULMAN, S. and EDIDIN, M. Redistribution of membrane proteins in isolated mouse intestinal epithelial cells. *Journal of Cell Biology*, **86,** 849–857 (1980)

5
Immune mechanisms in the small intestine: Part 1

Roy G. Shorter and Thomas B. Tomasi, Jr.

INTRODUCTION

The gastrointestinal tract is a major immune organ of the body and its degree of exposure to environmental antigens makes it a key factor in host defenses against pathogenic micro-organisms and in host reactivity to many nonviable materials, including potential carcinogens. The gut is a principal site for the sensitization of immunocytes which ultimately 'colonize' other mucosal sites, and serves as an initiation point for the cell traffic that occurs between various mucosae in the body. Such tissues have been termed the 'mucosal-associated lymphoid tissues' and a unitary concept of mucosal immune defenses is a theme of this chapter, with emphasis on its importance to the human. While a variety of other factors, for example mucus secretion and peristalsis, also provide vital mucosal defense functions acting in conjunction with the immune system, these have been reviewed elsewhere[27] and will not be detailed here.

THE GUT-ASSOCIATED LYMPHOID TISSUES (GALT)

Distribution

The lymphoid tissues of the wall of the gastrointestinal tract in man exist in four recognized anatomical locations:

(1) lymphocytes situated basally between the epithelial cells of the mucous membranes: the intraepithelial lymphocytes (IEL);
(2) lymphocytes loosely arranged in the connective tissues of the mucosal lamina propria, the lamina proprial lymphocytes (LPL);
(3) specialized nodules of lymphoid cells in the mucosa of the small intestine particularly the ileum, namely Peyer's patches (PP); and
(4) solitary mucosal lymphoid follicles.

Important additional features of the immunological 'apparatus' of the gastrointestinal tract are the salivary glands, pharyngeal tonsils, regional lymph nodes and the reticuloendothelial tissues of the liver.

Cell populations in GALT

Intraepithelial lymphocytes

Intraepithelial lymphocytes (IEL) are located basally between epithelial cells in essentially all human mucosal surfaces which have continuity with the external environment. Counts of IEL in human small bowel have ranged from 10 to 39 per 100 epithelial cells (mean: 21), and these lymphocytes vary in size, contain cytoplasmic granules and can cross the basement membrane in either direction[4, 9, 10, 15, 16, 18, 21, 23, 24]. Many of the granules in IEL resemble those in mast cells and one speculation is that granulated IEL are T cells which have a special relationship to the mucosal mast cells. T and B lymphocytes are present in the small intestinal IEL but precise definitions of subsets are lacking.

Lamina proprial lymphocytes

While small intestinal lamina proprial lymphocytes (LPL) have been studied more extensively than IEL, data on their characteristics are modest and somewhat conflicting and much further work is needed. In summary, the numbers of LPL in the small bowel mucosa of healthy humans range from 5000 to 11 000/square mm[9]. Among the B cells, normally there is a preponderance of IgA cells, and Bookman and Bull[1] concluded that human ileal LPL contain a lower proportion of B cells compared with the colon. T cells are present in the LPL of the human small bowel but little is known of the subsets, and null cells also have been detected.

Peyer's patches

Peyer's patches are organized aggregates of lymphoid cells in the submucosa of the small intestine, which lack afferent lymphatics and are 'peripheral' rather than 'central' lymphoid organs. In man they are present throughout the small bowel, although principally in the ileum, and are first identifiable at the 24th week of fetal development[5]. The epithelial cells overlying PP are a specialized type (M cells) which lack well developed microvilli but are pinocytic and can transport particulates and macromolecules from the intestinal lumen to the lymphocytes in the patches[2, 12, 19, 20]. PP are poorly developed in germ-free animals, but with conventional feeding, follicles are present which are composed predominantly (50–70 percent) of B lymphocytes[14]. However, PP also contain 11–40 percent T cells which are situated largely in interfollicular sites, and in the mouse the ratio of T:B cells in PP is greater in the neonatal period than in adult life[14]. As for other lymph nodes, approximately 80 percent of the B cells bear IgD[14]. PP have been found not to show natural killer activity and several groups reported that the B cells of PP could not be induced to plasma cells by immunization *in vitro*, and that T cells from PP were not stimulated to become cytotoxic cells whether the antigen was given orally or parenterally[14]. However, Kagnoff and Campbell[13] noted that antigen-reactive precursors of T or B effector cells were demonstrable in PP *in vitro* if the cultures were supplemented by peritoneal macrophages or with 2-mercaptoethanol (2ME). Thus the the apparent lack of ability of B cells from PP to form antibody may result from a relative lack of macrophages, and this 'feeder' function can be replaced by 2ME. As Kagnoff stressed, there is considerable evidence that PP are involved in the 'sampling' of antigens from the intestinal lumen and that they can be primed by the feeding of antigens, although this may occur without the induction of effector function[14]. Also, antigen-primed B cells migrate from PP to other sites, including the intestinal lamina propria, and there achieve effector function with the secretion of IgA[3,6]. Thus it may be that PP are a prerequisite for specific IgA responses in the intestinal lamina propria, although it is possible that the scattered lymphoid follicles in the intestinal mucosa also provide IgA precursor cells to the LPL. Some of these points will be considered later in greater detail.

Solitary lymphoid follicles

These are present in the mucosa and submucosa of the gut and lack the special epithelial relationship shown by PP. They contain T cells, B cells and macrophages[14] but little is known of their subsets or functional properties in man.

'HOMING' AND OTHER MIGRATORY PATTERNS OF GUT-ASSOCIATED LYMPHOID CELLS

Following antigen sensitization of PP, lymphocytes migrate to the mesenteric lymph nodes and thence, via the thoracic duct, to the systemic circulation and then to the lamina propria of the intestinal tract[26]. The observation that the migration of gut-associated lymphocytes occurs to the lamina propria of antigen-free explants of bowel suggests that such 'homing' is specific, although the qualities of the receptors on the lymphocytes and in the gut mucosa which are involved have not been defined. While specific 'homing' may occur in the absence of gut-luminal derived antigen(s), there is evidence that normally these play a major role in determining the extent of local immune responses[26]. Although large lymphocytes from the thoracic duct migrate to the lamina propria independently of antigen and may be responsible for the early antibody response, in the absence of antigen such cells may die *in situ*. However, if antigen either persists or is reintroduced at the site of the original mucosal challenge, these lymphocytes are stimulated and clonal expansion occurs. Later, small lymphocytes recirculating in the thoracic duct are recruited into the area where the antigen is present. Also it has been shown that isolated populations of T cells from the mesenteric lymph nodes of mice 'home' specifically to intraepithelial locations[11].

In addition to 'homing' and 'antigen-driven' clonal expansion, specific antibodies are formed at mucosal sites distant from the original site of antigen sensitization, and this has been reported from several animal models. For example, in the lactating animal, lymphoid cells sensitized in the gut migrate to the breast, so the IgA antibodies found in the milk may stem from this mechanism[22]. In studies in which pregnant rabbits were immunized with dinitrophenylated pneumococci, if the antigen was given orally then specific antibodies appeared in breast milk but not in the serum, implying that there was a migration of sensitized cells from the gut to the breast rather than absorption of the antigen. Had the latter occurred it could have been expected to induce a serum antibody response. Another migration pattern was found following enteric immunization of humans with killed *Streptococcus mutans*[17]. This immunization led to the appearance of strain-specific antibodies in the saliva and tears within a week of ingestion of the organisms. These were restricted to the IgA class and significant titers of specific antibodies were not found in the serum. Secondary challenge with the bacterium caused a rapid increase in salivary-specific antibodies which was characteristic of an anamnestic response. These findings imply that migration of antigen-sensitized cells occurs from the gut mucosa following enteric immunization by bacteria, and that specific antibody which appears in other external secretions such as saliva and tears results from this. In addition to their migration to salivary and lacrimal tissues, there is evidence that sensitized cells migrate from the gut to the mucosae of the bronchial, urinary and genital tracts, although this is less well established. Thus, it is likely that there is considerable traffic of immunocytes between various mucosal secretory sites which supports the concept of a general system of mucosal-associated lymphoid tissues and may have important clinical potential. For example, oral immunization by antigens of pathogenic organisms perhaps could be used in prophylaxis against certain local diseases in other mucosal sites; e.g. genital infections due to gonorrhea or ophthalmic infections by herpes viruses. However, it has not been established that there is cellular traffic between *all* mucous membranes. For example, does immunization via the eye result in immune responses in the vagina or urinary bladder? Also, migration patterns largely have been studied using B cells and relatively little is known about the mucosa to mucosa migration of T cells. More information is needed to answer the important question of whether transfer of cell-mediated immune reactions occurs from one mucosal site to another.

ANTIGENIC UPTAKE BY INTACT MUCOSAL SURFACES

The intestinal mucosa in the healthy adult mammal forms an incomplete block to the uptake of intraluminal antigens and many such materials may enter the intestinal wall and subsequently be found intact in the circulation. For example, antigens such as botulinus toxin and bovine serum albumin (BSA) gain access to the intestinal wall and to the intestinal lymph after their ingestion. Feeding BSA to hamsters is followed by its early appearance in intestinal submucosal mononuclear cells[7,8] and Warshaw *et al.*[28] suggested that the route of mucosal absorption of antigens may be the 'anatomical antithesis' of the secretion of IgA. Some organisms, such as *Salmonella typhi,* can penetrate the intact adult intestinal epithelium and gain access to the lamina propria, Peyer's patches and regional nodes although, as shown by Staley, Jones and Corley[25], intragastrically administered *E. coli* penetrated the intestinal epithelium in colostrum-deprived but *not* in colostrum-fed neonatal pigs. The structure and dose of the antigen, the age and the previous immunological experience of the animal with the antigen all appear to determine the nature and degree of the host's immunological response following its ingestion. Some of these points will be considered later but, parenthetically, much more work is needed to determine the mechanisms and control of antigenic absorption by the bowel in the human at various chronological stages of postuterine life and to define the factors influencing the resulting immunological responses. This information might provide greater insight into the mechanisms of certain human diseases which are of unknown etiopathogenesis, especially those with 'autoimmune' or 'allergic' features. It is particularly important to determine the immunological effects of feeding human infants with diets other than maternal breast milk[29].

Acknowledgements

This work was supported in part by a grant from the National Foundation for Ileitis and Colitis.

References

1 BOOKMAN, M. A. and BULL, D. M. Characteristics of isolated intestinal mucosal lymphocytes in inflammatory bowel disease. *Gastroenterology*, **77,** 503–510 (1979)

2 CARTER, P. B. and COLLINS, F. M. The route of enteric infection in normal mice. *Journal of Experimental Medicine*, **139,** 1189–1203 (1974)

3 CEBRA, J. J., GEARHARDT, P. J., KAMAT, R., ROBERTSON, S. M. and TSENG, J. Origin and differentiation of lymphocytes involved in the secretory IgA responses. *Cold Spring Harbor Symposium on Quantitative Biology*, **XIL,** 201–215 (1976)

4 COLLAN, Y. Characteristics of nonepithelial cells in the epithelium of normal rat ileum. *Scandinavian Journal of Gastroenterology*, **7** (Suppl. 18), 1–66 (1972)

5 CORNES, J. S. Number, size and distribution of Peyer's patches in the human small intestine. I. The development of Peyer's patches. *Gut*, **6,** 225–229 (1965)

6 CRAIG, S. W. and CEBRA, J. J. Peyer's patches: an enriched source of precursors for IgA-producing immunocytes in the rabbit. *Journal of Experimental Medicine*, **134,** 188–200 (1971)

7 DOLEZEL, J. and BIENENSTOCK, J. Immune response of the hamster to oral and parenteral immunization. *Cellular Immunology*, **2,** 326–334 (1971)

8 DOLEZEL,.J. and BIENENSTOCK, J. γA and non-γA immune response after oral and parenteral immunization of the hamster. *Cellular Immunology*, **2,** 458–468 (1971)

9 FERGUSON, A. Celiac disease and gastrointestinal food allergy. In *Immunological Aspects of the Liver and Gastrointestinal Tract*, edited by A. Ferguson, R. N. M. MacSween, 153–202. Lancaster, MTP Press Ltd (1976)

10 GLAISTER, J. R. Light, fluorescence and electron microscopic studies of lymphoid cells in the small intestinal epithelium of mice. *International Archives of Allergy and Applied Immunology*, **45,** 854–867 (1973)

11 GUY-GRAND, D., GRISCELLI, C. and VASSALI, P. The mouse gut T lymphocyte, a novel type of T cell. Nature, origin, and traffic in mice in normal and graft-versus-host conditions. *Journal of Experimental Medicine*, **148,** 1661–1677 (1978)

12 JOEL, D. D., SORDAT, B., HESS, M. W. and COTTIER, H. Uptake and retention of particles from the intestine by Peyer's patches in mice. *Experientia*, **26,** 694 (1970) (abstract)

13 KAGNOFF, M. F. and CAMPBELL, S. Functional characteristics of Peyer's patch lymphoid cells. I. Induction of humoral antibody and cell-mediated allograft reactions. *Journal of Experimental Medicine*, **139,** 398–406 (1974)

14 KAGNOFF, M. F. The gut-associated lymphoid tissue. In *Inflammatory Bowel Disease* (2nd Edn.), edited by J. B. Kirsner and R. G. Shorter, 71–85. Philadelphia, Lea and Febiger (1980)

15 MARSH, M. N. Studies of intestinal lymphoid tissue. I. Electron microscopic evidence of blast transformation in epithelial lymphocytes of mouse small intestinal mucosa. *Gut*, **16,** 665–682 (1975)

16 MEADER, R. D. and LANDERS, D. F. Electron and light microscopic observations on relationships between lymphocytes and intestinal epithelium. *American Journal of Anatomy*, **121,** 763–774 (1967)

17 MESTECKY, J., McGHEE, J. R., ARNOLD, R. R., MICHALEK, S. M., PRINCE, S. J. and BABB, J. L. Selective induction of an immune response in human external secretions by ingestion of bacterial antigen. *Journal of Clinical Investigation*, **61(3),** 731–737 (1978)

18 ORLIC, D. and LEV, R. An electron microscopic study of intraepithelial lymphocytes in human fetal small intestine. *Laboratory Investigation*, **37,** 554–561 (1977)

19 OWEN, R. L. and JONES, A. L. Epithelial cell specialization within human Peyer's patches: an ultrastructural study of intestinal lymphoid follicles. *Gastroenterology*, **66,** 189–203 (1974)

20 OWEN, R. L. Sequential uptake of horseradish peroxidase by lymphoid follicle epithelium of Peyer's patches in the normal unobstructed mouse intestine: an ultrastructural study. *Gastroenterology*, **72,** 440–451 (1977)

21 ROPKE, C. and EVERETT, N. B. Proliferative kinetics of large and small intraepithelial lymphocytes in the small intestine of the mouse. *American Journal of Anatomy*, **145,** 395–408 (1976)

22 ROUX, M. E., McWILLIAMS, M., PHILLIPS-QUAGLIATA, J. M., WEISZ-CARRINGTON, P. and LAMM, M. E. Origin of the IgA-secreting plasma cells in the mammary gland. *Journal of Experimental Medicine*, **146,** 1311–1322 (1977)

23 RUDZIK, O. and BIENENSTOCK, J. Isolation and characteristics of gut mucosal lymphocytes. *Laboratory Investigation*, **30,** 260–266 (1974)

24 SEELIG, L., Jr. and BILLINGHAM, R. E. Intraepithelial lymphocytes. *Journal of Investigative Dermatology*, **75,** 83–88 (1980)

25 STALEY, T. E., JONES, E. W. and CORLEY, L. D. Attachment and penetration of *Escherichia coli* into intestinal epithelium of the ileum in newborn pigs. *American Journal of Pathology*, **56,** 371–392 (1969)

26 TOMASI, T. B., Jr., LARSON, L. A., CHALLACOMBE, S. J. and McNABB, P. C. Mucosal immunity: the origin and migration patterns of cells in the secretory system. *Journal of Allergy and Clinical Immunology*, **65,** 12–19 (1980)

27 TOMASI, T. B., Jr. and McNABB, P. C. Host factors in mucosal disease. *Annual Review of Microbiology*, (in press)

28 WARSHAW, A. L., WALKER, W. A., CORNELL, R. and ISSELBACHER, K. J. Small intestinal permeability to macromolecules: transmission of horse-radish peroxidase into mesenteric lymph and portal blood. *Laboratory Investigation*, **25,** 675–684 (1971)

29 WATSON, D. W., BARTNIK, W. and SHORTER, R. G. Lymphocyte function and chronic inflammatory bowel disease. In *Inflammatory Bowel Disease* (2nd Ed.), edited by J. B. Kirsner and R. G. Shorter, 121–137. Philadelphia, Lea and Febiger (1980)

5
Immune mechanisms in the small intestine: Part 2

Roy G. Shorter and Thomas B. Tomasi, Jr.

THE MUCOSAL (SECRETORY) IMMUNE SYSTEM

Because mucosal surfaces, including the gut, are major sites of antigenic exposure in man, their external secretions form an immunological panoply which contributes to host defense. The clinical importance of immunological mechanisms functioning in these secretions first was suggested by the observation that titers of specific antibodies in mucosal fluids correlated better with host resistance to certain infections than did those of serum antibodies. In addition, antibody responses in secretions are regulated independently of those in the serum and there is evidence for a similar dichotomy in the regulation of cell-mediated immunity. These factors are critical to the concept of an immunological defense system involving all mucosal surfaces, including the alimentary tract, which has been termed the 'mucosal' or 'secretory' immune system.

The relative concentrations of various immunoglobulins show some differences between external (e.g. the gut) and internal secretions (e.g. serum). In the former there is a predominance of IgA, the IgG/IgA ratio often being less than 1, in contrast to 4:1 or 5:1 in serum, while IgM, IgD and IgE also are present in small amounts. However, internal secretions contain IgG as their major immunoglobulin class.

Although certain species differences exist, several features of external secretions are shared by all the various mammals that have been studied. This review will emphasize the findings in humans, and the gut and the other mucosal sites will be considered as a unitary system.

Structure of secretory IgA

Secretory IgA is a complex molecule composed of an IgA dimer (MW 300 000 daltons), a molecule of secretory component (SC; MW 70 000), and a molecule of J chain (MW 15 000). The entire sIgA molecule has a sedimentation coefficient of

11S and a molecular weight of approximately 385 000 daltons. SC binds to dimeric and polymeric IgA but not to 7S IgA, IgG or IgE, although the IgM in secretions also contains SC. A small amount of SC is present in free form in most normal external fluids but SC is entirely free in the external secretions of neonates or patients with IgA deficiency. Free SC binds to dimeric IgA *in vitro* and in the human this binding involves hydrophobic and disulfide bonds[33]. The relationship between SC and dimeric IgA may account for the increased stability of sIgA which makes it less susceptible to the action of various proteolytic enzymes[31,38]. This greater resistance of sIgA to proteolysis compared to other immunoglobulin molecules may result in a selective advantage to the survival and, thus, to the functional activities of such antibodies in external secretions.

Secretory component

Secretory component is a glycoprotein (MW 80 000), structurally unrelated to the immunoglobulins. Unlike IgA and J chain, which are produced by lamina proprial plasma cells, SC is synthesized by glandular epithelial cells and is present in fetal tissues as early as 8 weeks of age. Cells of the acini and ducts of human salivary and lacrimal glands, of the gastrointestinal tract epithelia (including the biliary ducts and gallbladder), of the respiratory mucosa, and of the epithelia of the uterine cervix, fallopian tubes and ureters all produce SC[37]. Isolated case reports have indicated that a deficiency of SC may be associated with a deficiency of sIgA in mucosal fluids, in some instances despite the presence of normal blood levels of IgA. This provides indirect support that SC is necessary for the transport of IgA across mucosal epithelia. Also there is good evidence in some species (mouse, rat) that SC also acts as a receptor for the transport of serum dimeric IgA across hepatic parenchymal cells and into the bile. Lastly, it was speculated that SC deficiency may be a common factor in the sudden death of infants, an hypothesis worthy of further study[22].

J chain

J chain is a glycopeptide (MW 15 000) which is disulfide-bonded to polymeric IgA and IgM but is absent from 7S monomeric IgA, IgG, IgD, or IgE[41]. It is incorporated into IgA and IgM immediately prior to the secretion of the polymer and because of its association with polymeric immunoglobulins, J chain may function *in vivo* by inducing correct polymerization of the subunits of IgA and IgM[15].

Higher polymers of IgA and IgM are disulfide-bonded to J chain such that only two of the monomeric units of IgA or IgM are bound to it, the remainder being bound to each other by disulfide bonds without the involvement of J chain. J chain is bound to the penultimate carboxy terminus cysteine of α and μ chains and may confer to IgA and to IgM the ability to bind SC, although SC does not complex directly to the J chain. Secretory component, residing in epithelial cell membranes, may act as a receptor for the transport of polymeric (mainly dimeric) IgA and IgM containing J chain. These immunoglobulins either are synthesized in the lamina propria or diffuse, via capillaries or sinusoids, to the epithelial surfaces which contain SC. Subsequently, they are transported into the secretions, probably by a 'coated pit-coated vesicle' mechanism[12].

IgA subclasses

Two subclasses of IgA (IgA1 and IgA2) have been identified in the serum and in secretions. IgA1 accounts for approximately 90 percent of the total serum IgA[32] while, in contrast, in certain secretions the IgA2 subclass comprises 40–60 percent of the total IgA. These subclasses are antigenically distinct and differ in their galactosamine content, hinge region length, the number of interchain disulfide bonds and their metabolic properties. Furthermore, the IgA2 subclass can be subdivided by allotypic markers into two types: A2m(1) and A2m(2). These markers have different incidences in various races as illustrated by the finding that A2m(1) is predominant in Caucasians whereas A2m(2) prevails in Negroid and in Mongoloid peoples[35].

Of clinical interest is the fact that the class and subclass antigens on the IgA molecule may be responsible for anaphylactic tranfusion reactions in those patients with selective IgA deficiency who develop antibodies against antigenic determinants of IgA following multiple blood transfusions. Antiboaies to allotype specificity also have been found to cause urticarial reactions in some of these individuals. These IgA subclasses also may be of clinical importance because certain pathogenic microorganisms, especially *Neisseria gonorrhoeae* and *Neisseria meningitidis*, produce enzymes capable of cleaving human IgA1[21,24]. These proteases are highly selective and cleave a single peptide bond in the hinge region of the heavy chain of the IgA1 subclass[25]. After this action the IgA1 antibodies lose some of their biological properties, including the ability to agglutinate the bacteria. In contrast, IgA2 is resistant to these proteases, as are all other proteins which have been studied.

Origin of IgA in secretions

It has been postulated that the majority of sIgA is produced within the various secretory mucosal tissues and some support for this was provided by studies described earlier in this review. Plasma cells in mucosal sites elaborate primarily dimeric IgA which then appears in the secretory fluids. The lamina propria of the human gastrointestinal tract contains approximately 20–30 IgA cells per IgG cell which differs from the peripheral lymph nodes and spleen in which the ratio is 1:4 (IgA:IgG). It has been concluded that only small amounts of IgA pass from the serum into the external secretions under normal circumstances. However, Halsey, Johnson and Cebra[14] tested the capacity of the lactating murine breast to transport labelled IgA dimers, other immunoglobulins or bovine serum albumin and found that immunoglobulins containing oligomeric J chain were transferred selectively from the serum into the colostrum. They stressed that a significant role for extraglandular synthesis of the IgA found in colostrum is worthy of consideration. However, their experiments did not determine the relative importance of the two possible mechanisms for the provision of maternal Ig to colostrum, i.e. the local synthesis of immunoglobulin by cells migrating from the gut, versus the production of Ig at distant mucosal sites, especially the gut lamina propria, followed by its passage via the circulation and transport into the mammary secretions. Nevertheless, in cattle and pigs there is strong evidence that a significant proportion of the IgA in breast milk is derived from the serum.

In mice and rats polymeric IgA is transported from the serum into the bile via the liver[17, 18, 23]. In these animals, experimental ligation of the bile duct results in a rapid increase of dimeric IgA in the systemic circulation. If the obstruction is relieved before permanent liver damage ensues, there is a rapid fall to normal of the serum level of IgA. Human dimeric IgA, derived either from monoclonal or polyclonal sources and containing J chain, binds specifically to plasma membranes of normal human hepatocytes. Therefore in man it is likely that the liver cell plays important roles in extracting polymeric IgA from the serum and in its transport into the bile, thus increasing the amount of sIgA arriving in the gut lumen. However, the amount of this contribution has yet to be determined.

Origins of IgG, IgE and IgM in secretions

It is generally accepted that a major proportion of the IgG in external secretions normally is derived by transudation from the serum, although some local synthesis occurs. Serum IgG gains the interstitial fluid of the lamina propria of the bowel by permeating the capillary walls, but the precise route of its transport across the gut epithelium into the mucosal secretion is unknown. In the small bowel it is probable that some passes into the lumen at the tips of the villi. When inflammation occurs in a mucous membrane, such as the gut, there is not only increased transudation of IgG from serum but also invasion of the mucosa by IgG-producing plasma cells, and these antibodies may be of clinical importance to host recovery from mucosal infections.

IgE is present only in very low concentrations in most secretory fluids but these are greater than can be explained by transudation from the serum, indicating local synthesis. Approximately 5 percent of the B cells in the lamina propria of the gastrointestinal and respiratory mucosae are IgE-producing cells, in contrast to the spleen and peripheral lymph nodes, in which only a few (<1 percent) are present[30]. The IgE in external secretions contains no SC and physicochemically and antigenically is similar to that in the serum. The route of its transport into secretions is unknown. This topic has been reviewed recently by Bienenstock and Befus[3].

IgM is synthesized in secretory tissues and the human gastrointestinal tract contains approximately five times more IgM-producing than it does IgG-producing cells. Also, IgM is present in parotid fluid in a higher concentration than IgG. Furthermore, patients with selective IgA deficiency have large numbers of

IgM-producing submucosal plasma cells and large amounts of IgM in their external secretions. Like IgA, the IgM molecule can bind secretory component and most sIgM contains noncovalently bound SC. Perhaps IgM also is transported across hepatocytes since SC binds IgM with high affinity in man[28]. Secretory IgM, and to a lesser extent IgG, can serve to replace IgA as the predominant secretory immunoglobulin in some individuals with selective IgA deficiency[29]. The extent of this replacement may be a major reason why certain IgA-deficient patients are asymptomatic while others suffer from recurrent infections.

Route of transport of sIgA and sIgM

The quantity of polymeric versus monomeric IgA synthesized by a mucosal tissue, e.g., the gut lamina propria, may depend largely on the production of cells containing J chain. Dimeric IgA complexed with J chain diffuses through the interstitium of the lamina propria, crosses the basement membrane and enters the intercellular space. However, because the apical portions of adjacent epithelial cells are in close apposition (tight junction), large molecules of the size of IgA or IgM cannot gain direct access to the lumen. Secretory component present on the lateral and basal aspects of the membranes of the epithelial cells may act as a receptor for Ig. By complexing with dimeric IgA or IgM, SC facilitates their transport into the epithelial cells by an endocytotic process involving the invagination of the cell membrane and the enclosure of the sIgA and sIgM molecules in membrane-bound vesicles. These vesicles then are transported to the apical (luminal) membrane of the epithelial cell and extruded by reverse pinocytosis[4].

Origin of serum IgA

Serum IgA is synthesized in amounts almost as great as IgG (approximately 2.5 g/day in human adults) but because of its shorter half-life, which is 6 days compared with 22 for the IgG1 subclass, its concentration is much lower, being only about 2 mg/ml compared with 12 mg/ml for IgG. Neither the origin nor the biological role of serum IgA have been fully defined in man. However, there is evidence that the secretory lymphoid tissues, particularly in the gastrointestinal tract, are major sources of circulating IgA in various animal species: firstly, oral immunization of mice with ferritin elicits circulating antiferritin antibodies which are largely of the IgA class. In contrast, parenteral immunization with this antigen results in the production of IgM and IgG antibodies by the lymph nodes and spleen. Such observations indicate that serum IgA antibodies to ferritin are derived from cells originating in the gut. These cells either may reside in the gastrointestinal tract or migrate from the gut to other lymphoid tissues such as the spleen. Secondly, mice exposed to whole body X-irradiation rapidly develop a marked deficiency of serum IgA but not of IgG or IgM, and shielding the gastrointestinal tract from the irradiation prevents this. Thirdly, in rats and dogs, most of the proteins found in mesenteric lymph are derived from the serum by transudation across the intestinal capillaries, but IgA is a striking exception and over 80 percent of the lymphatic IgA results from local synthesis by plasma cells in the intestinal lamina propria.

Unfortunately the contribution of the gut to circulating IgA in the human is less clear. It is important to appreciate that 90 percent of the total serum IgA in man is monomeric (7S) and only 10 percent polymeric, whereas in many other animals 10S (dimeric) IgA is predominant. In several species there is evidence that most of the IgA synthesized in the gut is dimeric which complicates the question of the sources of the serum 7S IgA in man. It is possible that monomeric and polymeric IgA are synthesized in secretory sites in the human intestine and then either diffuse or are transported in two different directions. Perhaps monomeric IgA diffuses into the lymphatics and thence into the circulation, while the dimer is transported into the intestinal lumen because SC in the epithelial cells acts as a receptor which preferentially binds polymeric IgA. The smaller size of 7S IgA compared to 10S IgA might facilitate its diffusion into lymphatics although a small amount of dimer also may gain the circulation by this route. In addition, dimeric IgA may be removed from the blood by the hepatic transport mechanisms mentioned earlier. In contrast to these concepts, it has been suggested that the bone marrow is a major source of serum IgA in the human. However, direct measurements of the contributions of the bone marrow and other lymphoid tissues to the total serum IgA pool are unavailable so no precise definitions exist for the origins of serum IgA in man.

FUNCTIONS OF THE MUCOSAL (SECRETORY) IMMUNE SYSTEM

Antiviral activity

The induction of virus-specific secretory antibodies is determined, firstly, by the nature of the viral antigen (i.e. whether it is live and virulent, attenuated or inactivated) and, secondly, by the dose and route of immunization (parenteral or local). These points are illustrated by studies using poliovirus in which similar levels of IgM, IgG, and IgA antibodies occurred in the serum after the immunization of humans either orally with live attenuated poliovaccine (Sabin) or parenterally with activated vaccine (Salk). However, marked secretory antibody responses in the alimentary tract were found only after oral immunization with the Sabin vaccine, and these persisted for as long as 5 years. In addition, when infants with double-barrelled colostomies were locally immunized in the distal colon, this led to a predominantly IgA antibody response and only the immunized segments were capable of preventing subsequent colonization by poliovirus. These and other experiments demonstrated that the poliomyelitis virus-neutralizing immunoglobulins, induced locally in secretions either by natural infection or by the viral vaccine, are largely sIgA antibodies. Furthermore, the antibody titers in secretions show a better correlation with resistance to reinfection by the live virus than do serum titers.

In general, two types of viral infection exist with respect to the relative importance to the protection of the host provided by secretory versus serum antibodies. In the first, the virus replicates in the mucosa at the portal of entry, e.g., the gastrointestinal tract, and a secretory antibody response occurs. Examples include infections by rhinovirus, myxoviruses and some types of adenovirus, in all of which the organism remains localized superficially in the mucosa. The second type is illustrated by infections due to poliovirus in which following an initial mucosal phase, systemic viral spread occurs and circulating antibody is important to the host's defences against this dissemination. In the prophylaxis of poliomyelitis, if Salk poliovaccine (a killed virus) is given parenterally then the major antibody induced is serum IgG, with little or no secretory response. This humoral response protects against systemic spread if subsequent natural exposure to virulent virus occurs, although the patient may become a temporary carrier (with virus persisting at the portal of entry) until the local secretory antibody responses develop. In contrast, as emphasized above, oral immunization by the Sabin poliovaccine induces a secretory antibody response which prevents not only local viral replication and mucosal penetration on any subsequent natural exposure to live virulent virus, but also the establishment of the carrier state.

Antitoxin activity

In infections by microorganisms which act primarily by secretion of exotoxins (e.g. cholera), the local action of mucosal antitoxin antibodies in the gut contributes significantly to the host's defenses against disease.

Antibacterial activity

Observations in humans immunized orally with killed cholera organisms suggest that immunity to cholera is mediated largely by intestinal secretory immunoglobulins. It is known also that the adherence of *Vibrio cholerae in vivo* to the mucosa of intestinal loops in rabbits is decreased markedly by the local presence of cholera-specific coproantibodies. Similar modifications of the adherence of *E. coli* to gut and urinary tract epithelial cells, of the adherence of gonococci to uterine cervical and vaginal mucosae and of streptococci to buccal epithelium also have been demonstrated. It is essential for their colonization of mucous membranes that the bacteria selectively adhere to epithelial surfaces. It is apparent that surface antigens of bacteria influence their adherence to mucosal surfaces and thus their colonization properties. However, also influencing adherence are host factors concerned with cleansing these membranes, including peristalsis in the bowel, rapid fluid flow, epithelial cell desquamation and the secretion of mucus[36]. Secretory IgA antibodies augment these cleansing effects by binding to antigenic components on the surface of bacteria, thereby inhibiting their adherence to and resulting colonization of the mucosa[11,42]. An illustration of this action of the mucosal immune system in the prevention of disease caused by bacteria is found in experimental caries. Certain strains of *Streptococcus mutans* are cariogenic and produce dextran polymers from sucrose. These polymers enable the organisms to adhere to and to colonize the smooth surfaces of teeth, which are requirements for the formation of dental plaque and caries. Antisera for *S. mutans* inhibit their adherence to teeth, independently of bacterial killing. For certain antibodies the inhibition of adherence correlates with inhibition of the synthesis of cell-associated polysaccharide by the bacterial enzyme glucosyltransferase (dextran sucrase) rather than the direct blocking of the surface structures involved in adherence. Importantly, rats immunized locally with *S. mutans* and subsequently infected orally with the live organisms, develop specific antibodies of the IgA class in the saliva which inhibit bacterial glucosyltransferase activity, decrease bacterial adherence and reduce the production of caries compared to control animals. Therefore it seems that oral immunization against dental caries may be possible in the human and methods to achieve this are being developed.

Lysis and killing of bacteria involves complement fixation but IgA does not fix complement via the classic pathway as do IgG and IgM. Although IgA can fix complement via the alternative pathway, it is unknown whether the very small amounts of complement and alternative pathway components in external secretions are sufficient to be biologically effective. Thus whether activation of the alternative pathway by sIgA is important to host defenses against bacteria is an unanswered question.

The ability of phagocytes to engulf microbia is enhanced by the presence of specific antibody, with or without the presence of complement. However, although secretory IgA antibodies can coat bacteria *in vivo*, the evidence is inconclusive that this leads to enhanced phagocytosis of the organisms.

Absorption inhibition of non-viable antigens by the gastrointestinal mucosa

As emphasized earlier, healthy adults of most mammalian species absorb immunologically significant quantities of macromolecular antigens across mucosal epithelial cells. Furthermore, studies in the rat showed that oral immunization either with bovine serum albumin or horseradish peroxidase inhibited the uptake of the immunizing protein but not that of the unrelated antigen[39]. Accordingly, local immune reactions may provide a normal control mechanism for limiting the intestinal absorption of intact macromolecules and perhaps this is mediated by an action of secretory antibodies. Thus, this 'immune exclusion' function of such antibodies may protect the host against harmful luminal antigens by forming non-absorbable complexes which then are degraded on the surface of the intestinal mucosa by luminal proteolytic enzymes. Malfunction of immune exclusion might be important to some human diseases. Germane to such a concept are features of patients with selective deficiency of IgA, many of whom have high titers of serum antibodies directed against milk and food antigens[16]. Their gastrointestinal tracts are 'leaky' and excessive amounts of gut luminal antigens are absorbed which then induce serum IgM and IgG antibody responses. In certain of these individuals, circulating immune complexes composed of milk proteins (casein, bovine albumin, etc.) complexed with specific antibodies, can be found within an hour of drinking 100 ml of milk[9]. The ready occurrence of immune complexes containing exogenous antigens may explain in part the apparent susceptibility of patients with selective IgA deficiency to certain autoimmune diseases. However, an alternative explanation involves excessive and continued absorption of foreign antigens which cross-react with 'self-antigens'. Cross-reactivities between the antigens of microbia and mammals and their possible pathogenetic roles in a number of human diseases have been reviewed by Lyampert and Danilova[19] and stressed by others in idiopathic inflammatory bowel diseases[40].

Local cell-mediated immunity

T cells, B cells and macrophages, all of which may participate in cell-mediated reactions, are present in the gut mucosae. It is unfortunate that relatively little is known of such immune reactions in the gastrointestinal tract because they are important to the control of certain infections, to the mechanisms of some 'hypersensitivity' diseases (e.g. celiac disease) or diseases with autoimmune features[40], and perhaps to the emergence and growth of some malignant tumors.

The oral induction of tolerance (oral tolerance)

While enteric immunization may induce both secretory and systemic immune responses, the feeding of some antigens, especially in small doses, can result in an antigen-specific state of non-reactivity (oral tolerance) that lasts a variable period of time, depending on the dose and type of antigen administered[7,34]. As an example, mice given a single dose of ovalbumin (OVA) enterically prior to systemic challenge by the same antigen remained tolerant to OVA for longer than 3 months. Not only may the systemic antibody response be abrogated following certain types of oral immunization, but contact sensitivity also may be affected. This was recognized in the older literature as the 'Sulzberger-Chase phenomenon'.

While the mechanisms involved in the induction of oral tolerance are not explained, the liver may play an important role, at least with antigenic materials that are absorbed and then transported via the portal circulation. However, it is possible also that many proteins are absorbed directly via the lymphatics into the systemic circulation, thus bypassing the liver. For those situations in which the liver seems critical to the induction of oral tolerance, perhaps the Kupffer cells remove immunogenic aggregates and permit 'tolerogenic' monomers or fragments to reach the peripheral lymphoid tissues. Many studies have been made of oral tolerance to a number of different antigens and tolerance to heterologous erythrocytes has been variably reported to be due to the action of suppressor T cells (Ts) or to the presence of inhibitory serum factors, i.e. antibody or antigen-antibody complexes[1,20]. As indicated above, the feeding of contact-sensitizing agents to experimental animals may lead to systemic unresponsiveness although skin painting with the same agent causes hypersensitivity. The outcome of such feeding is dependent upon the dose and, in general, smaller doses administered repeatedly are more 'tolerogenic'. It appears that the immunological status of the animal following either painting or feeding of contact-sensitizing agents is delicate and could depend upon a balance between effector and suppressor cells which may be critically affected both by the dose of the antigen and by its route of immunization.

At least two types of suppressor cells were demonstrated in mice following the feeding of haptens. Firstly, suppressor B cells (Bs), which inhibited the adoptive transfer of contact sensitivity, appeared in Peyer's patches and mesenteric nodes about 4–7 days after a single feed and later were present in the spleen. Secondly, the spleens and peripheral lymph nodes of mice which had been fed contact-sensitizing agents and subsequently skin painted with the same materials, contained suppressor T cells which limited the synthesis of DNA by lymph node cells. In adoptive transfer experiments Bs were inhibitory for as long as 20 weeks after cessation of feeding with the sensitizing antigen. There is evidence suggesting that Bs exert their inhibiting effect by the production of IgG and, if so, the mechanism would be identical to the phenomenon of antibody-mediated suppression of immune responses. Tolerance resulting from the intravenous injection of haptens is induced most efficiently if the hapten has been conjugated *in vitro* to syngeneic cells. The mechanisms of induction of tolerance by *free* hapten initially may involve its 'complexing' *in vivo* with surface antigens of cells such as lymphocytes and macrophages. Following oral administration it is possible that this 'complexing' process occurs locally in the gastrointestinal tract, with subsequent development of suppressor cells in the gut-associated lymphoid tissues. However, it has not been shown that suppressor cells are obligatory for the initiation and/or maintenance of oral tolerance to such chemicals and the uptake of the hapten by the liver may be a critical step in the 'tolerogenic' mechanisms.

Orally induced tolerance to soluble proteins has been studied extensively and the results can be summarized as follows: systemic tolerance follows either a single large dose of ovalbumin or human globulin (HGG) or the repeated feeding of smaller doses over several weeks. Small doses given over prolonged periods generally are much more effective than the same total dose given as a single feeding. Specific tolerance lasts for as long as 3–4 months and the efficiency of its production is generally as good as that resulting from the same dose of antigen given systemically. Importantly, tolerance is induced only in T cells[8]. Using adoptive transfer, suppressor T cells (Ts) have been demonstrated in the mesenteric nodes and spleens of animals rendered tolerant by the oral administration of various soluble proteins[7]. However, although the period of time for which Ts persist after oral immunization with soluble proteins has not been studied extensively, one report indicated that they disappeared from the spleen by 30 days, even though the animals remained tolerant for several months. This is reminiscent of findings in systemic tolerance induced parenterally in which its presence was noted in the apparent absence of suppressor cells. These observations suggest that suppressor mechanisms may *not* be critical either to the induction or the persistence of this oral tolerance, although active suppression may be present for periods longer than adoptive transfer studies indicate. In this regard, suppressor factors have been found in splenic extracts from animals tolerant to HGG as long as 3 months after induction of the tolerant state. It is possible that only low levels of suppressor activity are necessary to maintain T cell unresponsiveness late in tolerance. Significant differences have been found between murine strains in their susceptibility to the oral induction of tolerance to HGG, but whether this follows the genetic patterns and three-gene control (one of which is linked to H-2) postulated for systemically induced tolerance, has yet to be determined.

Systemic tolerance in mice can be induced not only by feeding 'classical' soluble proteins such as ovalbumin or human gamma globulin but also by ragweed antigens, including short ragweed and purified antigen E, and bacteria such as S mutans or cell wall preparations from these organisms. The systemic tolerance resulting from oral immunization with these antigens affects humoral antibody responses and T cell-mediated immunity. However, tolerance to streptococci or their cell walls is of short duration, with a return to normal responsiveness by one month. Importantly, such antigens given orally elicited systemic hyporesponsiveness accompanied by the production of specific IgA antibodies in saliva (i.e. mucosal immunity) in the absence of a serum antibody response. Thus, there was complete dissociation between the mucosal and systemic systems such that systemic tolerance coexisted with an active secretory antibody response. The mechanisms involved are unknown but one reasonable explanation is that the gut-associated lymphoid tissues (GALT) produce suppressor T cells for the IgM and IgG antibody responses as well as for delayed hypersensitivity, while for the IgA system the balance is in favor of the production of helper T cells.

In summary, currently it is impossible to reconcile some of the observations described above with any concept of a unified mechanism for the oral induction of tolerance. Although species differences and varied methodologies may account for some of the discrepancies, probably different mechanisms are involved which depend on the chemical structure of the antigen, and regulatory mechanisms may shift with time during the induction and maintenance of tolerance. A critical point is that the immunological status of an animal to a particular antigen determines the effect of subsequent feeding of the antigen. Thus, if it is first administered parenterally, subsequent feeding either does not induce tolerance or, in the case of soluble proteins, actually may boost the titers of IgG and IgE antibodies to the antigen. In part this may be due to the fact that immune exclusion is not fully operative following the systemic immunization, and so enterically absorbed antigen induces a secondary splenic response. To our knowledge no experiments have been reported which have tested whether continued feeding of an antigen, particularly in small doses, leads to tolerance in parenterally primed animals. Since absorption of the antigen progressively decreases with oral immunization, it may be that systemic tolerance would develop eventually, despite the initial parenteral priming. This point is critical to any clinical potential for treating already sensitized individuals by feeding with the antigen. Lastly, it must be stressed that oral tolerance has not been achieved either for transplantation or tumor antigens.

An exciting concept is that in the human the existence of an active secretory immune response concomitantly with systemic tolerance may serve as a normal control mechanism to inhibit the mucosal absorption of antigens which are potentially allergenic or autoantigenic. If this were so, then the systemic tolerance could be a host defense against the development of certain hypersensitivity and autoimmune diseases by preventing reactions to antigens which have escaped immune exclusion. This thesis is supported by evidence that the sensitization of patients with atopic allergies occurs early in life when the secretory immune system is immature and permits more ready access of allergens to the systemic lymphoid tissues than in the adult. Furthermore, as mentioned earlier, individuals with defective secretory IgA systems have a high incidence of associated allergies and autoimmune diseases. In addition, the apparent absence of systemic tolerance to food proteins in many of these patients implies a major role for the gut-associated lymphoid tissues in the mechanisms of orally induced tolerance. This thesis could be tested by experiments using animals rendered selectively deficient of IgA.

Thus, further studies of oral tolerance may lead to improved methods of prophylaxis of certain infectious states in the human and to a greater understanding of the pathogenesis of some diseases with allergic or autoimmune features.

HOST RESPONSES TO INTESTINAL PARASITIC INFECTIONS

Askenase[2] has reviewed extensively the responses of intestinal mast cells to nematode infections and their possible role in host rejection of these parasites. He emphasized that mast cells are present in the small intestinal wall in two groups: first, those in the serosal connective tissue and, secondly, those in the mucosa of which some are intraepithelial and others are in the lamina propria. Mucosal mast cells have features which differ from those in the serosa, including their sensitivity to steroids or X-irradiation, the presence of IgE in their cytoplasm as well as on their surfaces, their inability to bind bee venom-peptide, a lack of heparin and a lower sulfonated proteoglycan constituting the matrix of their granules[2]. Furthermore, mucosal mast cells are relatively resistant to degranulation and mediator release when stimulated by antigen. As a result, Askenase[2] concluded that these cells are poorly adapted for involvement in 'anaphylactic-type' responses but might participate in delayed hypersensitivity reactions which depend upon the activation of T cells by antigenic stimuli. Importantly, Guy-Grand, Griscelli and Vassalli[13] suggested that there is a relationship between intestinal intraepithelial T lymphocytes and mucosal mast cells such that the latter either are derived from these T cells or are dependent upon them for differentiation.

An increased number of intestinal mucosal mast cells is a consistent feature of host responses to nematode infestation, and Ruitenberg and Elgersma[26] showed in mice that this is thymic dependent. An accelerated mast cell response to nematode infections can be transferred adoptively not only by the injection of the T cell fraction from thoracic duct lymph but also by immune serum, so perhaps it is also antibody dependent. However, although this mucosal mast cell response is well recognized, its functional role in the host's defenses against nematodes is controversial and there are arguments for and against its direct action in their elimination. Askenase[2] developed three hypotheses for the mechanisms of local immune rejection of nematodes by the host which included roles for T cell-dependent recruitment and activation of mast cells in the intestinal mucosa, for T cell-induced modifications of the secretion of mucus by intestinal goblet cells and for local actions of IgA and IgE.

It is possible that mast cells also participate in local immune defenses to other parasitic infections, such as *Schistosoma mansoni*, since these cells augment the killing of schistosomules *in vitro* in an eosinophil-mediated IgG_{2a} antibody-dependent cytotoxic system involving complement[5]. In this reaction, IgG antibodies attach to antigenic determinants on the parasite, leading to the adherence of eosinophils via their surface receptors for IgG. Thus, eosinophils may mediate killing of the parasite *in vivo* by this or related mechanisms[10], perhaps involving secretion of the major basic protein of eosinophils, although this is not established[27]. Other immune responses directed towards Schistosoma involve neither mast cells nor eosinophils. For example, anti-schistosome IgE antibody in rats can complex with schistosomal antigens and then attach to macrophages via their membrane receptors for the Fc portion of IgE. This leads to macrophage activation and resultant killing of the schistosomules[6].

Lastly, IgA may be significant in immunity to some intestinal parasitic infections (e.g. coccidia in fowl) but its precise role is yet to be defined[3].

In summary, intestinal mucosal immune mechanisms may be major factors in defense against certain parasitic infestations but further data are needed to establish this.

CONCLUSIONS

Much further work is needed to increase the knowledge of mucosal immunity in the gut and other epithelial surfaces in contact with the external environment, including the influences of dietary factors[3]. Such information is important because of the potential roles for abnormalities of the mucosal immune system in the mechanisms of many human diseases. Lastly, it is possible also that the manipulation of mucosal immunity may extend and facilitate the prophylaxis and treatment of certain infectious diseases in man.

References

1 ANDRE, C., HEREMANS, J. F., VAERMAN, J. P. and CAMBIASO, C. L. A mechanism for the induction of immunological tolerance by antigen feeding: antigen-antibody complexes. *Journal of Experimental Medicine*, **142,** 1509–1519 (1975)

2 ASKENASE, P. W. Immunopathology of parasitic diseases: involvement of basophils and mast cells. *Springer Seminars in Immunopathology*, **2,** 417–442 (1980)

3 BIENENSTOCK, J. and BEFUS, A. D. Mucosal immunology. *Immunology*, **41,** 249–270 (1980)

4 BRANDTZAEG, P. Mucosal and glandular distribution of immunoglobulin components: differential localization of free and bound secretory component in secretory epithelial cells. *Journal of Immunology*, **112,** 1553–1559 (1974)

5 BUTTERWORTH, A. E., STURROCK, R. F., HOUBA, V., MAHMOUD, A. A. F., SHER, A. and REES, P. H. Eosinophils as mediators of antibody dependent damage to schistosomula. *Nature*, **256,** 727–729 (1975)

6 CAPRON, A., DESSAINT, J. P., JOSEPH, M., ROUSSEAUX, R., CAPRON, M. and BAZIN, H. Interaction between IgE complexes and macrophages in the rat: a new mechanism of macrophage activation. *European Journal of Immunology*, **7,** 315–322 (1977)

7 CHALLACOMBE, S. J. and TOMASI, T. B. Jr. Systemic tolerance and secretory immunity after oral immunization. *Journal of Experimental Medicine*, **152,** 1459–1472 (1980)

8 CHILLER, J. M., TITUS, R. G. and ETLINGER, H. M. Cellular dissection of tolerant states induced by the oral route or in neonatal animals. In *Immunological Tolerance and Macrophage Function*, edited by P. Baram, J. R. Battisto and C. W. Pierce, 195–200. New York, Elsevier Publishing Company (1979)

9 CUNNINGHAM-RUNDLES, C., BRANDEIS, W. E., GOOD, R. A. and DAY, N. K. Milk precipitins, circulating immune complexes and IgA deficiency. *Proceedings of the National Academy of Sciences of the United States of America*, **75,** 3387–3389 (1978)

10 DAVID, J. R., VADAS, M. A., BUTTERWORTH, A. E., De BRITO, P. A., CARVALHO, E. M., DAVID, R. A., BINA, J. C. and ANDRADE, Z. A. Enhanced helminthotoxin capacity of eosinophils from patients with eosinophilia. *New England Journal of Medicine*, **303,** 1147–1152 (1980)

11 FUBARA, E. S. and FRETER, R. Source and protective function of coproantibodies in intestinal disease. *American Journal of Clinical Nutrition*, **25,** 1357–1363 (1972)

12 GOLDSTEIN, J. L., ANDERSON, R. G. W. and BROWN, M. S. Coated pits, coated vesicles, and receptor-mediated endocytosis. *Nature*, **279,** 679–685 (1979)

13 GUY-GRAND, D., GRISCELLI, C. and VASSALLI, P. The gut-associated lymphoid system: nature and properties of the large dividing cells. *European Journal of Immunology*, **4,** 435–443 (1974)

14 HALSEY, J. F., JOHNSON, B. H. and CEBRA, J. J. Transport of immunoglobulins from serum into colostrum. *Journal of Experimental Medicine*, **151,** 767–772 (1980)

15 HAUPTMAN, S. P. and TOMASI, T. B. Jr. Mechanism of immunoglobulin A polymerization. *Journal of Biological Chemistry*, **250,** 3891–3896 (1975)

16 HUNTLEY, C. C., ROBBINS, J. B., LYERLY, A. D. and BUCKLEY, R. H. Characterization of precipitating antibodies to ruminant serum and milk proteins in humans with selective IgA deficiency. *New England Journal of Medicine*, **284,** 7–10 (1971)

17 KAARTINEN, A. M. Liver damage in mice and rats causes tenfold increase of blood immunoglobulin. *Scandinavian Journal of Immunology*, **8,** 161 (1978)

18 LEMAITRE-COELHO, I., JACKSON, G. D. F. and VAERMAN, J. P. High levels of secretory IgA and free secretory component in the serum of rats with bile duct obstruction. *Journal of Experimental Medicine*, **147,** 934–939 (1978)

19 LYAMPERT, I. M. and DANILOVA, T. A. Immunological phenomena associated with cross-reactive antigens of micro-organisms and mammalian tissues. *Progress in Allergy*, **18,** 423–477 (1975)

20 MATTINGLY, J. A. and WAKSMAN, B. Immunologic suppression after oral immunization of antigen. 1. Specific suppressor cells formed in rat Peyer's patches after oral administration of sheep erythrocytes and their system migration. *Journal of Immunology*, **121,** 1878–1883 (1978)

21 MULKS, M. H. and PLAUT, A. G. IgA protease production as a characteristic distinguishing pathogenic from harmless Neisseriaceae. *New England Journal of Medicine*, **299,** 973–976 (1978)

22 OGRA, P. L., OORA, S. S., COPPOLA, P. R. Secretory component and sudden-infant-death syndrome. *Lancet*, **2,** 387–390 (1975)

23 ORLANS, E., PEPPARD, J., REYNOLDS, J. and HALL, J. Rapid active transport of immunoglobulin A from blood to bile. *Journal of Experimental Medicine*, **147,** 588–592 (1978)

24 PLAUT, A. G., GENCO, R. J. and TOMASI, T. B. Jr. Isolation of an enzyme from *Streptococcus sanguis* which specifically cleaves IgA. *Journal of Immunology*, **113,** 289–291 (1974)

25 PLAUT, A. G., GILBERT, J. V., ARTENSTEIN, M. S. and CAPRA, J. D. *Neisseria gonorrhoeae* and *Neisseria meningitidis*: extracellular enzyme cleves human immunoglobulin A. *Science*, **190,** 1103–1105 (1975)

26 RUITENBERG, E. J. and ELGERSMA, A. Absence of intestinal mast cell response in congenitally athymic mice during *Trichinella spiralis* infection. *Nature*, **264,** 258–260 (1976)

27 SAMTER, M. Eosinophils–nominated but not elected. *New England Journal of Medicine*, **303,** 1175–1176 (1980)

28 SOCKEN, D. J., UNDERDOWN, B. J. Comparison of human, bovine and rabbit secretory component-immunoglobulin interactions. *Immunochemistry*, **15,** 499–506 (1978)

29 STOBO, J. D. and TOMASI, T. B. A low molecular weight immunoglobulin antigenically related to 19S IgM. *Journal of Clinical Investigation*, **46,** 1329–1337 (1967)

30 TADA, T. and ISHIZAKA, K. Distribution of γE-forming cells in lymphoid tissues of the human and monkey. *Journal of Immunology*, **104,** 377–387 (1970)

31 TOMASI, T. B. Jr. and CZERWINSKI, D. S. Immunological deficiency diseases in man. In *The National Foundation, Birth Defects–Original Article Series*, edited by D. Bergsma, 270–272. New York (1968)

32 TOMASI, T. B. Jr. and GREY, H. M. Structure and function of immunoglobulin A. In *Progress in Allergy*, edited by P. Kallos and B. Waksman, **16,** 81–213. New York, S. Karger (1972)

33 TOMASI, T. B. Jr. *The Immune System of Secretions*. 1–161. Englewood Cliffs, New Jersey, Prentice-Hall, Inc. (1976)

34 TOMASI, T. B. Jr Oral tolerance. *Transplantation*, **29,** 353–355 (1980)

35 TOMASI, T. B. Jr. and McNABB, P. C. The secretory immune system. In *Basic and Clinical Immunology*, (3rd Edn.) edited by H. H. Fudenberg, D. P. Stittes, J. L. Caldwell and J. V. Wells, 240–250. Los Altos, Lange Medical Publications (1980)

36 TOMASI, T. B. Jr. and McNABB, P. C. Host factors in mucosal disease. *Annual Review of Microbiology* (in press)

37 TOURVILLE, D., ADLER, R., BIENENSTOCK, J. and TOMASI, T. B. Jr. The human secretory immunoglobulin system–immunohistological localization of γA, secretory 'piece', and lactoferrin in normal human tissue. *Journal of Experimental Medicine*, **129,** 411–429 (1969)

38 UNDERDOWN, B. J. and DORRINGTON, K. J. Studies on the structural and conformational basis for the relative resistance of serum and secretory immunoglobulin A to proteolysis. *Journal of Immunology*, **112,** 949–959 (1974)

39 WALKER, A. W. and ISSELBACHER, K. J. Intestinal antibodies. *New England Journal of Medicine*, **297,** 767–773 (1977)

40 WATSON, D. W., BARTNIK, W., SHORTER, R. G. Lymphocyte function and chronic inflammatory bowel disease. In *Inflammatory Bowel Disease*, (2nd Ed.) edited by J. B. Kirsner and R. G. Shorter, 121–137. Philadelphia, Lea and Febiger (1980)

41 WILDE, C. E. and KOSHLAND, M. E. Molecular size and shape of the J chain from polymeric immunoglobulins. *Biochemistry*, **12,** 3218–3224 (1973)

42 WILLIAMS, R. C. and GIBBONS, R. J. Inhibition of bacterial adherence by secretory immunoglobulin A: a mechanism of antigen disposal. *Science*, **177,** 697–699 (1972)

6
Endocrine functions and disorders of the small intestine

T. E. Adrian, J. M. Polak and S. R. Bloom

INTRODUCTION

The correct functioning of the small intestine in the digestion, absorption and subsequent assimilation of ingested nutrients is of paramount importance. It is perhaps not surprising therefore that the control mechanisms for these processes are complex, involving the interaction between several circulating hormones and the enteric nervous system. We only have a sketchy view of this integrated control of intestinal function and the role of the gut in the subsequent metabolism of ingested food.

Knowledge of the role of regulatory peptides in gastrointestinal disease lags even further behind investigation of their physiology. While it is clear that the early diagnosis of pancreatic endocrine tumours is greatly aided by the availability of assays for the causative agents, other areas, that are particularly interesting as potential regulatory defects such as the very common disorders of intestinal motility, peptic ulceration and infections, have been little studied. The known abnormalities in gut peptide secretion noted so far are secondary changes in circulating hormone concentrations but the role of the peptidergic neurones in gut disorders has not been investigated. It is likely that gut hormones are causally involved in disease and our failure to recognise these disorders thus reflects our lack of understanding of the control mechanisms involved.

In this review the regulatory peptides which are predominantly localised in the small intestine will be considered in turn; they are listed in *Table 6.1*.

The other regulatory peptides found in the upper small intestine: secretin, cholecystokinin, somatostatin, bombesin, enkephalin and thyrotrophin releasing hormone, were considered in the previous volume of this series (*Foregut*). The authors recognise, however, that as the distribution of several peptides overlaps, this is a somewhat arbitrary split and suggest the two chapters be read side by side, if possible.

Table 6.1 Major biological effects of the regulatory peptides of the small intestine

Peptide	*Probable Mode of Action*	*Major Actions*
Secretin	Circulating hormone	Pancreatic bicarbonate secretion
Cholecystokinin	Circulating hormone	Gall bladder contraction, pancreatic enzyme secretion
Gastric inhibitory polypeptide (GIP)	Circulating hormone	Insulin release, inhibition of gastric acid secretion
Motilin	Circulating hormone	Stimulation of gastric emptying and intestinal motility, initiation of interdigestive motor complexes
Neurotensin	Circulating hormone	Inhibition of gastric acid and motility, stimulation of pancreatic secretion, release of pancreatic polypeptide from pancreas
Enteroglucagon	Circulating hormone	Trophic to small intestinal mucosa, slows intestinal transit time
Vasoactive intestinal polypeptide (VIP)	Neurotransmitter	Stimulates intestinal secretion, pancreatic secretion, release of insulin, inhibits gastric acid secretion and causes vasodilatation
Substance P	Neurotransmitter	Contracts smooth muscle, stimulates pain perception, pancreatic and salivary secretion and causes vasodilatation

GASTRIC INHIBITORY POLYPEPTIDE

While investigating the pharmacological properties of different preparations of cholecystokinin Brown and Pederson observed that impure preparations appeared to contain an inhibitor of acid secretion[25]. Brown further demonstrated the existence of a side fraction without CCK activity, produced by gel filtration, which strongly inhibited acid secretion from canine Heidenhain pouches. Subsequent purification, utilising this inhibitory effect on acid secretion, revealed a peptide to which the name gastric inhibitory polypeptide or GIP was given[23].

Chemistry

GIP is a 42 amino acid, straight-chained peptide which has considerable sequence homology with the classical hormones glucagon and secretin. Other peptides such as vasoactive intestinal polypeptide (VIP), enteroglucagon and PHI (*see* p.112) are further members of this family.

Several authors have noted the existence of a larger molecular form of GIP in both the small intestine and in the plasma[22,66]. Although this molecule has immunological similarity to GIP its chemical nature is as yet unknown. Brown *et al.* have recently reported that even highly purified preparations of natural GIP contain a minor component which, unlike GIP, is without insulinotropic activity[22].

Localisation

GIP-like immunoreactivity can be demonstrated throughout the small intestine but concentrations are highest in the duodenum and jejunum[26]. The anatomical distribution of the GIP-producing K cells correlates well with the functional localisation, assessed by intestinal glucose perfusion, in man[76].

Release

GIP circulates in plasma and levels rise in response to ingested nutrients, fat and glucose in particular, but some amino acids also evoke a response[66,77].

Actions

Although originally purified as a substance which inhibited gastric acid secretion GIP has several other biological actions. In the presence of moderate hyperglycaemia GIP greatly potentiates the release of insulin from the pancreas[37]. In addition GIP stimulates small intestinal secretion, stimulates mesenteric blood flow, reduces lower oesophageal sphincter pressure, delays gastric emptying and stimulates lipoprotein lipase activity[22]. Antral somatostatin release by GIP has recently been described and this could account for its influence on gastric acid secretion[57].

Physiology

Studies in man demonstrated an acid inhibitory effect of exogenously administered GIP although the levels of immunoreactive GIP achieved greatly exceeded those normally seen postprandially[68]. Recent studies using more physiological doses of GIP, have failed to show a convincing enterogastrone effect on pentagastrin stimulated acid secretion in man[55].

It is well established that glucose taken orally results in a far greater insulin response than the same amount of glucose administered intravenously. The term 'incretin' was coined by La Barre for the humoral factor from the gut responsible for the mediation of this enteroinsular axis. Dupré *et al.* demonstrated that in human subjects infusion of purified GIP with glucose caused far greater insulin response than intravenous glucose alone[37]. Soon GIP became the prime candidate to fit the role of 'incretin'. In addition, much circumstantial evidence has accumulated which supports this theory. Responses of insulin and GIP are reduced in parallel in malabsorption states such as coeliac disease and tropical sprue[5,6]. Similar blunted responses of both hormones follow the use of non-absorbable carbohydrates, such as guar, or sucrase inhibitors such as acarbose[49]. In addition the enteroinsular axis ceases to function in patients who have undergone jejuno-ileal bypass for morbid obesity. In these patients no GIP response to food is seen and the insulin response is greatly obtunded[7].

A recent study was undertaken in which the insulin response to oral glucose was compared with a GIP infusion together with intravenous glucose to mimic plasma levels during the oral test. The insulin response to oral glucose was far higher than that obtained after glucose and GIP infusion even though glucose and GIP concentrations were similar on the two days[67]. These findings suggest that other factors, possibly neural, are components of the enteroinsular axis and that GIP alone cannot account for the incretin effect.

Clinical significance

As the enteroinsular axis appears to be impaired in maturity-onset diabetes it was clearly of interest to study GIP secretion in this condition. The results so far have been conflicting, some workers reporting an increased GIP response to a meal or oral glucose[34], others finding a significantly lower response[50], and still others detecting no difference from normal[17,41].

MOTILIN

Motilin was discovered after the observation that chemical stimulation of the canine duodenum caused contractions in denervated fundic pouches[24]. The responsible hormonal mediator was subsequently purified from porcine intestine and called motilin[21].

Chemistry

Motilin is a 22 amino acid peptide which has only minor structural homology with gastrin and no similarity to other known peptide hormones[21]. Unlike most other peptide hormones the N-terminal region of motilin is important for biological activity.

A larger molecular form of motilin has been reported in both tissue and plasma[31]. The big motilin form is readily detected by N-terminal antibodies but is usually not fully detected by antibodies directed towards the C-terminal end of the motilin molecule[31].

Localization

Motilin is produced by a specific mucosal endocrine cell of the small intestine. This cell type sometimes also contains 5-hydroxytryptamine and is thus included amongst the enterochromaffin cells[59].

Highest concentrations of motilin are found in the proximal jejunum and duodenum with small amounts in the distal jejunum and gastric antrum. The relative ratio of the two molecular forms of motilin is constant throughout the intestine[26,31].

Release

Motilin circulates in plasma but fasting concentrations between individual healthy subjects vary considerably[30,78]. Motilin release appears to depend, in part, on cholinergic tone as atropine causes a marked suppression of plasma motilin levels.

After a small mixed meal there is a small transient rise of plasma motilin concentrations but this is followed by a rapid return to fasting levels. Interestingly, a high fat meal releases motilin whereas carbohydrates and protein suppress its release; it is therefore of no surprise that mixed meals have little overall effect[30]. Indeed plasma motilin concentrations are similarly affected by intravenous fat and glucose, a finding which has led to the speculation that motilin may regulate nutrient absorption by its influence on intestinal motility[30].

Motilin is also released in response to gastric distension whether stimulated by an oral water load or by an air-filled balloon.

Actions

Motilin causes tonic contraction of muscle strips of the small intestine and stomach, and on a molar basis has about 50 times the potency of acetylcholine[72]. In addition motilin potentiates the action of acetylcholine on the pylorus[71].

Studies on the isolated stomach and duodenum have shown that motilin increases electrical spike activity[44]. In the whole animal motilin induces formation of the interdigestive myoelectric complex[47,83]. In a recent study motilin was shown to increase gallbladder pressure in healthy, conscious pigs[3].

Physiology

Motilin infusion at physiological doses in healthy subjects caused a significant increase in the rate of gastric emptying of both solids[33] and liquids[32]. In addition similar doses of exogenous motilin increase electrical and mechanical activity of the human colon[62]. Thus motilin may be a physiological agent for the control of gastric emptying and colonic motility.

The physiological importance of motilin in the initiation of the phase three electrical spike activity of the interdigestive myoelectric complex is not clear. Phase three is a contractile activity front which arises in the foregut and migrates distally down the small intestine about every two hours in the fasting state. As one cycle reaches the distal ileum another originates in the stomach. Infusion of motilin in both dog and man can initiate a new complex in the quiescent post-complex period. However, the doses used result in plasma motilin concentration higher than those seen physiologically [47,83]. Futhermore, infusion of pancreatic polypeptide causes a marked suppression of circulating motilin levels but has no significant influence on the interdigestive motor complex indicating that new complexes are still formed in the relative absence of motilin[48].

Clinical significance

Little is known about the role of motilin in human disease. Motilin levels are elevated in patients with diarrhoea whether caused by acute infection, Crohn's disease, ulcerative colitis, tropical sprue or tumours[18]. Concentrations return to normal following successful treatment of these conditions.

Motility disorders of the gut are very common, however, and further investigation of motilin may be extremely rewarding.

The production of motilin by a tumour has not so far been described.

NEUROTENSIN

Neurotensin, a 13 amino acid peptide, was discovered during the purification of substance P from bovine hypothalamus[28]. This peptide caused vasodilatation and hypotension and was named because of this latter property.

Distribution and chemistry

In the small intestine neurotensin is found in discrete endocrine cells called the N cells which are most numerous in the ileal mucosa[60]. In addition neurotensin is found throughout the central nervous system with highest concentrations in the hypothalamus and basal ganglia[79]. Neurotensin has recently been isolated from the human small intestine and this material is identical to that originating from bovine hypothalamus[45]. Biological activity resides in the C-terminal end of the peptide.

Release

Ingestion of food releases neurotensin and plasma concentrations rise in response to food, particularly fat[10, 54]. Like most other regulatory peptides of the gut, neurotensin is released during infusion of bombesin and is suppressed by somatostatin[2, 10]. The molecular forms of neurotensin in the circulation which are detected in present radioimmunoassays show some variation. C-terminally directed antisera appear to pick up fragments of this end of the neurotensin molecule; similarly N-terminally directed antisera also show a small molecular form in the circulation which is probably not biologically active[10]. With an antiserum requiring the entire neurotensin sequence there appear to be two molecular forms in the circulation, one emerging at the void volume of Sephadex G-50 columns and a second co-eluting with pure neurotensin. Following a meal stimulus it is only the smaller molecular form which increases in concentration in the plasma[10].

Physiology

Neurotensin has widespread pharmacological actions which include vasodilatation, peripheral hypotension, smooth muscle contraction, hyperglycaemia and insulin release[28]. Little is known about the physiological role of neurotensin, however. Low dose infusion studies in man failed to reveal any cardiovascular effects[15]. When infused into mildly hyperglycaemic calves neurotensin caused a pronounced insulin release[11] although this effect was not seen in man. Pancreatic polypeptide release invariably follows neurotensin infusion (*Figure 6.1*) and suggests that this ileal peptide may play a role in the entero-pancreatic polypeptide axis[11, 15].

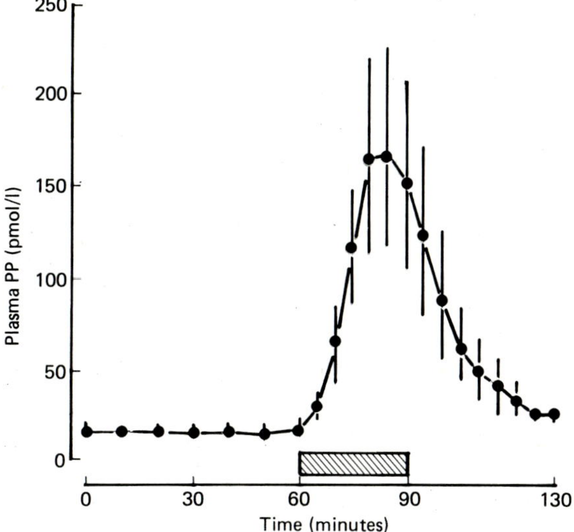

Figure 6.1 Plasma pancreatic polypeptide (PP) concentrations during neurotensin infusion (shaded area) in 6 healthy volunteers

Neurotensin has inhibitory effects on both the motor and secretory functions of the stomach[14], and in addition causes watery bicarbonate secretion from the pancreas[42].

Clinical significance

A greatly enhanced neurotensin release is seen in patients who suffer the complications of unduly rapid gastric emptying (the dumping syndrome) following gastric surgery for duodenal ulcer[13].

Although large doses of neurotensin can cause hypotension, a rise in haematocrit and an increase in heart rate, which are all symptoms of 'dumping', it is probable that the rise of neurotensin in this condition is a secondary response to ileal nutrients rather than a cause of the syndrome. Indeed neurotensin release is enhanced in other conditions where food reaches the terminal ileum, as is found after ileo-jejunal bypass[7].

More recently neurotensin has been found in pancreatic endocrine tumours and their metastases, and is particularly frequent in VIP-producing tumours of the pancreas[12] (*Figure 6.2*).

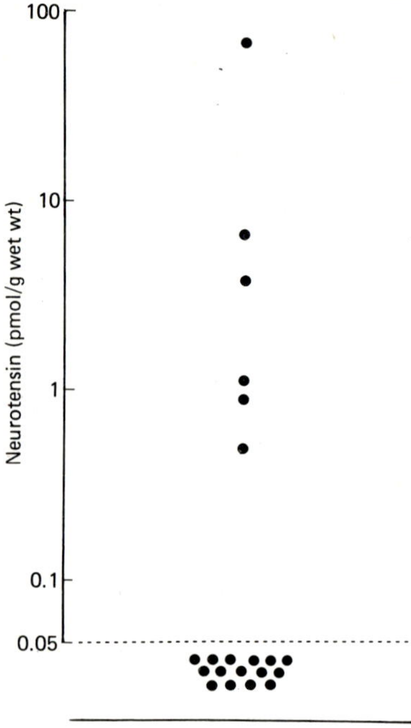

Figure 6.2 Neurotensin-like immunoreactivity in extracts of 21 pancreatic VIPomas

This neurotensin is released into the circulation as plasma levels are grossly elevated in these patients. The significance of the relationship between neurotensin and VIP-production by tumours is not known but it is of interest since neurotensin is not found in normal pancreas[12]. Pancreatic endocrine tumours often contain more than one cell type (*Figure 6.3*) and release different hormones into the circulation.

ENTEROGLUCAGON

Enteroglucagon was first discovered when the antisera used in early radioimmunoassays for glucagon detected immunoreactive material in the gut as well as in the pancreas[80, 81]. Indeed most antibodies raised to pancreatic glucagon detect the intestinal material but a small proportion are specific for pancreatic glucagon[46]. Studies of antibody specificity with synthetic glucagon fragments have revealed that antisera directed towards the N-terminal and mid-region of the glucagon molecule crossreact with enteroglucagon, whereas C-terminally directed antisera are more specific for pancreatic glucagon[4, 43].

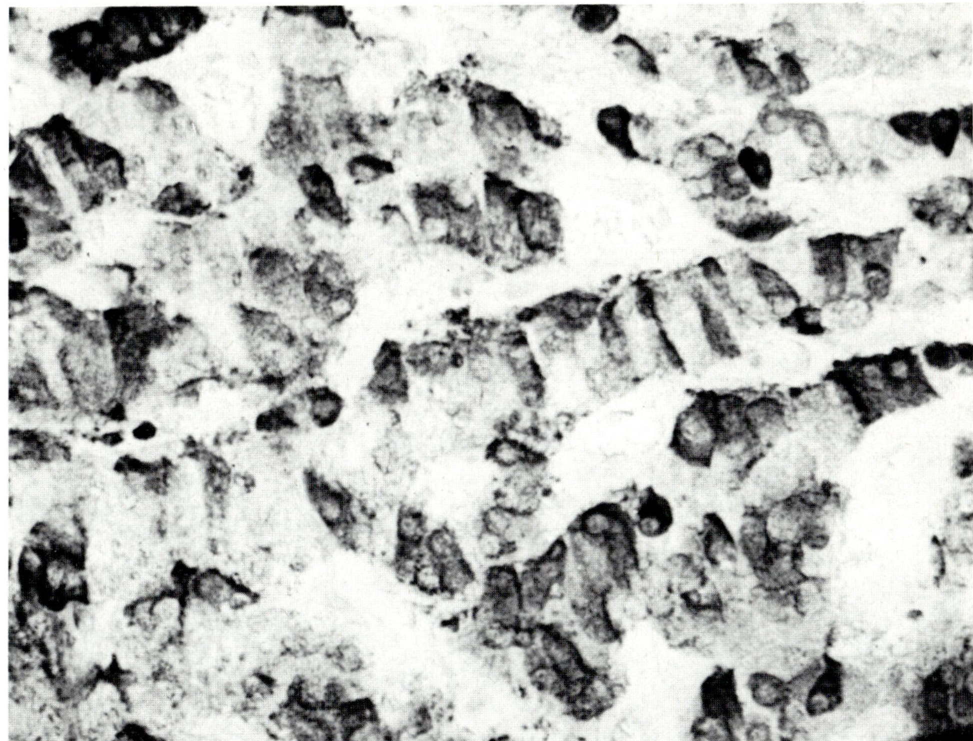

Figure 6.3 Neurone-specific enolase (NSE) staining of a mixed pancreatic apudoma. NSE is a recently discovered non-specific marker for neuroendocrine tumours. (×300)

Chemistry

Early studies demonstrated several molecular forms of enteroglucagon, both in the small intestine and in the circulation[82]. More recently the major form of porcine enteroglucagon was isolated from intestinal extracts. As it was originally thought to comprise of 100 amino acids it was called glicentin (from GLI: glucagon-like immunoreactivity), however, subsequent sequence analysis has revealed that glicentin has only 69 amino acid residues[75]. This peptide contains the entire amino acid sequence of pancreatic glucagon (resídues 33–61). The C-terminal extension is probably the same as that described in 'proglucagon' which has been extracted from porcine pancreas[73]. It has been suggested that an enteroglucagon-like molecule is synthesised in both the A cells of the pancreas and the enteroglucagon cells of the gut. In the pancreas, however, this molecule is split by intracellular enzymes to yield pancreatic glucagon and the N-terminal fragment. The latter can be detected with glicentin antisera in normal pancreas.

Distribution

Enteroglucagon in the gut is synthesised in a specific mucosal endocrine cell called the EG cell. Enteroglucagon is found throughout the gut with the highest concentrations in the ileum and colon in man[43]. The most abundant molecular form of enteroglucagon in human gut and plasma elutes from a gel column in an identical position to porcine glicentin[43].

Release

Plasma enteroglucagon concentrations rise substantially following ingestion of fat, particularly long chain triglycerides, or carbohydrate, although the response to a small mixed meal is often mediocre[43]. This reflects the distribution of the EG cells in the ileum and colon, which normally receive little chemical stimulation, as most nutrients are absorbed in the proximal small intestine.

Physiology

Insufficient enteroglucagon has been purified to undertake pharmacological studies and the only clues as to its physiological role stem from the study of a single patient with an enteroglucagon-producing tumour. This patient had marked small intestinal villous hypertrophy and a greatly increased intestinal transit time[16]. These symptoms disappeared promptly following the removal of the tumour and the plasma enteroglucagon level returned to normal. It is probable that enteroglucagon therefore slows transit and causes mucosal growth in the intestine. Indeed it is well established that intestinal hypertrophy results from distal small intestinal resection and a humoral factor is thought to be responsible as villous hypertrophy can be detected even in an isolated loop of bowel[63]. These surgical manoeuvres are always accompanied by elevated enteroglucagon concentrations[63]. Neonatal enteroglucagon levels rise promptly after birth although this rise is dependent on enteral feeding[43].

It would thus appear that enteroglucagon is the most likely candidate to fulfil the role of the trophic hormone of the gut.

Clinical significance

The symptoms of an enteroglucagon-producing tumour are described above. It is clear that because of the biosynthetic relationship between enteroglucagon and glucagon, production of enteroglucagon-like material might result from A cell tumours of the pancreas. Indeed mucosal hypertrophy has been described in several patients with the glucagonoma syndrome[53].

High circulating concentrations of enteroglucagon are seen in patients with coeliac disease, postinfective tropical malabsorption (*Figure 6.4*), cystic fibrosis,

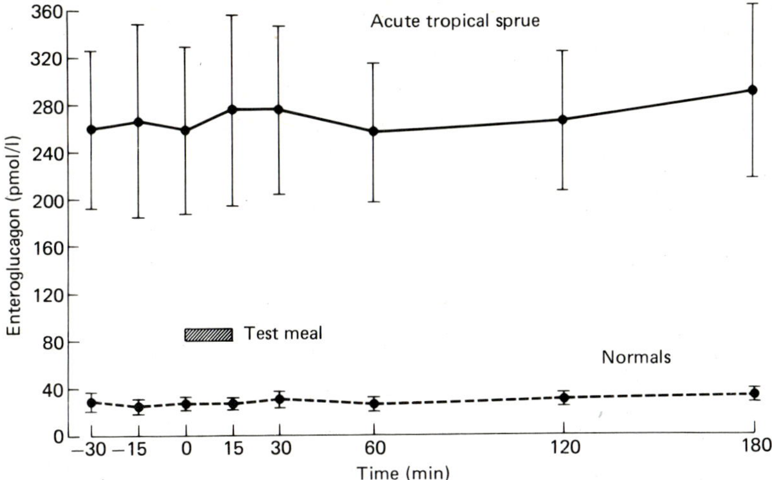

Figure 6.4 Plasma enteroglucagon concentrations in 8 patients with tropical malabsorption and 12 controls. (From Besterman *et al.*[6], courtesy of the Editor and Publishers, *British Medical Journal*)

and in other conditions associated with a loss of effective small intestinal mucosal absorptive surface area[5,6]. As enteroglucagon would appear to be trophic to the gut, its elevation in these diseases would seem to be appropriate.

VASOACTIVE INTESTINAL POLYPEPTIDE

Vasoactive intestinal polypeptide (VIP) was isolated from porcine small intestine, as a substance which caused prolonged peripheral vasodilatation[65]. In recent years it has become apparent that both the distribution and actions of this peptide are more widespread.

Chemistry

VIP is a straight-chained polypeptide of 28 amino acids which shows sequence homology with the classical hormones glucagon and secretin. Enteroglucagon, GIP and PHI are all members of this family of peptides which has undoubtedly stemmed from a common ancestor. There are several reports of different VIP-like components but the predominant molecular form in the human gut appears to be identical to porcine VIP[35].

Distribution

Although originally isolated from the small intestine, VIP is found in intrinsic neural elements throughout the alimentary tract from the oesophagus to the

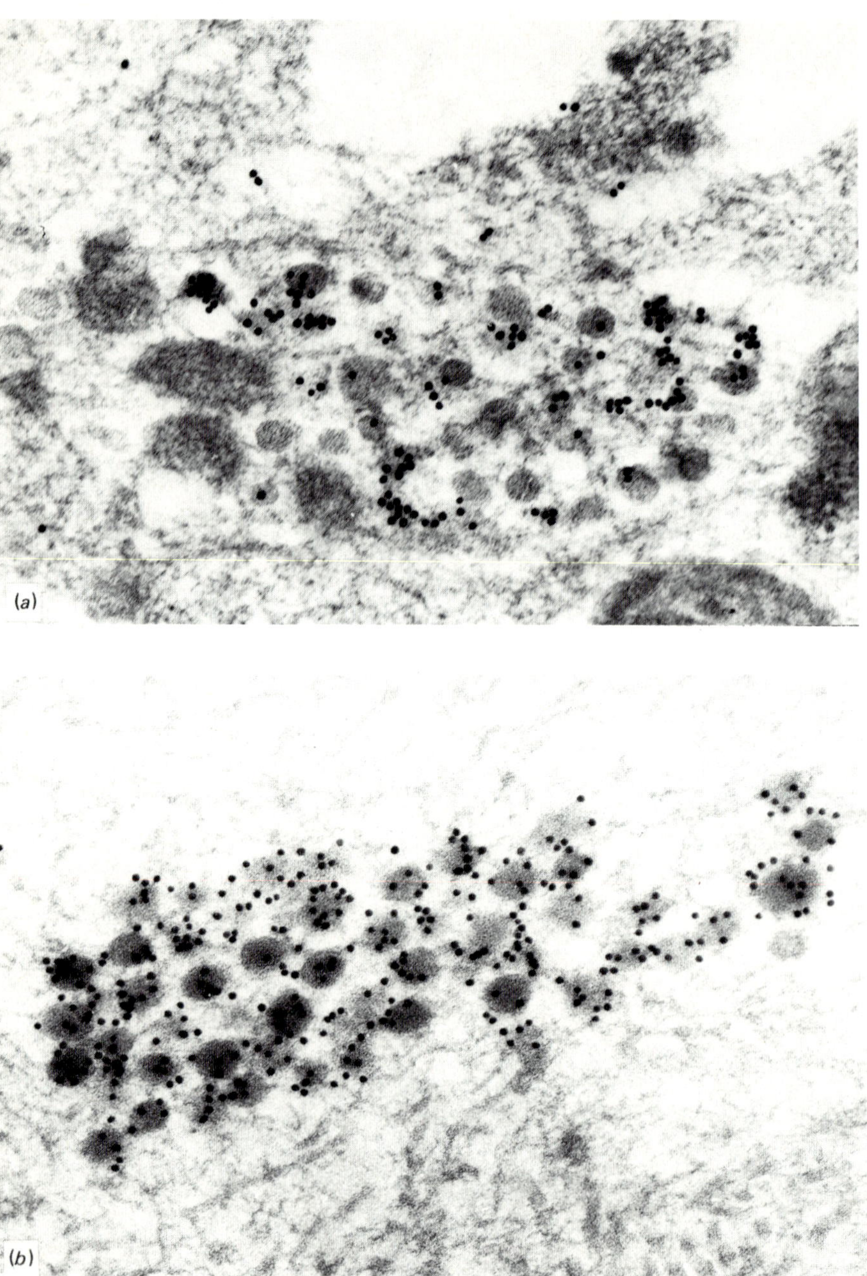

Figure 6.5 Immunogold staining procedure at the ultrastructural level distinguishing two sub-populations of P-type neurosecretory granules. (*a*) Substance P containing smaller (average size 85 nm diameter) neurosecretory granules. (*b*) Larger neurosecretory granules containing VIP (average size 92 nm). (× 68K)

rectum, including the salivary glands and pancreas[26]. In addition, VIP is found throughout the central nervous system and in other organs such as the lung and urogenital tract[27, 64]. Electron immunocytochemistry reveals that VIP is present in large, P type, neurosecretory granules (*Figure 6.5*).

Actions

VIP stimulates a net small intestinal fluid secretion, pancreatic bicarbonate secretion and a reduction in gastric acid secretion. VIP relaxes smooth muscle, for example in blood vessels where it causes vasodilatation and it also stimulates insulin secretion and hepatic glycogenolysis[64].

Physiology

It would appear that VIP functions as a neurotransmitter. Local release of VIP has been demonstrated following neural stimulation, for example, of the vagus and chorda tympani[19, 39]. Probable physiological roles in the gut include vasodilatation in the mesenteric and salivary gland vessels, regulation of gastric, small intestinal and pancreatic secretions and relaxation of the gallbladder and of sphincters such as the lower oesophageal sphincter.

Clinical significance

VIP is not normally found in the circulation to any significant extent, as would be expected of a neuropeptide with a short half life. High plasma VIP concentrations are, however, found in association with a VIP-producing tumour in the Verner-Morrison syndrome[20, 52] (*Figure 6.6*). The effect of elevated circulating VIP is

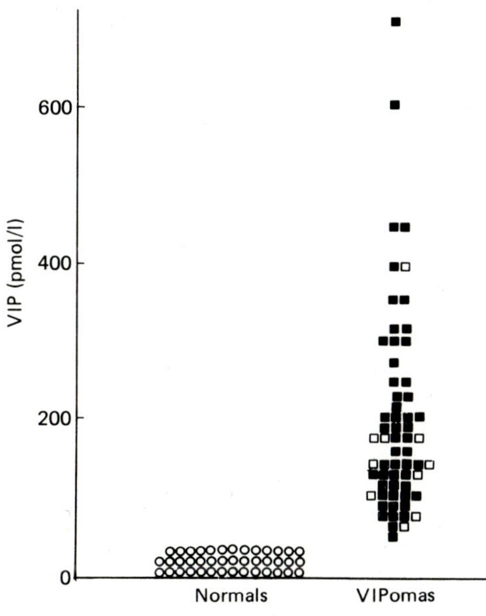

Figure 6.6 Plasma vasoactive intestinal peptide (VIP) concentration in the first received sample from 62 patients with the Verner-Morrison syndrome (mean = 203 ± 17 pmol/l) and 41 controls (mean = 3.4 ± 0.4 pmol/l). (■) Pancreas; (□) ganglioneuroblastoma. (From Long *et al.*[52], courtesy of the Editor and Publishers, *British Medical Journal*)

profound as the patients suffer from torrential diarrhoea (usually more than one litre per day) and hypokalaemia. Other symptoms include abdominal colic, weight loss and spontaneous flushing. Hypochlorhydria is frequently seen, a factor which distinguishes this syndrome from that of gastrinoma in which diarrhoea is also often seen. The primary VIPoma tumour is usually in the pancreas but ganglioneuroblastomas of the sympathetic chain (tumours which are more often seen in young children than in adults) may also produce VIP. The diagnosis can be confirmed by routine plasma VIP estimation[52].

Increased numbers of abnormal VIPergic neurons are seen in the diseased gut tissue from patients with Crohn's disease (*Figure 6.7*), and tissue VIP concentrations are similarly elevated. This abnormality is not seen in ulcerative colitis and it would therefore appear that Crohn's disease is associated with a VIP nerve disorder[9]. Reduction of VIP nerves is seen in the aganglionosis of both congenital (Hirschsprung's disease) and acquired (Chagas' disease) forms and tissue concentrations are low[8,51].

SUBSTANCE P

Substance P was the first peptide shown to have a dual localization in the brain and gut. Although its spasmogenic and vasodilatory properties were recognised in 1931[38], nearly 40 years passed before it was finally purified from bovine hypothalamus[29].

Chemistry and distribution

Substance P is a basic, straight-chained peptide of 11 amino acid residues with biological activity residing in the C terminal portion of the molecule[29]. Substance P neurones are found throughout the gastrointestinal tract in intrinsic neurones and nerve fibres. Immunocytochemistry at the ultrastructural level has shown substance P to be localized to large P-type neurosecretory granules, distinct from those storing VIP (*Figure 6.5*). In addition, it is present in autonomic fibres of a number of other peripheral organs, such as the pancreas, urogenital tract and the eye[58]. High concentrations of substance P are found in the brain, in areas known to be associated with pain perception, and in the dorsal horn of the spinal cord[61].

Physiology

The pharmacological actions of substance P have been thoroughly investigated although it is not clear, as yet, which of these actions are physiological. The localization of substance P and its apparent interaction with the enkephalins suggest a role in pain perception[61].

Several of the biological effects of substance P may be secondary to its potent spasmogenic and vasodilatory properties. Substance P causes hyperglycaemia

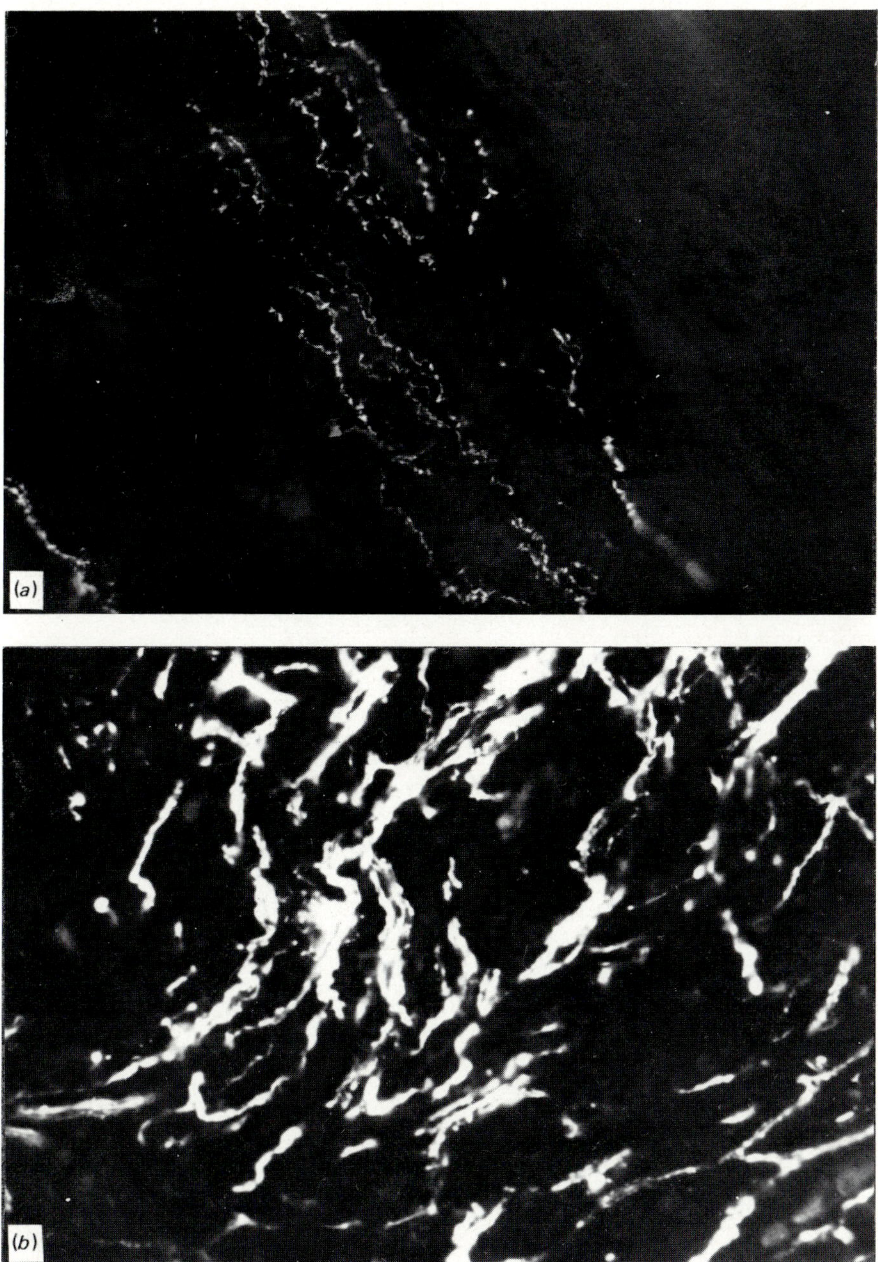

Figure 6.7 Immunostaining for vasoactive intestinal polypeptide (VIP) in a piece of normal bowel (*a*) and on tissue from a patient with Crohn's disease (*b*). Note the appearance of normal VIPergic nerves displaying varicosities. Note also that in Crohn's disease the nerves appear extremely hyperplastic, disorganised and thickened. (×210)

through an inhibition of insulin release and concomitant release of glucagon. It stimulates juice and enzyme secretion from the exocrine pancreas and salivary glands, but reduces hepatic bile output. Substance P contracts smooth muscle in all regions of the gastrointestinal tract and a recent study showed that it causes net water absorption in the small intestine[56].

Clinical significance

Substance P-like immunoreactivity has been detected in carcinoid tumours of the foregut, midgut and hindgut[69]. High circulating substance P concentrations have also been reported in some patients, which is of importance since substance P is capable of causing flushing, hypotension, bronchoconstriction and diarrhoea, all symptoms of the carcinoid syndrome[61]. It should be noted that there is increasing evidence of production of neurohormonal peptides by carcinoid tumours regardless of the site of the tumour. Pancreatic polypeptide, insulin, glucagon, somatostatin and enkephalins have all been reported in carcinoid tumours although the significance of these findings is unknown at present[1, 40, 70].

Local reductions in the substance P-containing intrinsic nerves of the intestine are seen in the aganglionosis associated with Hirschsprung's and Chagas' diseases[8, 51]

NEWLY DISCOVERED PEPTIDES OF THE SMALL INTESTINE

Using a novel method which identifies peptides with a C-terminal amide group Tatemoto and Mutt have recently isolated two biologically active peptides from small intestine[74]. The first is called PHI because it is of porcine origin and has an N-terminal histidine and a C-terminal isoleucine amide group. The N-terminal region of PHI has sequence homology with VIP and secretin and shares with these two peptides the ability to stimulate pancreatic bicarbonate secretion[36, 74]. The second peptide is called PYY as both the N-terminal and C-terminal residues are tyrosine, the latter of which is amidated. PYY has structural homology with pancreatic polypeptide and neurotensin[74]. Studies on the physiology of these two new regulatory peptides are awaited with interest.

CONCLUSIONS

Only a decade ago, the recognised gut hormones were gastrin, cholecystokinin and secretin. Since that time the list of such regulatory peptides of the gut has grown and with it our knowledge of the complexities of the release and biological effects of these substances. We are only slowly becoming aware, however, of the great importance of the neuroendocrine interactions which, it seems, control the secretory, absorptive and motor processes of the small intestine. It is hoped that continued effort in this field will soon yield information on the way in which control is lost or modified in disorders of the alimentary tract. The way will then be open for a more rapid therapeutic advance.

References

1 ADRIAN, T. E. Pancreatic polypeptide. *Journal of Clinical Pathology*, (Suppl. 8) 85–91 (1981)

2 ADRIAN, T. E., BARNES, A. J., LONG, R. G., O'SHAUGHNESSY, D. J., BROWN, M. R., RIVIER, J., VALE, W., BLACKBURN, A. M. and BLOOM, S. R. The effect of somatostatin analogs on secretion of growth, pancreatic and gastrointestinal hormones in man. *Journal of Clinical Endocrinology and Metabolism*, **53,** 675–681 (1981)

3 ADRIAN, T. E., MITCHENERE, P., SAGOR, G. R., CHRISTOFIDES, N. D. and BLOOM, S. R. Effect of motilin and other gut hormones on gall bladder pressure. *Regulatory Peptides*, **1,** (Suppl. 1) 1 (1980)

4 ASSAM, R. and SLUSHER, N. Structure/function and structure/immunoreactivity relationships of the glucagon molecule and related synthetic peptides. *Diabetes*, **21,** 843–853 (1972)

5 BESTERMAN, H. S., BLOOM, S. R., SARSON, D. L., BLACKBURN, A. M., JOHNSTON, D. J., PATEL, H. R., STEWART, J. S., MODIGLIANI, R., GUERIN, S. and MALLINSON, C. N. Gut hormone in profile in coeliac disease. *Lancet*, **1,** 785–788 (1978)

6 BESTERMAN, H. S., COOK, G. S., SARSON, D. L., CHRISTOFIDES, N. D., BRYANT, M. G., GREGOR, M. and BLOOM, S. R. Gut hormones in tropical malabsorption. *British Medical Journal*, **2,** 1252–1255 (1979)

7 BESTERMAN, H. S., SARSON, D. L., BLACKBURN, A. M., CLEARY, J., PILKINGTON, T. R. E., GAZET, T. C. and BLOOM, S. R. Gut hormone profile in morbid obesity and following jejuno-ileal bypass. *Gut*, **19,** A986 (1978)

8 BISHOP, A. E., POLAK, J. M., BRYANT, M. G. and BLOOM, S. R. Abnormalities of neural and hormonal peptides in Hirschprung's disease. *Regulatory Peptides*, **1,** (Suppl. 1) 11 (1980)

9 BISHOP, A. E., POLAK, J. M., BRYANT, M. G., BLOOM, S. R. and HAMILTON, S. Abnormalities of vasoactive intestinal polypeptide-containing nerves in Crohn's disease. *Gastroenterology*, **79,** 853–860 (1980)

10 BLACKBURN, A. M. and BLOOM, S. R. Neurotensin in man. In *Gut Hormones* Volume 2, edited by S. R. Bloom and J. M. Polak, 306–311. Edinburgh, Churchill Livingstone (1981)

11 BLACKBURN, A. M., BLOOM, S. R. and EDWARDS, A. V. Pancreatic endocrine responses to exogenous neurotensin in the conscious calf. *Journal of Physiology (London)*, **314,** 11–21 (1981)

12 BLACKBURN, A. M., BRYANT, M. G., ADRIAN, T. E. and BLOOM, S. R. Pancreatic tumours produce neurotensin. *Journal of Clinical Endocrinology and Metabolism*, **52,** 820–822 (1981)

13 BLACKBURN, A. M., CHRISTOFIDES, N. D., GHATEI, M. A., SARSON, D. L., EBEID, F. H., RALPHS, D. N. L. and BLOOM, S. R. Elevation of plasma neurotensin in the dumping syndrome. *Clinical Science*, **59,** 237–243 (1980)

14 BLACKBURN, A. M., FLETCHER, D. R., BLOOM, S. R., CHRISTOFIDES, N. D., LONG, R. G., FITZPATRICK, M. L. and BARON, J. H. Effect of neurotensin on gastrin function. *Lancet*, **1,** 987–989 (1980)

15 BLACKBURN, A. M., FLETCHER, D. R., ADRIAN, T. E. and BLOOM, S. R. Neurotensin infusion in man: pharmacokinetics and effect on gastrointestinal and pituitary hormones. *Journal of Clinical Endocrinology and Metabolism*, **51,** 1257–1261 (1980)

16 BLOOM, S. R. An enteroglucagon tumour. *Gut*, **13,** 520–523 (1972)

17 BLOOM, S. R. GIP in diabetes. *Diabetologia*, **11,** 334 (1975)

18 BLOOM, S. R., CHRISTOFIDES, N. D. and BESTERMAN, H. S. Raised motilin in diarrhoea. *Gut*, **19,** 959 (1978)

19 BLOOM, S. R. and EDWARDS, A. V. Vasoactive intestinal peptide in relation to atropine resistant vasodilatation in the submaxillary gland of the cat. *Journal of Physiology* (*London*), **300,** 41–53 (1980)

20 BLOOM, S. R., POLAK, J. M. and PEARSE, A. G. E. Vasoactive intestinal polypeptide and watery diarrhoea syndrome. *Lancet*, **2,** 14–15 (1973)

21 BROWN, J. C., COOK, M. A., and DRYBURGH, J. R. Motilin, a gastric motor activity stimulating polypeptide: the complete amino acid sequence. *Canadian Journal of Biochemistry*, **51,** 533–537 (1973)

22 BROWN, J. C., DAHL, M., KWAUK, S., McINTOSH, C. H. S., MULLER, M., OTTE, S. C. and PEDERSON, R. A. Properties and actions of GIP. In *Gut Hormones*, Volume 2, edited by S. R. Bloom and J. M. Polak, 248–255. Edinburgh, Churchill Livingstone (1981)

23 BROWN, J. C. and DRYBURGH, J. R. A gastric inhibitory polypeptide: the complete amino acid sequence. *Canadian Journal of Biochemistry*, **49,** 867–872 (1971)

24 BROWN, J. C., JOHNSON, L. P. and MAGEE, D. F. Effect of duodenal alkalinization on gastric motility. *Gastroenterology*, **50,** 333–339 (1966)

25 BROWN, J. C. and PEDERSON, R. A. A multiparameter study on the action of preparations containing cholecystokinin – pancreozymin. *Scandinavian Journal of Gastroenterology*, **5,** 537–541 (1970)

26 BRYANT, M. G. and BLOOM, S. R. Distribution of the gut hormones in the primate intestinal tract. *Gut*, **20,** 653–659 (1979)

27 BRYANT, M. G., BLOOM, S. R., POLAK, J. M., ALBUQUERQUE, R. H., MODLIN, I. and PEARSE, A. G. E. Possible dual role for vasoactive intestinal peptide as gastrointestinal hormone and neurotransmitter substance. *Lancet*, **1,** 991–993 (1976)

28 CARRAWAY, R. and LEEMAN, S. E. The isolation of a new hypotensive peptide, neurotensin, from bovine hypothalami. *Journal of Biological Chemistry* (*Baltimore*), **248,** 6854–6861 (1973)

29 CHANG, M. M. and LEEMAN, S. E. Isolation of a sialogogic peptide from bovine hypothalamic tissue and its characterisation as substance P. *Journal of Biological Chemistry* (*Baltimore*), **245,** 4784–4790 (1970)

30 CHRISTOFIDES, N. D., BLOOM, S. R., BESTERMAN, H. S., ADRIAN, T. E. and GHATEI, M. A. Release of motilin by oral and intravenous nutrients in man. *Gut*, **20,** 102–106 (1978)

31 CHRISTOFIDES, N. D., BRYANT, M. G., GHATEI, M. A., KISHIMOTO, S., BUCHAN, A. M. J., POLAK, J. M. and BLOOM, S. R. Molecular forms of motilin in the mammalian and human gut and human plasma. *Gastroenterology*, **80,** 292–300 (1981)

32 CHRISTOFIDES, N. D., LONG, R. G. FITZPATRICK, M. L., McGREGOR, G. P. and BLOOM, S. R. Effect of motilin on the gastric emptying of glucose and fat in humans. *Gastroenterology*, **80,** 456–460 (1981)

33 CHRISTOFIDES, N. D., MODLIN, I. M., FITZPATRICK, M. L. and BLOOM, S. R. Effect of motilin on the rate of gastric emptying and gut hormone release during breakfast. *Gastroenterology*, **76,** 903–907 (1979)

34 CREUTZFELDT, W. The incretin concept today. *Diabetologia*, **16,** 75–85 (1979)

35 DIMALINE, R. and DOCKRAY, D. J. Multiple immunoreactive forms of vasoactive intestinal peptide in human colonic mucosa. *Gastroenterology*, **75,** 387–392 (1978)

36 DIMALINE, R. and DOCKRAY, G. J. PHI: A new gut peptide with vasoactive intestinal peptide (VIP)-like actions on the pancreas in birds and mammals. *Regulatory Peptides*, **1,** (Suppl. 1) 527 (1980)

37 DUPRÉ, J., ROSS, S. A., WATSON, D. and BROWN, J. C. Stimulation of insulin secretion by gastric inhibitory peptide in man. *Journal of Clinical Endocrinology*, **37,** 826–827 (1973)

38 VON EULER, U. S. and GADDUM, J. M. An unidentified pressor substance in certain tissue extracts. *Journal of Physiology* (*London*), **72,** 74–87 (1981)

39 FAHRENKRUG, J., GALBO, H., HOLST, J. J. and SCHAFFALITZKY DE MUCKADELL, O. B. Influence of the autonomic nervous system on the release of vasoactive intestinal polypeptide from the porcine gastrointestinal tract. *Journal of Physiology* (*London*), **280,** 405–422 (1978)

40 FALKMER, J., ALUMETS, J., HAKANSON, R., LJUNGBERG, O., SUNDLER, F. and TIBBLIN, S. Occurrence of pancreatic polypeptide (PP), somatostatin, glucagon, insulin, enkephalin, β-endorphin and substance P in rectal carcinoids. A preliminary report of nineteen cases. In *Gut Peptides, Secretion, Function and Clinical Aspects*, edited by A. Miyoshi, 351–355. Amsterdam, Elsevier (1977)

41 FINKE, Y., EBERT, R. and CREUTZFELDT, W. GIP secretion in juvenile onset diabetes following maximal oral stimulation. *Diabetologia*, **19,** 273–274 (1980)

42 FLETCHER, D. R., BLACKBURN, A. M., ADRIAN, T. E., CHADWICK, V. S. and BLOOM, S. R. Effect of neurotensin on pancreatic function in man. *Life Sciences*, **29,**2157–2161 (1981)

43 GHATEI, M. A. and BLOOM, S. R. Enteroglucagon in man. In *Gut Hormones*, Volume 2, edited by S. R. Bloom and J. M. Polak, 332–338. Edinburgh, Churchill Livingstone (1981)

44 GREEN, W. E. R., RUPPIN, H., WINGATE, D. L., DOMSCHKE, W., WÜNSCH, E., DEMLING, L. and RITCHIE, H. D. Effects of 13 NLE motilin on the electrical and mechanical activity of the isolated perfused canine stomach and duodenum. *Gut*, **17,** 362–370 (1976)

45 HAMMER, R. A., CARRAWAY, R., WILLIAMS, R. H. and LEEMAN, S. E. Isolation of human intestinal neurotensin. *Gastroenterology*, **76,** 1150 (1979)

46 HEDING, L. G. Radioimmunological determination of pancreatic and gut glucagon in plasma. *Diabetologia*, **7,** 10–19 (1971)

47 ITOH, Z., AIWAWA, I., TAKEUCHI, S. and COUCH, E. F. Hunger contractions and motilin. In *Proceedings of the Fifth International Symposium on Motility*, edited by G. Vantrappen, 48–55. Herentals, Typoff Press (1975)

48 JANSSENS, J., HELLEMANS, J., ADRIAN, T. E., BLOOM, S. R., PEETERS, T. L., CHRISTOFIDES, N. D. and VANTRAPPEN, G. R. Pancreatic polypeptide is not involved in the regulation of the migrating motor complex in man. *Regulatory Peptides*, **3,** 41–49 (1981)

49 JENKINS, D. J. A. J., TAYLOR, R. H., NINEHAM, R., GOFF, D. V., BLOOM, S. R., SARSON, D. L. and ALBERTI, K. G. M. M. Combined use of guar and acarbose in reduction of postprandial glycaemia. *Lancet*, **2,** 924–927 (1979)

50 KARUP, T., MOODY, A. J., and SESTOFT, L. Diminished gastric inhibitory polypeptide (GIP) secretion in newly diagnosed insulin dependent diabetics (IDD). *Diabetologia*, **19,** 292 (1980)

51 LONG, R. G., BISHOP, A. E., BARNES, A. J., ALBUQUERQUE, R. H., O'SHAUGHNESSY, D. J., McGREGOR, G. P., BANNISTER, R., POLAK, J. M. and BLOOM, S. R. Neural and hormonal peptides in rectal biospy specimens from patients with Chagas' disease and chronic autonomic failure. *Lancet*, **1,** 559–562 (1980)

52 LONG, R. G., BRYANT, M. G., MITCHELL, S. J., ADRIAN, T. E., POLAK, J. M. and BLOOM, S. R. Clinicopathological study of pancreatic and ganglioneuroblastoma tumours secreting vasoactive intestinal peptide (VIPomas). *British Medical Journal*, **282,** 1767–1771 (1981)

53 MALLINSON, C. N., BLOOM, S. R., WARIN, A. P., SALMON, P. R. and COX, B. A glucagonoma syndrome. *Lancet*, **2,** 1–5 (1974)

54 MASHFORD, M. L., NILSSON, G., RÖKAEUS, A. and ROSSELL, S. The effect of food ingestion on circulating neurotensin-like immunoreactivity in the human. *Acta Physiologica Scandinavica* (*Stockholm*), **104,** 244–246 (1976)

55 MAXWELL, V., SHULKES, A., BROWN, J. C., SOLOMON, T. E., WALSH, J. H. and GROSSMAN, M. I. The effect of gastric inhibitory polypeptide on pentagastrin-stimulated acid secretion in man. *Digestive Diseases and Sciences,* **25,** 113–116 (1980)

56 MITCHENERE, P., ADRIAN, T. E., KIRK, R. M. and BLOOM, S. R. Effect of gut regulatory peptides on intestinal luminal fluid in the rat. *Life Sciences*, **29,** 679–688 (1981)

57 McINTOSH, C. H. S., PEDERSON, R. A., KOOP, H. and BROWN, J. C. Inhibition of GIP-stimulated somatostatin-like immunoreactivity (SLI) by acetylcholine and vagal stimulation. In *Gut Peptides*, edited by A. Miyoshi, 100–104. Amsterdam, Elsevier (1974)

58 NILSSON, G. and BRODIN, E. Tissue distribution of substance P-like immunoreactivity in the dog, cat, rat and mouse. In *Substance P*, edited by U. S. von Euler and B. Pernow, 49–54. New York, Raven Press (1977)

59 POLAK, J. M. and BUCHAN, A. M. J. Motilin immunocytochemical localisation indicates possible molecular heterogeneity or the existence of a motilin family. *Gastroenterology*, **76,** 1065–1066 (1979)

60 POLAK, J. M., SULLIVAN, S. N., BLOOM, S. R., BUCHAN, A. M. J., FACER, P., BROWN, M. R. and PEARSE, A. G. E. Neurotensin in human intestine: radioimmunoassay and specific localisation in the N cell. *Nature*, **270,** 183–185 (1977)

61 POWELL, D. and SKRABANEK, P. Substance P. In *Gut Hormones* Volume 2 edited by S. R. Bloom and J. M. Polak, 396–401. Edinburgh, Churchill Livingstone (1981)

62 RENNIE, J. A., CHRISTOFIDES, N. D., BLOOM, S. R. and JOHNSON, A. G. Stimulation of human colonic motility by motilin. *Gut*, **20,** 912 (1979)

63 SAGOR, G. R., Al MUKHTAR, M. Y. J., GHATEI, M. A., WRIGHT, N. A. and BLOOM, S. R. The effect of altered luminal nutrition on cellular proliferation and plasma concentrations of enteroglucagon and gastrin after small bowel resection in the rat. *British Journal of Surgery*, **69,** 14–18 (1982)

64 SAID, S. I. VIP overview. In *Gut Hormones* Volume 2, edited by S. R. Bloom and J. M. Polak, 379–384. Edinburgh, Churchill Livingstone (1981)

65 SAID, S. I. and MUTT, V. Isolation from porcine intestinal wall of vasoactive octacosapeptide related to secretin and to glucagon. *European Journal of Biochemistry*, **28,** 199–204 (1972)

66 SARSON, D. L., BRYANT, M. G. and BLOOM, S. R. A radioimmunoassay for gastric inhibitory polypeptide in human plasma. *Journal of Endocrinology*, **85,** 487–496 (1980)

67 SARSON, D. L., WOOD, S. M., HOLDER, D. and BLOOM, S. R. The effect of glucose-dependent insulinotropic polypeptide infused at physiological concentrations on the release of insulin in man. *Diabetologia*, **22,** 33–36 (1982)

68 SIMMONS, T. C., MAXWELL, V. L., TAYLOR, I. L. and GROSSMAN, M. I. Effect of GIP on gastric acid secretion in vagotomised human subjects. *Gastroenterology*, **78,** 1260 (1980)

69 SKRABANEK, P., CANNON, D., KIRRANE, J. and POWELL, D. Substance **P** secretion by carcinoid tumours. *Irish Journal of Medical Science (Dublin)*, **147,** 47–49 (1978)

70 SPORRONG, B., FALKMER, S., ROBBOY, S. J., ALUMETS, J., HAKANSON, R., LJUNBERG, O. and SUNDLER, F. Evidence for neurohormonal peptides in ovarian carcinoids: a preliminary report of immunohistochemical findings. In *Cellular Basis of Chemical Messengers in the Digestive System*, edited by M. I. Grossman, 257–265. New York, Academic Press (1981)

71 STRUNZ, U., DOMSCHKE, W. DOMSCHKE, S., MITZNEGG, P., WÜNSCH, E., JAEGER, E. and DEMLING, L. Potentiation between 13-Nle-Motilin and acetylcholine on rabbit pyloric muscle *in vitro*. *Scandinavian Journal of Gastroenterology*, **12,** (Suppl. 39) 29–35 (1976)

72 STRUNZ, U., DOMSCHKE, W., MITZNEGG, P., DOMSCHKE, S., SCHUBERT, E. WÜNSCH, E., JAEGER, E. and DEMLING, L. Analysis of the motor effects of 13-norleucine motilin on the rabbit, guinea pig, rat and human alimentary tract *in vitro*. *Gastroenterology*, **68,** 1485–1491 (1975)

73 TAGER, H. S. and STEINER, D. F. Isolation of a glucagon-containing peptide: primary structure of a possible fragment of proglucagon. *Proceedings of the National Academy of Sciences of the United States of America*, **708,** 2321–2325 (1973)

74 TATEMOTO, K. and MUTT, V. Isolation of two novel candidate hormones using a chemical method for finding naturally occurring polypeptides. *Nature*, **285,** 417–418 (1980)

75 THIM, L. and MOODY, A. J. The primary structure of porcine glicentin (proglucagon). *Regulatory Peptides*, **2,** 139–150 (1981)

76 THOMAS, F. B., SHOOK, D. F., O'DORISIO, T. M., CATALAND, S., MEKHJIAN, H. S., CALDWELL, J. H. and MAZZAFERRI, E. L. Localisation of gastric inhibitory polypeptide release by intestinal glucose perfusion in man. *Gastroenterology*, **72,** 49–54 (1977)

77 THOMAS, F. B., SINAR, D., MAZZAFERRI, E. L., CATALAND, S., MEKHJIAN, H. S., CALDWELL, J. H. and FROMKES, J. J. Selective release of gastric inhibitory polypeptide by intraduodenal amino acid perfusion in man. *Gastroenterology*, **74,** 1261–1265 (1978)

78 TRACK, N. S., WATTERS, L. M. and GAULDIE, J. Motilin, human pancreatic polypeptide and gastrin, plasma concentrations in fasting subjects. *Clinical Biochemistry*, **12,** 109–117 (1979)

79 UHL, G. R. and SNYDER, S. H. Regional and subcellular distributions of brain neurotensin. *Life Sciences*, **19,** 1827–1832 (1976)

80 UNGER, R. H., EISENTRAUT, A. M., SIMS, K., McCALL, M. S. and MADISON, L. L. Sites of origin of glucagon in dogs and humans. *Clinical Research*, **9,** 53 (1961)

81 UNGER, R. H., KETTERER, H. and EISENTRAUT, A. M. Distribution of immunoassayable glucagon in gastrointestinal tissues. *Metabolism*, **15,** 865–867 (1966)

82 VALVERDE, I., RIGOPOULOU, D., MARCO, J., FALOONA, G. R. and UNGER. R. H. Characterisation of glucagon-like immunoreactivity (GLI). *Diabetes*, **19,** 614–623 (1970)

83 VANTRAPPEN, G., JANSSENS, J., PEETERS, T. L., BLOOM, S. R., CHRISTOFIDES, N. D. and HELLEMANS, J. Motilin and the interdigestive migrating motor complex in man. *Digestive Diseases and Sciences*, **24,** 497–500 (1979)

7
Motility of the small intestine

David L. Wingate

INTRODUCTION

The motility of the small intestine is a subject which was ill-understood by scientists and clinicians alike until little more than a decade ago. Recent scientific advances have revealed clear patterns of organization of intestinal motility and these in turn have advanced the understanding of the control mechanisms which are involved. Because these advances have not yet led to significant changes in the management of the disease state, they are not widely known to clinicians. Therefore, any attempt to describe the clinical aspects of small intestinal motility at the present time must be prefaced by a description of the physiology of motility. Whereas the early concept of intestinal motility, which even today influences the thinking of clinicians on this subject, was of a simple tube which merely responded to the presence of intraluminal content by the movement of peristalsis, it is now clear that the regulation of motility is highly complex. It depends on an intrinsic nervous system with multiple neurotransmitters and is modulated by extrinsic nervous controls. The small intestine receives digesta mixed with digestive juices; this chyme must be moved along the intestine at a rate to allow intraluminal digestion, followed by adequate exposure to the surface of the bowel for the final stage of digestion by brush-border enzymes and subsequent absorption, while at the same time continual mixing of the chyme takes place. Finally, when the nutrients have been absorbed, the non-absorbable residue must be passed to the large intestine. In addition, it seems likely that it is the motor activity of the small intestine which serves to prevent the oral migration of colonic bacteria. Whereas the digestive and absorptive functions of the small bowel have a considerable functional reserve (as evidenced by the fact that loss of a significant proportion of the small intestinal mucosa or pancreas does not lead to an absorptive or secretory deficit), it is clear that the transit function of the small bowel must be continually capable of precise adaptation to an input which is highly variable in volume, consistency and chemical content. These considerations alone imply the existence of a sophisticated control system; the significant advance of recent years is that such a control system is no longer an indirectly inferred entity but a reality, defined at least in part.

MOTOR ANATOMY OF THE SMALL INTESTINE

The structures conferring the property of motility on which the small bowel depends are the layers of smooth muscle and their nervous connections.

Muscle

The smooth muscle of the small intestine is arranged in three layers. An outer layer of longitudinal muscle is separated by the neural myenteric plexus from an inner layer of circular muscle; both layers completely invest the small intestine along its entire length. The names of these layers reflect both the orientation of the smooth muscle fibres and the direction of their contractile activity. The third muscle layer of the small bowel is less well understood; this is the thin layer of muscularis mucosae which underlies the mucosa, and which sends muscle fibres into the villus cores; activity of this muscle layer presumably alters the conformation of the absorptive surface.

Nerve

The innervation of intestinal smooth muscles comprises extrinsic and intrinsic nerves. Extrinsic innervation consists of vagal parasympathetic and splanchnic sympathetic nerves. The intrinsic innervation is composed of the intrinsic nerve plexuses (myenteric and submucous). Vagal innervation is mainly in the proximal bowel, and the majority of vagal fibres are afferent fibres projecting to the nucleus tractus solitarius in the medulla. The efferent vagal fibres arise in the dorsal vagal nucleus close to the nucleus tractus solitarius, and vago-vagal reflexes appear to be mediated through interneurones connecting these two nuclei. The intrinsic nerve plexus contain numerous ganglia, and there are extensive intrinsic nerve connections between the two plexuses, and also between the plexuses and the muscle and mucosal layers. The intrinsic nerve plexuses are the only nerve networks apart from the brain itself which contain a supporting network of glial cells.

MOTOR PHYSIOLOGY OF THE SMALL INTESTINE

Electrophysiology

Muscle

The smooth muscle fibres are arranged in a syncytium, with the fibres in electrical contact through plexuses, allowing the spread of depolarization to take place virtually synchronously through a mass of fibres; in this respect intestinal smooth muscle appears to resemble myocardium. It is currently believed that co-ordination of muscle fibres occurs by this type of direct contact, although there is morphological evidence that a network of fine conducting tissue, the interstitial cells of Cajal, may be an essential co-ordinating element[47]. The syncytial property of the tissue also allows areas to act as electrical pacemakers with the spread of depolarization from pacemakers to drive other cells at the speed of the pacemaker.

The other fundamental property which the intestinal smooth muscle cell shares with the myocardium is that of spontaneous rhythmic depolarization. As shown in *Figure 7.1*, the smooth muscle cell undergoes regular depolarization and repolarization. This may be detected *in vitro* by intracellular recording of membrane potential by a micro-electrode, but (as also depicted in *Figure 7.1*), the synchronous depolarization of cells in a given area creates electrical changes which can be detected by a large volume extracellular electrode placed on the muscle mass; this type of extracellular recording resembles the electrocardiogram, and results from similar electrical changes in the tissue. This electrical phenomenon was first described by Alvarez and Mahoney in 1921[1] as the 'electroenterogram'.

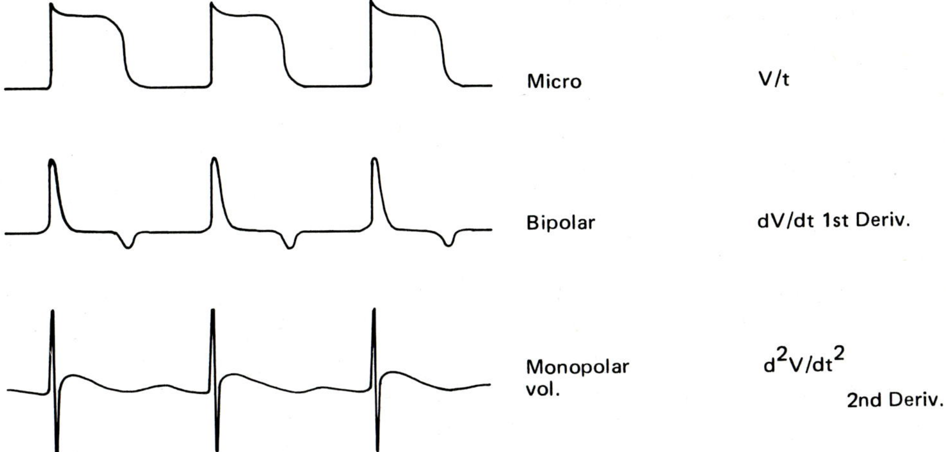

Figure 7.1 Schematic representation of the slow wave of the small intestine as recorded by (above) an intracellular electrode, (middle) a bipolar external large volume electrode, and (below) a monopolar external large volume electrode. The relationship between signal voltage and time is given at the right of each trace.

Intestinal smooth muscle differs from myocardium in one crucial respect. The contractile work of myocardium is modulated by changes in the repetition rate of depolarization (heart rate), since each depolarization is associated with a contraction. In contrast, the repetition rate of intestinal smooth muscle is remarkably regular, varying by little more than 10 per cent, but each cycle of depolarization does not imply a contraction. Only (*Figure 7.2*) when action potentials are superimposed on the depolarization plateau is there tension change; conversely, action potentials and, hence, tension change can only occur at the time of depolarization. Alvarez[1] was initially baffled by the apparent lack of close association between the electroenterogram and muscle contraction, because he was initially unable to record the spike potentials which are the electrical signals of

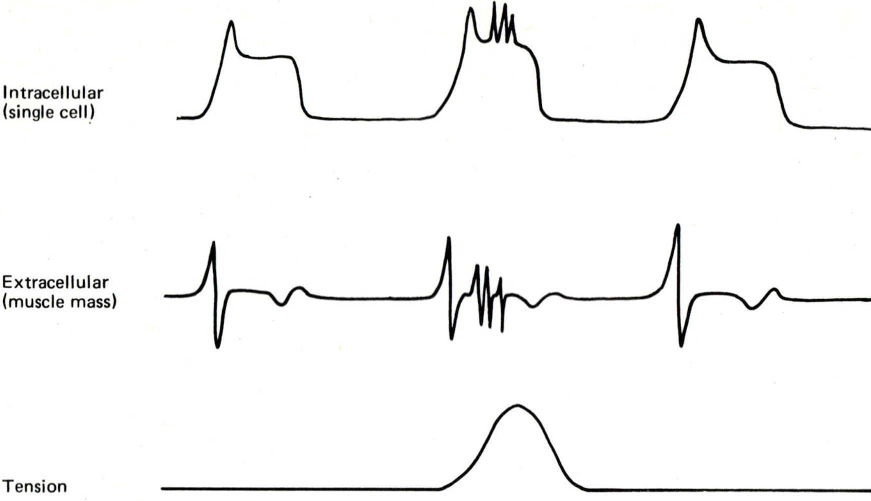

Figure 7.2 Schematic representation of the relationship between the slow and fast electrical activity and the tension change in the smooth muscle of the small intestine. In the upper trace, action potentials are seen superimposed on the plateau of depolarization, and these are reflected as a burst of spike activity phase-locked to the extracellularly recorded slow wave (middle) and local tension change (below)

tension change. Because of the synchrony of adjacent fibres, the onset of depolarization can be picked up by an external electrode, giving a signal resembling the QRS wave of the ECG, and this allows spike bursts to be recorded in the same way; as shown by Ambache[2], these spike bursts are summed action potentials from adjacent individual muscle cells. Because the electrical changes in the externally recorded electroenterogram preserve the temporal relationship between depolarization and action potential, spike bursts are said to be phase-locked to the slow wave; the latter is the term which is generally used to denote the regular rhythmic externally recorded electrical change in the smooth muscle. The sequence of slow waves is also commonly termed the basic electrical rhythm or BER. The slow wave is sometimes termed the pacesetter potential, since the slow wave reflects the opportunities that the muscle has to contract. Contraction with every slow wave occurs infrequently, but the basic electrical rhythm serves to define the maximal rate at which contraction may occur. In any area of the small intestine, the number of contractions per minute cannot exceed the number of slow waves, but is usually very much less. The ability of the bowel to modulate its contraction rate in this way allows infinite variations of contractile activity. Unlike the electrocardiogram, however, the electroenterogram cannot be recorded from the body surface; the electrical change in the long and convoluted intestine lacks the vectorial quality of myocardial depolarization.

The intestinal smooth muscle also shares the property of pacemaking with the myocardium. The intrinsic rate of repetition of depolarization varies along the small intestine; electrical coupling of the cells allows the faster cells to drive the slower cells, and hence (as in the heart) the region with the fastest rate dominates the remainder and serves as a pacemaker. Hermon-Taylor and Code[22] showed that the pacemaker of the small intestine is situated immediately distal to the pylorus; the pacemaking rate is 36 per minute in the rat, 17 per minute in the dog, and 11 per minute in man. This pacemaking frequency is maintained over the proximal small intestine but declines distally. When the continuity of the intestine is broken by transection, the bowel proximal to the section is still driven by the duodenal pacemaker, but distal to the section, the proximal cut end becomes the pacemaker for the remaining distal bowel at a lower frequency. Although anastomosis following transection restores the anatomical continuity of the bowel, electrical coupling of smooth muscle across the anatomosis does not occur because of the interposition of fibrous tissue; hence the site of an anastomosis is permanently marked by an abrupt change in the slow wave frequency.

Nerve

The neurophysiology of the intrinsic and extrinsic innervation is complex; for detailed accounts, readers are referred to recent reviews by Wood[57] and Roman and Gonella[34]. The extrinsic efferent innervation is composed of the cholinergic parasympathetic vagal input which is excitatory to smooth muscle, and the adrenergic sympathetic splanchnic input which is inhibitory. The classic view of intestinal innervation, derived largely from *in vitro* studies of smooth muscle, was that the innervation consisted only of a balance between adrenergic and cholinergic nerves, but the advances in smooth muscle physiology revealed the existence of non-adrenergic non-cholinergic (NANC) innervation. This discovery has led to the continuing search for 'the NANC neurotransmitter', at first thought to be adenosine triphosphate (ATP). Subsequent studies of the enteric nerves has shown that the concept of a single NANC neurotransmitter is probably illusory. *Figure 7.3* summarises present evidence on the possible identity of NANC neurotransmitters within the intrinsic plexuses, based on evidence derived from electrophysiology, morphology, and immunocytochemistry, but it would be foolish to regard this as more than an interim summary; some of these putative transmitters will not be finally validated, and doubtless other candidates will emerge. The strongest case at present can be made for 5-hydroxytryptamine[20], but although there is little doubt of the existence of serotoninergic nerves, there is very little evidence to show what function these nerves serve. All that can be said with any confidence at this point is that our appreciation of the complexity of the enteric innervation has considerably outstripped our capacity to understand the function of the component parts. Our present concept of the role of the enteric nerves, and their relation to the extrinsic nerves is summarised in *Figure 7.4* in which it can be seen that they serve as a link between receptor and effector, and in addition embody an intrinsic programme of organised motor activity; the relationships between receptor, effector, and motor programme are modulated by the influence of extrinsic innervation.

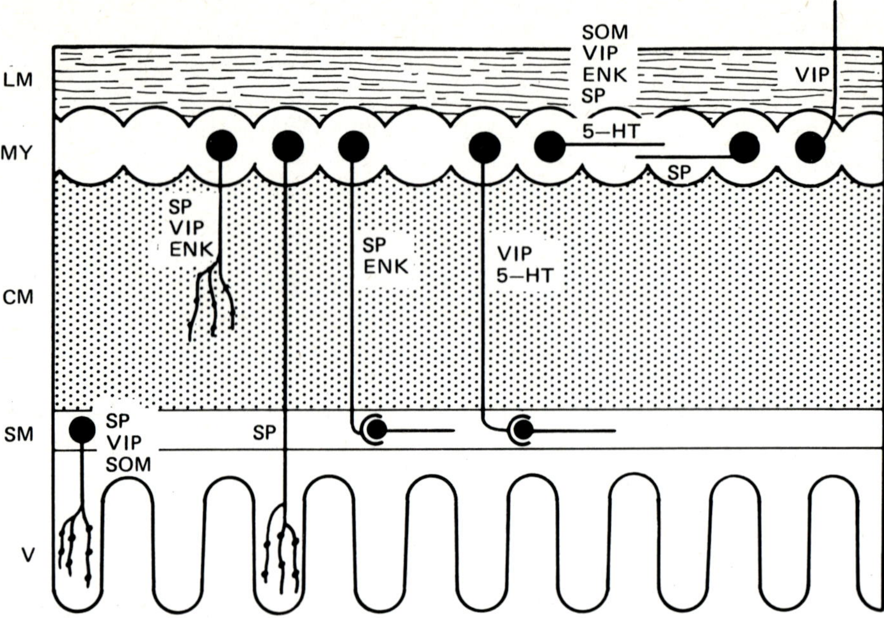

Figure 7.3 Schematic representation of the neuroanatomy and putative neurotransmitters of the small intestine. The myenteric plexus (MY) is shown between the longitudinal (LM) and circular (CM) muscle, and the submucous plexus (SM) between the circular muscle and the villous layer (V). (Putative neurotransmitters: SOM = somatostatin, VIP = vasoactive intestinal peptide, ENK = encephalin, SP = Substance P, 5-HT = 5-hydroxytryptamine)

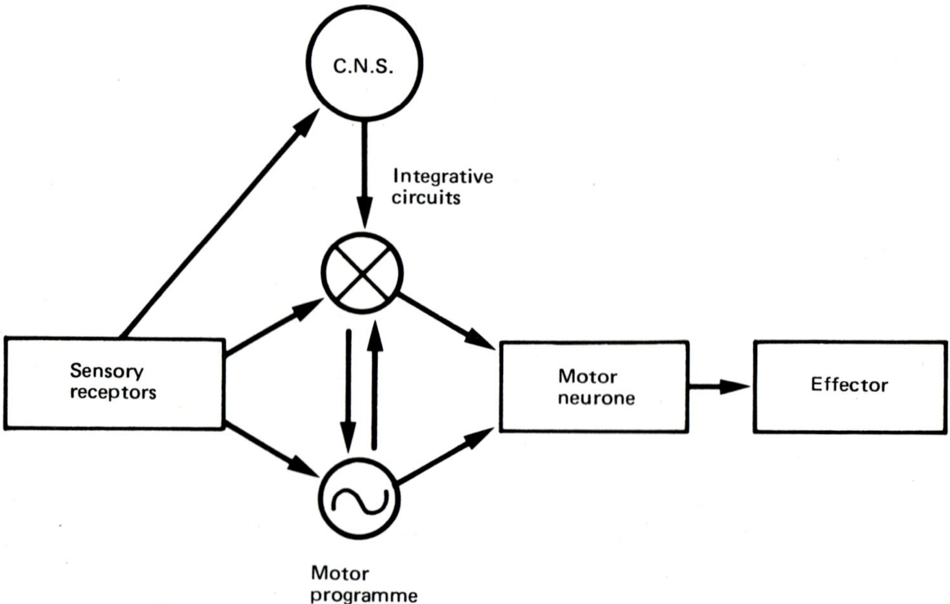

Figure 7.4 Functional interconnections between sensory receptors and motor effectors in the small intestine.

ENDOCRINOLOGY

The classical view of gut hormones, exemplified by the role of secretin shown by Bayliss and Starling[4], as humoral agents released from mucosal sites to activate distant target cells, has been destroyed by the discovery of numerous gastrointestinal peptides which are not only not confined to the mucosa, but which are also not confined to the digestive tract. These peptides, which are, for the most part, best reclassified as neuropeptides or 'brain-gut peptides' are intimately associated with the extrinsic and intrinsic nerves of the gut; since it is clear that much of the innervation of the gut is concerned with the regulation of motility, a role for gut peptides in the regulation of motility seems highly probable. However, it is also probable that this role is not endocrine; for the most part, the peptides probably act as neurotransmitters or neuromodulators. Experimental infusions of peptides have shown numerous effects on motility, but for the most part there is little evidence that these effects are physiological. Some possible effects of peptides will be mentioned in context in the description of organized motility below, but there is no good evidence that any of these effects are endocrine in the true sense of substances acting as humoral agents.

Comparative physiology

The inaccessibility of the small bowel to systematic study without surgical intervention has dictated that much pertinent research, particularly in recent years, has been carried out in animal models. Fortunately, species differentiation of the small intestine among mammals is less than that found at the proximal and distal ends of the digestive tract; in particular, canine small intestine seems to provide a good model for the study of motility in relation to man. The major differences in the organization of motility reside in the dietary intake of different species. In general, carnivores (as exemplified by man, rat and dog) consume infrequent meals which are relatively low in bulk, high in nutrient content, and which are digested by endogenous catalytic enzymes; in contrast, herbivores (cows, sheep and horses) pass much of their waking time consuming food which is rich in bulk, low in nutrient density, and which requires bacterial digestion. Ruckebusch and Bueno have emphasised the importance of diet in determining the pattern of small bowel motility in their studies of the pig, an omnivore, in which patterns of small bowel motility can be manipulated by the choice of diet[35].

Methods of investigation

An ideal method for the study of motility would yield simultaneous information about the contractile activity of the individual muscle layers and the gross movements of the intestinal wall at multiple sites, the corresponding changes in intraluminal pressure, and the resulting patterns of transit of digesta, using non-invasive techniques in human subjects who are freely mobile and able to eat normally. No such technique exists, and consequently, the investigation techniques that are used provide only a fraction of the total required information. This requires both the scientific and the clinical investigator to formulate a specific question that requires solution and then to choose the technique that appears most likely to answer the question.

An important consequence of these technical limitations is that terms applied to one type of methodology do not have the same meaning in another context. To give one example; movements of the small bowel wall may be organised so as to retard the transit of digesta by standing contractions or to accelerate transit by propulsive contractions. To the scientist studying wall movements, any contractile activity is often referred to as 'motility', and for him, 'increased motility' means increased contractile activity irrespective of the consequent alterations of transit. For the radiologist studying transit, 'motility' often implies transit, and therefore 'increased motility' denotes 'increased transit'; but increased transit may be due to an alteration, even a reduction, in contractile work. Similar considerations bedevil the analysis of intraluminal pressure change. For this reason, care is required in reading the reports of individual research or diagnostic manoeuvres.

Electrophysiology

Strictly speaking, electrophysiological study of intestinal smooth muscle refers to the examination of the electrical changes of the smooth muscle cell, which requires the smooth muscle to be studied *in vitro*. Since *in vitro* tissue does not exhibit the patterns of motility observed in the tissue *in situ*, such techniques are not relevant to the investigation of intestinal motility, although they are of considerable importance to the smooth muscle physiologist or pharmacologist. The only electrophysiological technique available for the study of motility (in the sense of organised organ movement) is that of electromyography, in which the electrical changes of the muscle mass are recorded.

Electromyography

Much recent research is based on the results obtained from electromyography in conscious animals with implanted serosal electrodes. This was introduced more than two decades ago[3] in dogs, and since then has been used in other mammalian species, including rat[36], sheep[37], and pig[35]. The technique involves suturing silver or platinum electrodes, usually embedded in an acrylic base, on to the serosal surface of the small intestine at laparotomy. Sterile wires lead from the electrodes to a cannula in the abdominal wall, from which, after recovery, the animal can be connected to a polygraph. Useful though this may be for the study of experimental animals, it is clearly not easily applicable to man.

Although the electromyogram of the intestine originates from electrical changes within smooth muscle which are similar to those in the myocardium, the 'electroenterogram' cannot usefully be detected on the body surface; in particular, while skilful electronic signal analysis may allow detection of the slow wave on the body surface, the spikes which signal muscle contraction cannot be distinguished in this way. Electromyography has been attempted in two ways in man. First, using techniques similar to those used in animals, electrodes have been implanted on the bowel at laparotomy using catgut sutures which dissolve after five days; at this time, the electrodes are withdrawn. The disadvantage of this technique is that recordings obtained in this way[10, 43] reflect the immediate postoperative state during which motility is not normal. The second method that has been used is recording from the mucosal surface using either wick electrodes[13, 15] or ring electrodes wrapped around an intestinal tube[19]. The problem here is that of contact with the intestinal wall; while it is possible to get adequate recordings of the electromyogram from an electrode in firm contact with the mucosa, firm contact cannot be ensured with this method, and is probably confined to periods when the circular muscle of the gut is actively contracting. Perhaps for this reason, the technique has not been widely adopted.

In general, it is probably fair to say that, at the present time, electromyography is a technique of great importance in the study of animal intestinal motility, but not in man.

Contractile activity

Instead of direct recording of muscle activity, local contraction may be measured by means of a pressure sensor, such as a strain gauge transducer, applied directly to the muscle mass. The techique for this in animals is similar to that used for electromyography, as is the information obtained. This technique has been used particularly in dogs, especially by Itoh *et al.*[24] who have brought considerable refinement to the method. Using miniaturised sensors it has also been used in small animals such as the rat[41]. It has, as yet, no place in the study of human small intestine.

Intraluminal pressure change

The recording of intraluminal pressure change has been carried out in animals throughout the 20th century[5], but in recent decades has been less popular than electromyography. Except in the presence of a stoma or fistula, it is difficult to introduce a pressure recording sensor into the small intestine of laboratory animals, whereas co-operation for this procedure is more forthcoming from human subjects than it is for the implantation of serosal sensors. The introduction of intestinal intubation[11] made the recording of human intraluminal pressure change possible. Although early techniques used air-filled balloons connected by a lumen to the exterior as sensor, recent practice has been to use a column of water to transmit the pressure to an external pressure sensor; slow flow is maintained in the water column to ensure patency of the tube. A multi-lumen tube with ports at equispaced intervals allows recording of intraluminal pressure change at multiple sites, and the observation thereby of prograde or retrograde contractile activity. This technique gives a clear picture of patterns of motility[49], but again has certain disadvantages. The subject must tolerate the presence of an oral or nasal tube throughout the study, and is immobilised by attachment to a polygraph. Moreover, not only is the pressure record complicated by intra-abdominal extra-enteric pressure change but also by more subtle pressures such as oropharyngeal movement.

A variant of this technique is the use of strain-gauge transducers in place of perfused tubes. These may be used attached to an intestinal tube; in this case, they give data equivalent to that obtained with perfused lumens leading to external transducers[32]. An alternative is the use of strain gauges as sensors for one or more radiotelemetric pressure capsules[6, 48]; with this technique, the sensors are anchored in the lumen by a thread attached externally. Less detailed pressure data is available from this technique than from a multiple perfused tube system, but the technique may be used with ambulant subjects, and is better tolerated for longer periods of time than a perfused tube.

Radiology

Although radiology is clinically helpful in, for example, the assessment of subacute intestinal obstruction or crude assessments of transit rate, the transit of barium is not easily related to patterns of intestinal movement and is almost certainly a poor guide to the way in which digesta are moved.

Radionuclide scanning

The advent of radionuclides whose distribution in the small intestine may be followed with an external counter has provided crude estimates of small bowel transit of digesta, since, unlike barium sulphate, radionuclides such as 99-Technetium sulphur-colloid may be mixed with food without noticeably changing the composition of the meal. However, the passage of these substances along the small bowel has to be largely inferred from observations of their departure from the stomach and their arrival in the caecum, since the convoluted and varying contours of the small bowel do not allow precise or quantitative isotope location. It is possible, at least in theory, that scanning techniques employing nuclear magnetic resonance will solve the problem of accurate localization of markers within the small bowel without unacceptable radiation hazard, but this remains to be seen.

NORMAL MOTILITY OF THE SMALL INTESTINE

In man (and dog and rat), the patterns of motility exhibited in fasting and after food are entirely different. Fasting motor activity is cyclical or (more correctly) periodic; this has accounted for much confusion in the study of motility since the assumption that there is a steady state which is in any sense 'basal' has been shown to be incorrect. Feeding abolishes periodicity.

Fasting motor activity – the migrating myoelectric complex (MMC)

As early as 1905, it was noted that in fasted dogs, brief bouts of motor activity were separated by longer periods of motor quiescence[5]. The early history[51] of research into small bowel motility was dominated by the neglect of this early observation in favour of Bayliss and Starling's assertion that motility only occurred in response to the presence of intraluminal content[4]. However, in 1969, Szurszewski showed that, in dogs, fasting motility was characterised by what he termed a 'migrating myoelectric complex'[45]. At intervals of approximately 90 minutes, brief (3–7 mins) periods of contraction at the maximal frequency of the bowel recur. These episodes of regular contraction (or regular spike bursts) are preceded by a period of irregular contraction (or irregular spike bursts) and followed by a period of motor quiescence. The episodes of regular contraction, now more conveniently known as *activity fronts*, migrate relatively slowly down the entire small bowel from the antrum, duodenum, or proximal jejunum, to the terminal ileum taking about 90–120 minutes to migrate; it follows that a new migrating complex is usually arising proximally as one dies away distally. Subsequently, the term 'migrating myoelectric complex' – or MMC – was modified[9] to include all three activity types, *Phase I* being quiescence, *Phase II* the irregular activity, and *Phase III* the activity front itself. A fourth component (*Phase IV*) which is the transition from Phase III to Phase I, is inconstant and often absent.

The next major step was the demonstration that the MMC is a property common to most (if not all) mammalian species. The first clear demonstration of its existence in man was published in 1975 in an obscure journal[42]; effectively, the first systematic study to show human MMCs, and certainly the first study to document their interruption by food was published by Vantrappen *et al.* in 1977[49]. There appears to be little difference between human (*Figures 7.5 and 7.6*) and animal (*Figure 7.7*) MMCs; although human MMCs are apparently very much less regular[46], human subjects are usually only studied once or twice, whereas laboratory animals are trained and habituated to study.

The 'purpose' or 'function' of the MMC is obscure, at least in man and dog, although it has been postulated that it has a role in man in the prevention of bacterial overgrowth of the small bowel[49]. However, the value of the MMC is that it is a recurrent and consistent periodic pattern which is amenable to experimental challenge and to diagnostic evaluation.

Postprandial activity

In the dog, as shown by Code and Marlett[16], and later by Vantrappen *et al.*[49] in man, normal oral feeding interrupts the MMC sequence at all levels of the small bowel and replaces it with persistent but irregular contractile activity. This pattern of activity persists until the nutrient load has been delivered by the stomach; following this, the MMC sequence resumes. The irregular activity following food is not identical with that seen in the irregular phase of the fasting MMC, but sophisticated computer analysis is required to prove this point. Presumably this

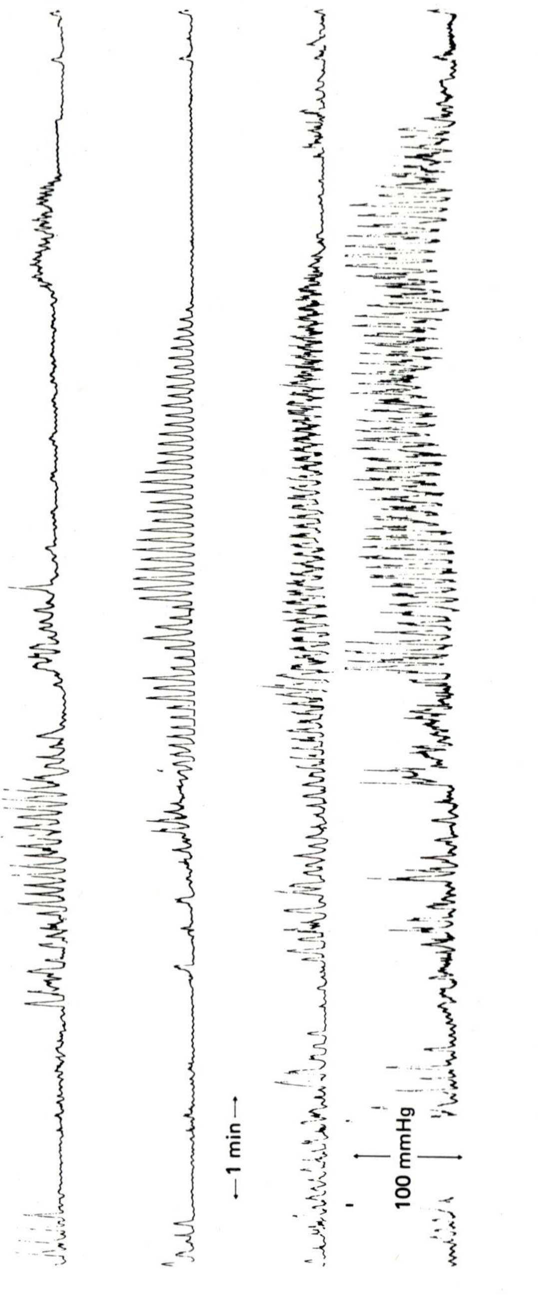

Figure 7.5 A human migrating motor complex (MMC) recorded by perfused tubes with four ports sited at 10 cm intervals between mid-duodenum (top) and jejunum (bottom). Note the characteristic phasic contraction of the activity front at the frequency of the small intestinal slow wave. (By kind permission of Ian Wilson FRCS, Charing Cross Hospital, London, UK)

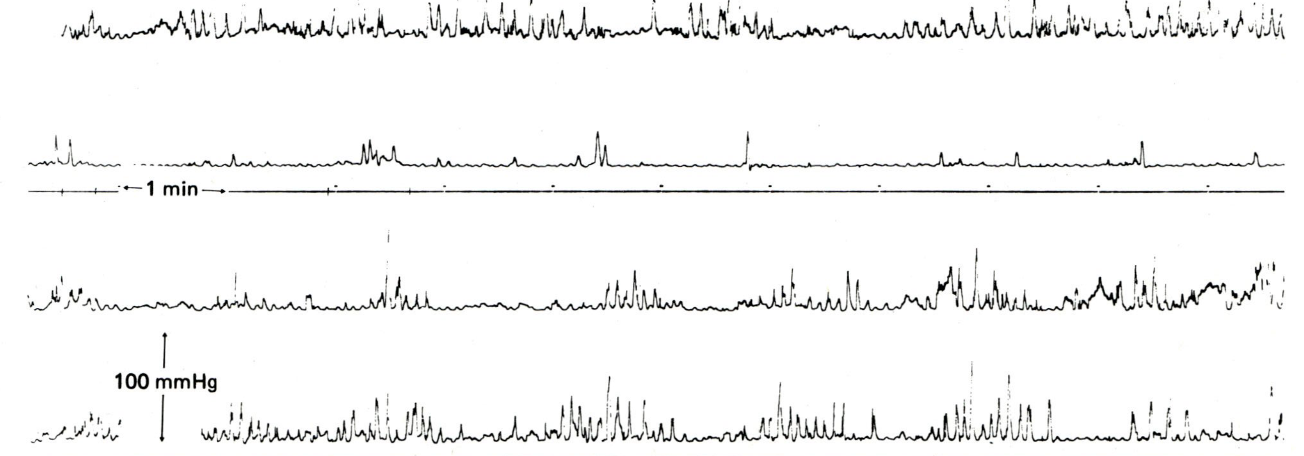

Figure 7.6 The irregular contractile activity (Phase II) of the complex shown in *Figure 7.5* shows a characteristic grouping of contractions into brief migrating bursts at intervals of about one minute; the so-called 'minute rhythm' (By kind permission of Ian Wilson FRCS, Charing Cross Hospital, London, UK)

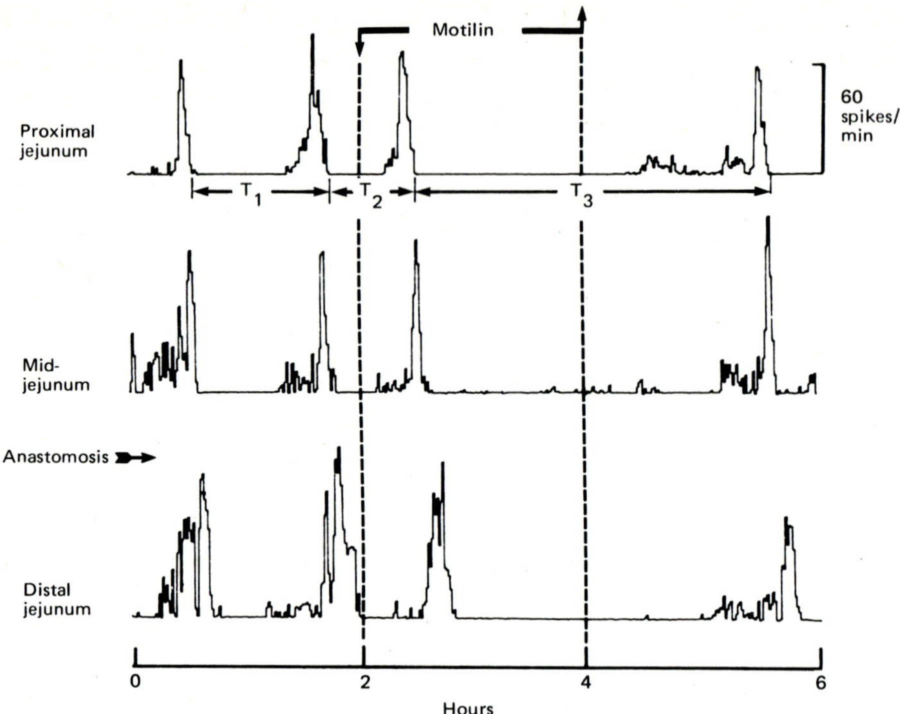

Figure 7.7 The effect of motilin on the integrated spike activity of the canine small intestine. The effect of a motilin infusion is to diminish the period between MMCs (T2) as compared with the period prior to infusion (T1); the after-effect of the infusion, possibly due to the unphysiological plasma level of motilin produced by the infusion, is a lengthening of the period (T3). Transection and reanastomosis of the intestine in the mid-jejunum as shown does not interfere with the orderly progression of the MMC, even though functional continuity is not re-established between muscle cells after anastomosis, only between intrinsic nerves. (By kind permission of Ms Julie Pinnington, Gastrointestinal Science Research Unit, London, UK)

postprandial activity corresponds to the gross movement of segmentation, by which mixing is accomplished. In herbivores, such as sheep[7], MMCs are not interrupted by feeding, but herbivores are constantly 'feeding', ingesting material which is high in bulk, and low in nutrient value. From this it would appear that MMCs are not *per se* 'interdigestive', but are interrupted in those species who feed rapidly and infrequently on meals which are low in bulk, and high in nutrient value.

CONTROL MECHANISMS OF NORMAL MOTILITY

The discovery of reproducible patterns of motor activity which are modulated by the presence or absence of food has, inevitably, led to a search for the underlying control mechanisms which engender the periodic rhythm, and for those which adjust it in accordance with feeding. Both nerves and gastrointestinal peptides appear to play a part in the control mechanisms.

Neural

Intrinsic nerves

The intrinsic nerves appear to control small bowel motility in two major respects. First, they appear to control the apparent propagation of the MMC. It is important to appreciate that the MMC is not a physical entity which is being propelled, bolus-like, down the bowel, but rather the sequential excitation of the muscle in a caudad direction. That this is a function of the intrinsic nerves can be shown by local intra-arterial selective blockade[39]. It had also been shown that MMC propagation is undisturbed when the extrinsic (but not the intrinsic) innervation is destroyed[8]. The second important property of the intrinsic nerves in the small bowel appears to be the ability to produce MMC-like activity in isolated lengths of small bowel. It has been shown that MMC-like activity appears in isolated lengths of small bowel which have been intrinsically and extrinsically denervated[8], or even autotransplanted to a different location[40]. The small bowel differs in this respect from the stomach, since the MMC-like activity of isolated bowel has a shorter period than that of the remaining bowel[40], whereas isolated autotransplanted gastric pouches exhibit activity fronts which are synchronous with the stomach. The co-ordinating role of the intrinsic nerves is seen following bowel resection. Following reanastomosis, there is no electrical continuity between the muscle layers, but after a recovery period[28], MMCs progress smoothly down the anastomosed bowel (*Figure 7.7*) because of fusion of the intrinsic nerves across the anatomosis.

Extrinsic nerves

The role of the extrinsic nerves appears to be important in ensuring that the motor activity is adapted to extraenteric events. In 1972, it was asserted[9] that MMCs traversed a Thiry-Vella loop in the correct temporal sequence, and this led to the concept of motility control, and hence MMC sequencing, by an extraenteric oscillator modulating regional excitation through the extrinsic nerves[50]. These observations were probably incorrect, in that Thiry-Vella loop MMCs are asynchronous, as discussed above, but the conceptual model is residually useful in ascribing to the extrinsic nerves the function of altering motility in response to feeding. Extrinsically denervated isolated loops do not show abolition of MMC-like activity on feeding[40], whereas normal Thiry-Vella loops excluded from the nutrient stream do show relatively normal postprandial motor activity[28]. Following vagotomy, the motor response of the small bowel to food is impaired[33]. Acute vagal blockade will convert postprandial to periodic fasting motor activity[17]. Presumably the modulation of MMC interval which is particularly evident in man[46] is controlled through the extrinsic nerves, but this has not been verified.

Endocrine

Many studies have been out to define the effect of peptides on motility, but these have, in general, involved systemic administration of peptides to give supraphysiological plasma peptide concentrations, and the interpretation of such studies in terms of physiology is difficult. The MMC is useful in this respect because it is an integrated physiological phenomenon; in this respect, only two peptides so far seem to be important.

Motilin

In 1976, it was clearly demonstrated by two independent groups of workers that the duodenal mucosal peptide motilin, if infused into a fasting animal, will induce a premature MMC, while being without apparent effect in the fed state[23, 56]. The idea that the origin of an MMC is associated with motilin release has been strengthened by the fact that MMCs in dog and in man are associated with a rise in the plasma concentration of endogenous motilin[12, 29]. The situation is not as simple as it might seem. It has become clear, from human studies[48, 49], that some MMCs arise distal to the stomach and duodenum, and such MMCs are not associated with changes in plasma motilin[31]. Moreover, motilin does not induce MMCs in jejunal Thiry-Vella loops[31]. The simplest interpretation of the present data is that gastroduodenal MMCs are associated with motilin release, but the uninterrupted onward progress of these MMCs is modulated by the intrinsic nerves, and not by motilin. Because of the shorter period of intrinsic jejunal MMC-like activity, absence of a gastroduodenal MMC produces an interval in which an autonomous jejunal MMC, unrelated to motilin release, can arise. Motilin release not only stimulates a gastroduodenal MMC but also appears to inhibit autonomous jejunal periodic activity as seen in a Thiry-Vella loop[30]. Further but fragmentary evidence of the importance of motilin are the observations of MMC suppression by the administration of motilin antiserum[27], and, in the presence of nerve damage, of absent gastroduodenal periodic activity and absent plasma motilin[52]. Whether or not motilin acts as a humoral or local agent has not been determined, but it is worth noting that almost alone among the ‘gut hormones’, motilin is not found in other body systems but is virtually confined to the duodenum.

Somatostatin

The only other peptide which seems to be clearly implicated in small bowel motility is somatostatin. Somatostatin infusion induces MMCs which start below the duodenum, and are similar to the spontaneous MMCs which are not associated with plasma motilin peaks[31]. It seems plausible to suppose that somatostatin is, in some way, involved in the periodic motor programme of the intestinal intrinsic nerves.

Other peptides

Although studies show an apparent effect of 'digestive' peptides such as gastrin and cholecystokinin on small bowel motility, it seems unlikely that this is a direct effect. It is more likely that these peptides directly control gastric, or gastroduodenal, motility, and that this effect is transmitted onwards. Neither CCK nor gastrin infusions have a consistent effect on the motility of the distal bowel[53]. Exogenous opioids exert an effect on small bowel motility[25], but it is not clear whether endogenous opioids play a physiological role.

ABNORMAL MOTILITY

The documentation of abnormal motility is fragmentary; a number of conditions in which motility is known to be abnormal have been recorded but, in general, studies of intestinal motility in these syndromes have been few, and it is not known whether there are indeed pathognomonic abnormal patterns.

Primary disorders

Chronic pseudo-obstruction

Disordered motility may result from primary disease of muscle or nerve. In general, the effect of such disease is delayed or obstructed transit, leading to the term 'pseudo-obstruction'. The majority of these cases, which are rare, are due to familial or idiopathic smooth muscle myopathy, which may affect the proximal bowel, the entire bowel, or even other smooth muscle such as the urinary tract[18]. In the few cases that have been fully studied, the motility disorder may range from hypomotility to hypermotility[26, 38], but the common result is delayed or absent transit of intestinal contents. The presentation depends upon the region initially or maximally affected; the first manifestation may be oesophageal dysfunction or alternatively, obstinate and progressive constipation. Although these syndromes appear, at present, to be uncommon, it is likely that many milder cases are classified as 'functional disorders' or 'irritable bowel'. It is a mistake to think that constipation denotes only colonic involvement; the small bowel may also be involved.

Paralytic ileus

Acute transient motor paralysis of the bowel occurs in association with acute intra-abdominal conditions such as perforation and peritonitis. It can also be produced by handling of the bowel during surgery. The condition is self-limiting provided that the cause is removed. Electromyography in animals following laparotomy reveals normal slow waves but complete absence of spike activity. The mechanism of paralytic ileus is not known; although adrenergic inhibition of motility is suspected, adrenergic blockers are therapeutically ineffective.

Secondary disorders

Autonomic neuropathy

DIABETES MELLITUS

The nature of disordered motility in small intestine in the presence of autonomic neuropathy due to diabetes is undefined, but slow, or even retrograde transit seems unlikely because of the frequent presence of bacterial overgrowth. Metoclopramide, which relieves some cases of diabetic gastroparesis, has not been shown to be beneficial in the small intestine. Antibiotic treatment is helpful if overgrowth is present.

PORPHYRIA

In patients with acute intermittent porphyria, MMC's may be abnormally frequent and the normal response to food may be impaired[21].

SHY-DRAGER SYNDROME

Abnormal intestinal motility in cases of generalised autonomic neuropathy is to be expected but has not been clearly defined.

CHAGAS' DISEASE

Chagas' disease, due to infection with a trypanosome, is endemic in South America; it has been estimated that in Brazil alone, there are 10 000 000 cases. Oesophageal and colonic involvement appears as achalasia and aganglionosis respectively; small bowel involvement is known to occur from autopsy evidence, but, again, is ill-defined. The clinical features of small bowel involvement are (probably) those of chronic pseudo-obstruction. The neuropathy is not due to the parasite itself, but to the immune response of the tissue to *T. cruzii*.

Thyroid disease

Hypothyroidism is associated with constipation, and, conversely, hyperthyroidism is associated with diarrhoea. It has been shown[14] that the basic electrical rhythm of the small intestine is altered by thyroid imbalance, this being presumably a metabolic effect. It is not known to what extent motility itself is affected.

Scleroderma

When the small bowel is involved in scleroderma, fibrosis of the smooth muscle occurs. The result is hypomotility, with diminution of migrating complexes and bacterial overgrowth. In the latter event, antibiotic treatment is indicated.

Mechanical obstruction

ACUTE AND SUB-ACUTE OBSTRUCTION

The effect of extrinsic obstruction on small bowel motility depends upon whether the obstruction is complete (acute) or partial (sub-acute). In partial obstruction, the normal pattern of motility proximal to the site of obstruction is replaced by more frequent bursts of powerful contractions, at intervals of 10–20 minutes which presumably represent an attempt by the bowel to propel content beyond the obstruction[44]. This abnormal pattern may prove to be of diagnostic value when, and if, facilities for recording motility become more generally available. As partial obstruction progresses to complete obstruction, so does the pattern of motility change to that of paralytic ileus.

THERAPY OF MOTILITY DISORDERS

The foregoing account shows that the characterization of abnormal motility is still rudimentary. It is, therefore, scarcely surprising that therapy is largely a matter of trial and error, and prescribed on the erroneous assumption that there is 'too little' or 'too much' motility which requires correction whereas, as has been shown, the problem is one of correct or incorrect patterns governed by complex neuroendocrine controls. Rational therapy must depend upon better knowledge of the physiology and pathophysiology of motility.

Cholinergic and related drugs

Metoclopramide

Metoclopramide, a procainamide analogue, may have some value as a cholinergic agent, but its effect on small bowel motility appears to be small[54]. It has been postulated that it is useful as a dopamine antagonist, but there is no evidence that dopaminergic transmission plays any significant part in normal or abnormal small bowel motility.

Domperidone

Domperidone is a newer agent with pharmacological properties similar to metoclopramide. The same considerations apply to its use as to the earlier drug.

Anticholinergic and related drugs

Anticholinergic agents will, in theory, diminish 'excessive motility', but the indication for this is obscure except for specific procedures, such as the use of anticholinergics to inhibit duodenal motility to allow endoscopic cannulation of the papilla of Vater.

Glucagon

Pancreatic glucagon is of some theoretical interest. Administered in bolus doses, it has a powerful anticholinergic effect on the small bowel, but this is almost certainly due to the ability of glucagon to release endogenous adrenaline. Low doses of glucagon, at least in the dog, stimulate small bowel motility[55]; this may prove therapeutically useful.

Future possibilities

Consideration of what is becoming known about the complexity of intestinal motility and its controls must lead to the realization that there are at present no therapeutic agents which are clearly related to the control processes which they are intended to influence. The therapeutic outlook must remain bleak for syndromes in which there is destruction of nerve or muscle. In contrast, in syndromes in which there are inappropriate patterns of motility, there are reasonable prospects that specific agents, probably analogues of endogenous peptides, will be found which will modulate incorrect patterns and responses towards normality.

References

1 ALVAREZ, W. C. and MAHONEY, L. J. Action current in stomach and intestine. *American Journal of Physiology*, **58,** 476–493 (1922)

2 AMBACHE, N. The electrical activity of isolated mammalian intestine. *Journal of Physiology*, **106,** 139–153 (1947)

3 BASS, P., CODE, C. F. and LAMBERT, E. H. Motor and electric activity of the duodenum. *American Journal of Physiology*, **201,** 287–291 (1961)

4 BAYLISS, W. M. and STARLING, E. H. The movement and innervation of the small intestine. *Journal of Physiology*, **24,** 99–143 (1899)

5 BOLDYREFF, W. N. Le travail periodique de l'appareil digestif en dehors de la digestion. *Archives des Sciences Biologique*, **11,** 1–157 (1905)

6 BROWNING, C., VALORI, R. M., WINGATE, D. L. and MacLACHLAN, D. A new pressure-sensitive ingestible radio-telemetric capsule. *Lancet*, **2,** 504–505 (1981)

7 BUENO, L., FIORAMONTI, J. and RUCHEBUSCH, Y. Rate of flow of digesta and electrical activity of the small intestine in dogs and sheep. *Journal of Physiology*, **249,** 69–85 (1975)

8 BUENO, L., PRADDAUDE, F. and RUCKEBUSCH, Y. Propagation of electrical spiking activity along the small intestine: intrinsic versus extrinsic neural influences. *Journal of Physiology*, **292,** 15–26 (1979)

9 CARLSON, G. M., BEDI, B. S. and CODE, C. F. Mechanism of propagation of intestinal interdigestive myoelectric complex. *American Journal of Physiology*, **222,** 1027 –1030 (1972)

10 CATCHPOLE, B. N. and DUTHIE, H. L. Postoperative gastrointestinal complexes. In *Gastrointestinal Motility in Health and Disease*, edited by H. Duthie, 33–42, Lancaster, MTP Press (1978)

11 CHAPMAN, W. P. and PALAZZO, W.-. Multiple-balloon-kymograph recording of intestinal motility in man with observations on the correlation of the tracing patterns with barium movements. *Journal of Clinical Investigation*, **28,** 1517–1525 (1949)

12 CHEY, W. Y., LEE, K. Y. and TAI, H. H. Endogenous plasma motilin concentration and interdigestive myoelectric activity of the canine duodenum. In *Gut Hormones*, edited by S. R. Bloom, 355–358, Edinburgh, Churchill Livingstone (1978)

13 CHRISTENSEN, J., CLIFTON, J. A. and SCHEDL, J. P. Variations in the frequency of the human duodenl basic electrical rhythm in health and disease. *Gastroenterology*, **51,** 200–206 (1966)

14 CHRISTENSEN, J., SCHEDL, H. P. and CLIFTON, J. A. The basic electrical rhythm of the duodenum in normal human subjects and in patients with thyroid disease. *Journal of Clinical Investigation*, **43,** 1659–1667 (1964)

15 CLIFTON, J. A., CHRISTENSEN, J. and SCHEDL, H. P. The human small intestinal slow wave. *American Climatological Association*, **77,** 217–225 (1965)

16 CODE, C. F. and MARLETT, J. A. The interdigestive myoelectric complex of the stomach and small bowel of dogs. *Journal of Physiology*, **246,** 298–309 (1975)

17 DIAMANT, N. E., HALL, K., MUI, H. and EI-SHARKAWY, T. Y. Vagal control of the feeding motor pattern in the lower oesophageal sphincter, stomach and upper small intestine of dog. In *Proceedings of the Seventh International Symposium on GI Motility*, edited by J. Christensen, 365–370. New York, Raven Press (1980)

18 FAULK, D. L., ANURAS, S. and CHRISTENSEN, J. Chronic intestinal pseudo-obstruction. *Gastroenterology*, **74,** 922–931 (1978)

19 FLECKENSTEIN, P. A probe for intraluminal recording of myoelectrical activity from multiple sites in the human small intestine. *Scandinavian Journal of Gastroenterology*, **13,** 767–770 (1978)

20 GERSHON, M. D. and ERDE, S. M. The nervous system of the gut. *Gastroenterology*, **80,** 1571–1594 (1981)

21 GORCHEIN, A., VALORI, R. M., WINGATE, D. L. and BLOOM, S. R. Abnormal gut motility in acute intermittent porphyria (AIP): a neuropathic model. *Gastroenterology*, **82,** 1070 (1982)

22 HERMON-TAYLOR, J. and CODE, C. F. Localisation of the duodenal pacemaker and its role in the organisation of duodenal myoelectric activity. *Gut*, **12,** 40–47 (1971)

23 ITOH, Z., HONDA, R., KIWATASHI, K., TAKEUCHI, S., AIZAWA, I., TAKAYANAGI, R. and COUCH, E. F. Motilin-induced mechanical activity in the canine alimentary tract. *Scandinavian Journal of Gastroenterology*, **11** (Suppl. 39), 93–110 (1976)

24 ITOH, Z., TAKEUCHI, S., AIZAWA, I. and TAKAYANAGI, R. Characteristic motor activity of the gastrointestinal tract in fasted conscious dogs measured by implanted force transducers. *American Journal of Digestive Diseases*, **23,** 229–238 (1978)

25 KONTUREK, S. J., THOR, P., KROL, R., DEMBINSKI, A. and SCHALLY, A. V. Influence of methionine-enkephalin and morphine on myoelectric activity of small bowel. *American Journal of Physiology*, **238,** G384–G389 (1980)

26 KUMPURIS, D. D., BRANNAN, P. G., GOYAL, R. K. Characterisation of motor activity in the jejunum of normal subjects and two patients with idiopathic intestinal pseudo-obstruction syndrome. *Gastroenterology*, **76,** 1177 (1979)

27 LEE, K. Y., CHANG, T. M. and CHEY, W. Y. Effect of rabbit anti-motilin serum on interdigestive myoelectric complex of the antrum and small intestine. *Digestive Diseases and Sciences*, **25,** 726 (1980) (abstract)

28 PEARCE, F. A. and WINGATE, D. L. Myoelectric and absorptive activity in the transected canine small bowel. *Journal of Physiology*, **302,** 11–12P (1980)

29 PEETERS, T. L., VANTRAPPEN, G. and JANSSENS, J. Fluctuations of motilin and gastrin levels in relation to the interdigestive complex in man. In *Gastrointestinal Motility*, edited by J. Christensen, 287. New York, Raven Press (1980)

30 PINNINGTON, J. and WINGATE, D. L. Motilin and the canine migrating myoelectric complex (MMC): a reassessment. *Journal of Physiology*, **319,** 49–50P (1981)

31 POITRAS, P., STEINBACH, J. H., VAN DEVENTER, G., CODE, C. F. and WALSH, J. H. Motilin-independent ectopic fronts of the interdigestive myoelectric complex in dogs. *American Journal of Physiology*, **239,** G215–G220 (1980)

32 REES, W. D. W., MILLER, L. J. and MALAGELADA, J. R. Role of gastric acid secretion in the generation of human interdigestive motor activity. *Gut*, **19,** A997 (1978)

33 REVERDIN, N., HUTTON, M., LING, A., THOMPSON, H. H., WINGATE, D. L., CHRISTOFIDES, N. ADRIAN, T. E. and BLOOM, S. R. Vagotomy and the motor response to feeding. In *Proceedings of the Seventh International Symposium on GI Motility*, edited by J. Christensen, 359–364. New York, Raven Press (1980)

34 ROMAN, C. and GONELLA, J. Extrinsic control of digestive tract motility. In *Physiology of the Gastrointestinal Tract*, edited by L. R. Johnson, 289–333, New York, Raven Press (1981)

35 RUCKEBUSCH, Y. and BUENO, L. The effect of feeding on the motility of the stomach and small intestine in the pig. *British Journal of Nutrition*, **35,** 397–405 (1976)

36 RUCKEBUSCH, Y. and FIORAMONTI, J. Electrical spiking activity and propulsion in small intestine in fed and fasted rats. *Gastroenterology*, **68,** 1500–1508 (1975)

37 RUCKEBUSCH, Y. and LAPLACE, J. P. La motricité intestinale chez le mouton: phenomenes mecaniques et electriques. **161**, 2517–2523 (1967)

38 SARNA, S. K., DANIEL, E. E., WATERFALL, W. E., LEWIS, T. D. and MARZIO, L. Post-operative gastrointestinal electrical and mechanical activities in a patient with idiopathic intestinal pseudo-obstruction. *Gastroenterology*, **74,** 112–120 (1978)

39 SARNA, S., STODDARD, C., BELBECK, L. and McWADE, D. Intrinsic nervous control of migrating myoelectrical complexes. *American Journal of Physiology*, **4,** G16–G23 (1981)

40 SARR, M. G., and KELLY, K. A. Myoelectric activity of the autotransplanted canine jejunoileum. *Gastroenterology*, **81,** 303–310 (1981)

41 SCOTT, L. D. and SUMMERS, R. W. Correlation of contractions and transit in rat small intestine. *American Journal of Physiology*, **230,** 132–137 (1976)

42 STANCIU, C. and BENNETT, J. R. The general pattern of gastroduodenal motility; 24 hour recordings in normal subjects. *Revištă Medico-chirurgicală a Societătii de Medici şi Naturalisti din Iaşi*, **79,** 31–36 (1975)

43 STODDARD, C. J., SMALLWOOD, R. H. and DUTHIE, H. L. Migrating myoelectrical complexes in man. In *Gastrointestinal Motility in Health and Disease*, edited by H. Duthie, 9–17, Lancaster, MTP Press (1978)

44 SUMMERS, R. W., ANURAS, S. and GREEN, J. Jejunal motility patterns in normal subjects and symptomatic patients with partial mechanical obstruction or pseudo-obstruction. *Zeitschrift fur Gastroenterologie*, **19,** 413 (1981) (abstract)

45 SZURSZEWSKI, J. H. A Migrating electric complex of the canine small intestine. *American Journal of Physiology*, **217,** 1757–1763 (1969)

46 THOMPSON, D. G., WINGATE, D. L., ARCHER, L., BENSON, M. J., GREEN, W. J. and HARDY, R. J. Normal patterns of human upper small bowel motor activity recorded by prolonged radiotelemetry. *Gut*, **21,** 500–506 (1980)

47 THUNEBERG, L., RUMESSEN, J. J. and MIKKELSEN, H. B. Interstitial cells of Cajal – an intestinal impulse generation and conduction system? *Scandinavian Journal of Gastroenterology*, **17**, (Suppl. 71) 143–144 (1982)

48 VALORI, R. M. and WINGATE, D. L. Evaluation of a dual pressure-sensitive radiopill in ambulant human subjects. *Gut*, **23,** A433 (1982)

49 VANTRAPPEN, G., JANSSENS, J., HELLEMANS, J. and GHOOS, Y. The interdigestive motor complex of normal subjects and patients with bacterial over-growth of the small intestine. *Journal of Clinical Investigation*, **59,** 1158–1166 (1977)

50 WINGATE, D. L. The eupeptide system: a general theory of gastrointestinal hormones. *Lancet*, **1,** 529–532 (1976)

51 WINGATE, D. L. Backwards and forwards with the migrating complex. *Digestive Diseases and Sciences*, **26,** 641–666 (1981)

52 WINGATE, D. L., BLOOM, S. R. and GORCHEIN, A. Absent nerves and absent motilin. *Scandinavian Journal of Gastroenterology*, **17,** (Suppl. 71) 139 (1982)

53 WINGATE, D. L., PEARCE, F. A., HUTTON, M., DAND, A., THOMPSON, H. H. and WUNSCH, E. Quantitative comparison of the effects of cholecystokinin, secretin and pentagastrin on gastrointestinal myoelectric activity in the conscious dog. *Gut*, **19,** 593–601 (1978)

54 WINGATE, D. L., PEARCE, E. A., HUTTON, M., and LING, A. Effect of metoclopramide on interdigestive myoelectric activity in the conscious dog. *Digestive Disease Science*, **25,** 15–21 (1980)

55 WINGATE, D. L., PEARCE, E. A. THOMAS, P. A. and BOUCHER, B. J. Glucagon stimulates intestinal myoelectric activity. *Gastroenterology*, **74,** 1152 (1978)

56 WINGATE, D. L., RUPPIN, H., GREEN, W. E. R., THOMPSON, H. H., DOMSCHKE, W., WUNSCH, E., DEMLING, L. and RITCHIE, D. H. Motilin-induced electrical activity in the canine gastrointestinal tract. *Scandinavian Journal of Gastroenterology*, **11,** (Suppl. 39) 111–118 (1976)

57 WOOD, J. D. Physiology of the enteric nervous system. In *Physiology of the Gastrointestinal Tract*, edited by L. R. Johnson, 1–37, New York, Raven Press (1981)

8
Interactions among micro-organisms and the host

P. D. Walker

INTRODUCTION

The interaction between the host and its microbes has recently been reviewed by Savage[54]. As this review deals comprehensively with the earlier literature only the salient points will be summarized here. The present chapter will concentrate on some of the adhesive mechanisms by which bacteria attach to animal tissues and parallels drawn with human situations. Examples will be given of some of the factors which result in autochthonous relationships becoming allochthonous. Finally, some recent work on the role of cellular immunity as a possible means of controlling populations will be reviewed.

Any discussion of the interactions of the organism and the host can only be understood in terms of ecological theory. Under normal conditions the gastrointestinal tract can be regarded as a balanced ecosystem within which there are numerous microbial interactions of benefit to the animal. According to modern ecological theory ecosystems are composed of habitats and niches. Habitats are physical spaces in the system and the way that an organism makes a living in the habitat defines its niches in the ecosystem[2].

Habitats are normally occupied by climax communities of autochthonous or indigenous microbial species. Each of these species occupies a niche in the habitat and thereby contributes in some way to the economy of the whole system. The species composition of these communities is maintained reasonably constant with the passage of time. During the development of the animal the gastrointestinal system is colonized by a series of different bacteria species. In the neonate organisms such as *Escherichia coli* and *Streptococcus faecalis* predominate while in the adult animal large populations of strict anaerobes are established corresponding to a decline in the population levels of coliforms and enterococci. Populations of bacteria may be as high as 10^{10}–10^{11} per gram in the large intestine of all vertebrate animals although the numbers in the small intestine of higher animals are much lower; up to 10^{8} per gram, but usually less, occur in the jejunum and ileum of man[54]. Such microbes assist their host to resist infectious disease through microbial interference activities and prepare their host to react immunologically to pathogens of numerous types by inducing natural antibodies which cross react with the antigens of the invaders[54].

Allochthonous or transient organisms are also frequently found in any given habitat but these normally contribute little to the economy of the ecosystem and in the case of the gastrointestinal tract may be merely in passage being derived from food or water, or from another habitat in the gastrointestinal system. Allochthonous microbes may colonize a habitat when it is vacated by an autochthonous resident; however, this only occurs if the system is disturbed. Although pathogens may temporarily colonize a habitat in this way, it is also evident that some pathogens are autochthonous to the gastrointestinal system and usually live in harmony with their hosts. Such microbes only become pathogenic when the ecosystem is seriously disturbed and the microbes are free from the restraints that regulate their localization and population levels. Examples of these are microbial overgrowth of the human small intestine and abscess formation when intestinal microbes gain access to parenteral tissues[54].

The consensus of opinion is that the numbers of organisms in the small intestine of humans is relatively small, 10^4 per gram of tissue. The numbers observed and the types of species isolated vary from worker to worker but these can, in part, be explained by differences in sampling and culture techniques[15, 20, 51]. Most workers agree that the upper and mid small intestine contain only small populations of predominantly Gram positive facultative aerobic organisms, together with small numbers of anaerobes, yeasts and fungi. Some increase in numbers occurs after consumption of food but declines after a few hours.

It is also clear that in various pathological conditions overgrowth of the small intestine can take place from regions more distal, resulting in a flora more akin to that observed in the large bowel[20]. Furthermore, it is evident that in the more distal portions of the small intestine, i.e. in the region of the ileo-caecal valve the flora observed is intermediate between that of the more proximal portion of the small intestine and of the colon[20]. As the flora, under these conditions, resemble the flora in the colon, the reader is referred to the appropriate chapter in this volume.

Association between microbes and the host can be luminal, epithelial or cryptal. A large number of associations are epithelial involving attachment of the organism to the surface. Some adhesive mechanisms by which bacteria attach to animal tissues will now be considered.

THE NEONATAL INTESTINE

Prior to the development of a normal flora the neonatal intestine is particularly susceptible to a number of pathogens. Normal hygiene as practised with young babies is normally sufficient to prevent such colonization but the conditions under which the neonates of large animals are raised provide no such protection. Two examples will be illustrated. Although these involve allochthonous organisms the mechanisms involved throw light on the more general aspects of attachment and colonization.

The neonates of sheep, cattle and pigs are susceptible to colonization by strains of *E. coli*. It has been shown that the first stage in *E. coli* infection is the adhesion of the organisms to the intestinal villi (*Figure 8.1*). Following adhesion proliferation and release of enterotoxins occur, resulting in a disturbance of the water and electrolyte balance causing diarrhoea, dehydration and death. The adhesion of these strains of *E. coli* to the intestine is mediated by specific adhesive factors elaborated by the organism. These are 'K' or capsular antigens which may be proteinaceous or polysaccharide in composition.

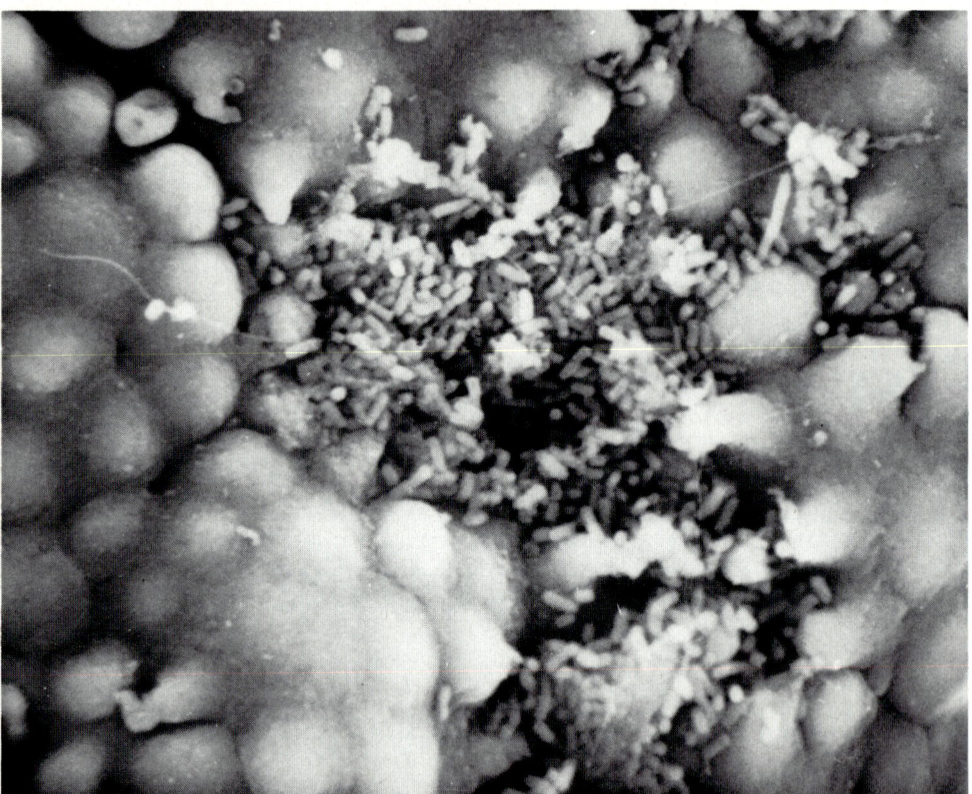

Figure 8.1 **Scanning electron micrograph of intestinal villi showing colonization with *E. coli* K99 positive organism. Note integrity of the villous surface. (× 1912)**

It has been shown in enteropathogenic strains of *E. coli* affecting sheep, cattle and pigs that proteinaceous surface antigens promoting colonization of the small intestine are under the control of transmissible plasmids. These are small irregular intracellular DNA molecules which multiply independently of chromosomal DNA. A large number of piglet enteropathogenic strains possess the 88 plasmid which controls the production of a proteinaceous surface antigen, the K88 antigen, facilitating the adherence of the organism to the intestinal villi[25, 56]. Similarly calf and lamb enteropathogenic strains and to a less extent piglet strains, produce a plasmid determined proteinaceous antigen designated K99[39, 49, 58]. The role of the various antigens in promoting colonization of the intestine can be analysed by implanting plasmids into non-pathogenic strains of *E. coli* or alternatively, by removal of these plasmids from pathogenic strains and subsequently feeding such modified strains to the neonate[56, 57, 58]. The intestine was divided into seven equal parts from stomach to colon and the numbers of adherent organisms from wall scrapings expressed in $\log_{10}$ per gram of tissue. The results of a typical experiment are illustrated in *Table 8.1*. It can be seen that addition of the 99 adhesin into a O−K−99− strain of *E. coli* results in enhanced colonization of the posterior portion of the small intestine. Addition of O antigen is without effect on

Table 8.1 Viability and distribution of *E. coli* 0149 in the digestive tract in piglets challenged with this organism from normal sows and sows vaccinated with K88 positive K88 negative vaccines*.

		Average number of viable E. coli *0149(×10⁸)***						
Group	*Vaccine given to dam*	*Stomach*	*Small intestine Contents*	*Small intestine Tissue*	*Large intestine*	*Faeces*	*Total*	*Change in counts in 48h(%)****
1	None (4 litters)	7.1	55.4	303.9	41.9	69.6	477.7	+377.7
2	K88-negative (6 litters)	6.0	11.5	91.8	27.6	11.9	148.8	+48.8
3	K88-enriched (6 litters)	2.6	6.5	0.6	17.1	0.01	26.8	−73.2

* Nursing piglets were exposed to 1×10^{10} *E. coli* strain 0149 orogastrically between 12 and 24 hours post-partum.
** Four hours after exposure one to three piglets per litter were sacrificed and the numbers of the challenge organism in various parts of the gastrointestinal tract and in the faeces were counted.
*** Change in counts were calculated by subtracting dose of challenge organism (1×10^{10}) from average total numbers of viable *E. coli* 0149. The difference was expressed as the per cent increase (+) or decrease (−) from the challenge dose.

colonization. Similarly the addition of the K30 polysaccharide antigen (O+K+99−) results in significant colonization of the small intestine but when this is combined with the K99 antigen (K+99+) then the resulting colonization is more effective than either alone. Addition of the 88 adhesion (K+99+88+) results in colonization of the anterior as well as the posterior portions of the piglet intestine. More recently it has been demonstrated that some 88 and 99 negative piglet enteropathogenic strains produce specific pili called 987P which permit them to adhere to the posterior small intestine[24, 42, 44].

The K88 antigen is a fibrous capsule surrounding the cells of the organism and the importance of this antigen and the role of adhesion in disease caused by enteropathogenic *E. coli* in piglets is shown clearly in *Table 8.1*. This table shows the number of organisms present in the small intestinal contents and on the tissues in piglets from normal sows and sows vaccinated with one of two vaccines, one K88 positive and one K88 negative. The latter vaccine contains only ‘O’ antigens and stimulates the production of ‘O’ or bactericidal antibodies, whereas the K88 positive vaccine stimulates the production of both ‘O’ and K88 antibodies. In these experiments piglets were infected with 10^{10} organisms of *E. coli* strain 0149, 12–18

Table 8.2 The concentration of organisms in different parts of the alimentary tract of a piglet given orally a mixture of forms of an 09ßK30,99 calf enteropathogenic strain possessing different combination of O, K, 88 and 99 antigens (Modified from Smith and Huggins[56])

	*Number of organisms of stated form (log_{10} per g) in wall scrapings of small intestine, part**					
Forms of strain in mixture	*Stomach contents*	*1*	*3*	*5*	*7*	*Colon contents*
O−K−99−	<2.0	2.0	2.0	5.7	3.3	3.6
O−K−99+	4.0	5.2	5.7	7.4	7.3	7.7
O+K−99−	<2.0	2.8	3.0	6.4	4.2	4.6
O+K−99+	7.2	5.5	5.9	7.3	7.9	6.6
O+K+99−	6.3	5.2	4.6	8.9	8.3	7.9
O+K+99+	6.6	6.2	6.2	9.9	9.9	9.9
O+K+99+88+	7.5	9.4	9.6	9.8	9.9	9.9

* The small intestine was divided into seven equal parts for counting; part 1 was nearest to the stomach and part 7 to the colon.

hours after birth. Four hours later the pigs were sacrificed and counts made of the numbers of the challenge organism in various parts of the gastrointestinal tract and in the faeces. Counts on the tissues were made after the tissue had been thoroughly washed with saline to remove non-adherent organisms.

The large reduction in the numbers of organisms adherent to the small intestine in piglets from gilts vaccinated with a K88 containing vaccine shows the importance of the anti-adhesion in affording protection against the disease[42]. Further data on the length of protection obtained with this vaccine are shown in *Figure 8.2*. In these experiments piglets from gilts vaccinated with the K88 containing vaccine were

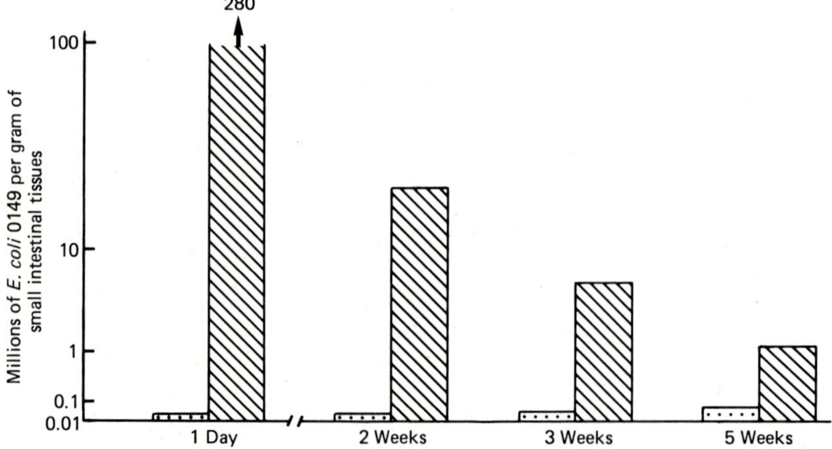

Figure 8.2 Extent of adhesion of *E. coli* 0149 to the small intestine of nursing and weaned piglets of various ages of K88 immunized sows. Each piglet received orally 10 000 million *E. coli* 0149 and was sacrificed 4 hours later. Each bar represents an average count of 10 piglets. (dotted bar) Nursing; (hatched bar) weaned

divided into two, one half being left on the dam and the other half weaned on to boiled milk. At the intervals shown in the figure, piglets were challenged with the enteropathogenic *E. coli* strain 0149, sacrificed at 4 hours and counts made on the numbers of organisms adhering to the small intestine. These histograms show the differences in count in the numbers of organisms adhering in the two groups.

It can be seen that throughout the whole of the nursing period there is a significant difference in the numbers of organisms adhering from vaccinated and unvaccinated litters. The protective effect of antibodies present in the milk of vaccinated gilts is lost when the piglets are weaned on to boiled milk. Furthermore, it can be seen that as the piglets increase in age progressively smaller numbers of K88 producing *E. coli* adhere to the small intestine although even at 6 weeks there is significant difference between the two groups[59].

A second species of organism to which the small intestine of large animal neonates is susceptible are clostridial species. For example, young piglets are susceptible to a profound haemorrhagic necrotic enteritis of the jejunum following infection with *Cl. perfringens* type C[3, 14, 22, 37, 38]. Again attachment of the organisms to the intestinal villi is an important first step[1] and following adhesion, proliferation and the elaboration of a necrotic toxin, β-toxin leads to extensive necrosis of the villi[59] (*Figure 8.3*).

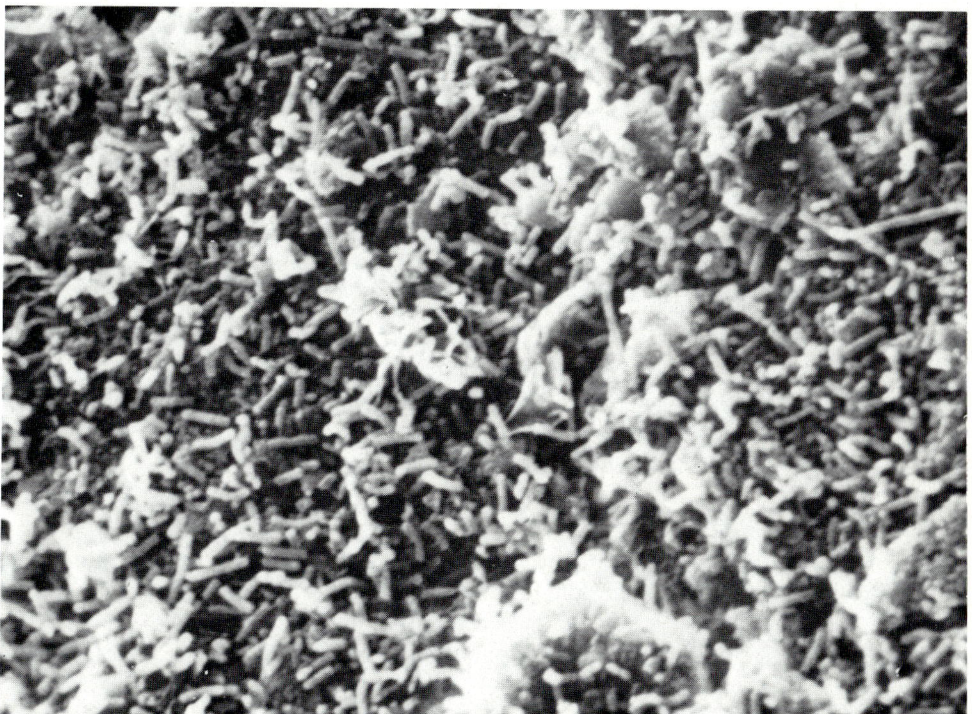

Figure 8.3 Scanning electron micrograph of the piglet jejunum following infection with *Cl. perfringens* type C. Note complete disintegration of the villous surface. (×1600)

Piglets are usually affected during the first week of life, blood is usually present in the faeces and most affected pigs die within 24–48 hours after the onset of the bloody diarrhoea. The essential pathogenesis of the infection is necrosis of the small intestine particularly severe in the upper jejunum, the lower half being affected with varying degrees of severity. Occasionally the ileum, caecum and colon may also be involved. After the initial necrotizing inflammation necrosis progresses through the mucosal crypts and sub-mucosa and extensive necrosis of the mucosa and muscularis mucosae occurs. The sub-mucosa is described as thickened oedematous and occasionally also emphysematous. In both naturally and experimentally infected animals the tissue is infiltrated and surrounded by masses of Gram positive bacteria forming a lining to the intestine.

These two examples have been treated in some detail as they illustrate certain principles and have clear parallels in the human situation. In the case of both these organisms attachment is a prerequisite for colonization of the intestine. If attachment is interfered with colonization does not occur. Not only can attachment be interfered with by specific antibody but also as the age of the piglet increases less and less K88 positive organisms attach to the intestine. Clearly physiological changes occur in receptor sites to which the K88 antigen can no longer attach. Possession of the K88 antigen no longer confers a selective colonization advantage. Furthermore, the secondary symptoms of infection depend on the nature of the toxins elaborated. In the case of autochthonous species the first stage of attachment is observed but colonization does not result in secondary symptoms and thus the basis for a stable relationship occurs. Changes in population may follow physiological changes in the intestine involving receptor sites.

Young babies are susceptible to disease caused by *E. coli* and specific protein adhesive antigens, 'P' antigens have been described[26]. Furthermore, infection with clostridia has been described in young children, particularly following artificial feeding and in cases involving congenital heart defects[23]. In the case of congenital heart defects it is clear that circulatory problems are experienced resulting in the creation of anaerobic conditions which favour the growth of any clostridia present. Artificial feeding may well cause interference with the important initial establishment of bifidobacteria due to the presence of lactoferrin and because of the lack of maternal antibodies which would be protective.

THE ADULT INTESTINE

Under normal conditions experimental infection in the adult animal presents considerable problems. Unlike the neonate which can be infected orally during the first few days of life before the development of stomach acidity, the adult intestine is protected both by stomach acidity and an indigenous microbiological flora. Enteric infections in adult animals can only be induced following the neutralization of stomach acidity and interference with the normal washing action of the intestine by substances such as opium and belladonna[4].

However, enteric infections of the small intestine do occur in the adult animal and this usually occurs following changes in feeding pattern. For example, adult sheep turned out to graze in the spring consume large quantities of grass from lush pasture. Intestinal stasis results from distension produced by the consumption of large quantities of food and gas formed due to fermentation of the high carbohydrate levels following change of diet. These conditions allow the proliferation of clostridial organisms present in the intestine leading to colonization and proliferation in the small bowel[8]. Symptoms of infection are caused by the β- and ε-toxins elaborated by the organisms.

Enterotoxaemias due to clostridial species are relatively uncommon in humans. However, when similar feeding patterns to those undertaken by animals are perceived then similar problems arise.

Pig-bel is a necrotizing enteritis of the jejunum in young adults in Papua New Guinea[40,41]. *Clostridium perfringens* type C is widely distributed in the environment and is present in the intestine in normal individuals[32]. Under these conditions it is autochthonous to the intestinal system. The changes that lead to its role as an allochthonous organism are complex and involve several different factors[30,31].

The staple diet of the population is primarily sweet potato and only rarely is meat eaten. Meat is consumed on various ceremonial occasions such as weddings, births, and other epochal events and following these a proportion of the young adult population experience the disease with varying symptoms. Due to malnutrition the population exhibits varying degrees of protein starvation resulting in low levels of pancreatic enzymes. Furthermore, sweet potato contains trypsin inhibitors as do various round worms with which infestation is common. Following consumption of

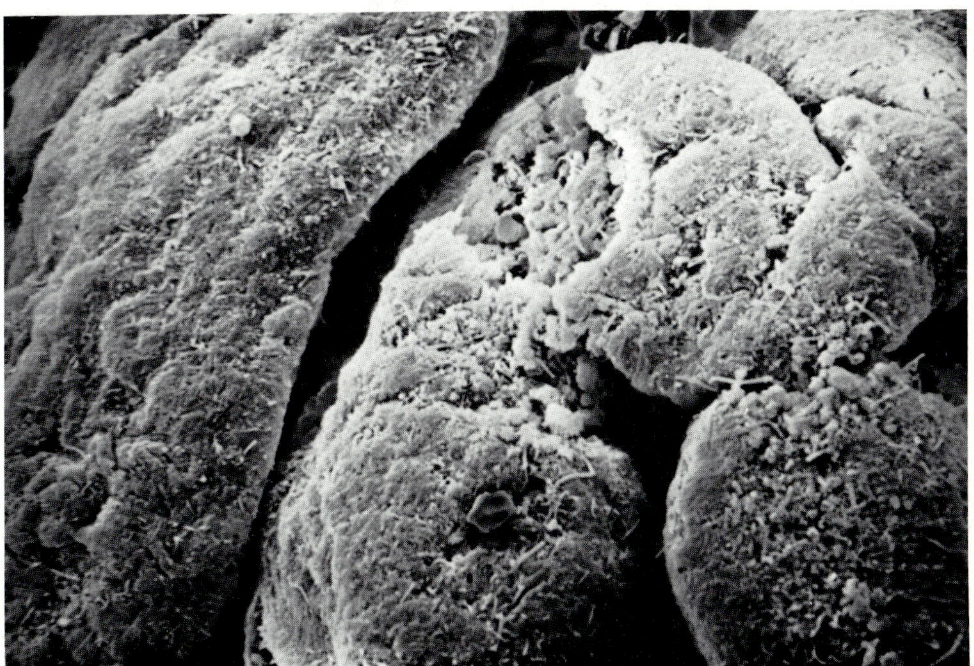

Figure 8.4 **Scanning electron micrograph of the jejunum from a case of pig-bel in a young adult.** Note necrosis of the villous surface. (×600)

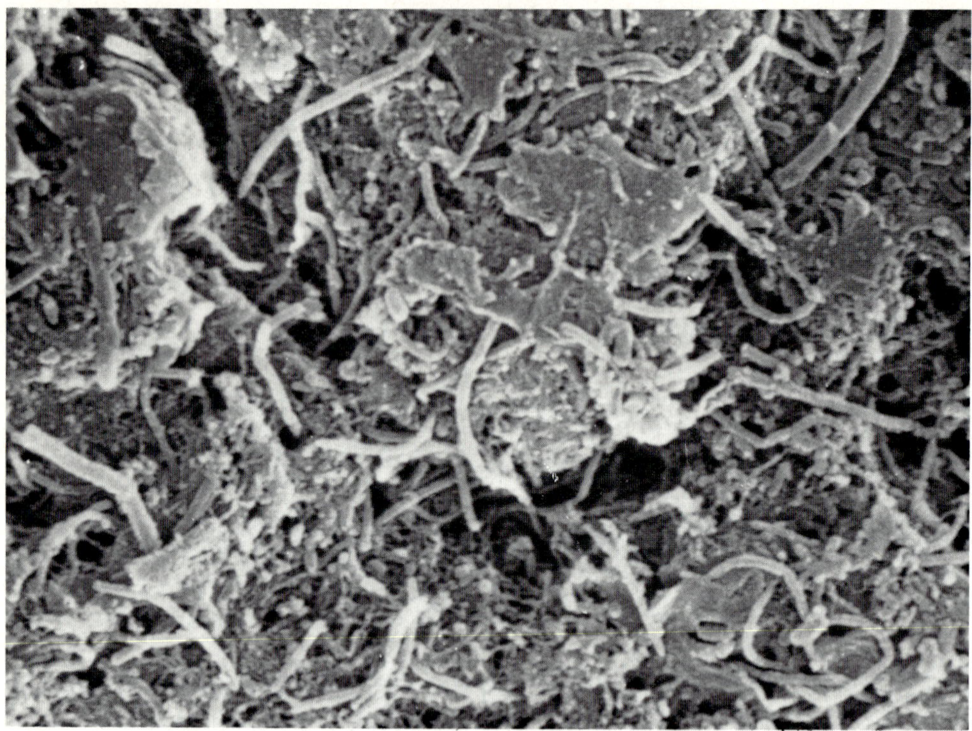

Figure 8.5 Scanning electron micrograph of the jejunum from a case of pig-bel in a young adult. Note necrosis of villous and adherent organisms. (×3125)

a meat meal *Cl. perfringens* type C organisms either introduced with the meat or present as part of the normal flora multiply in the new environment created by the consumption of meat producing β-toxin. The low levels of pancreatic enzymes, together with the trypsin inhibitors present, are unable to destroy the toxin. One of the actions of β-toxin is to paralyse villi and the normal motility of the intestine is interfered with[50]. Under such conditions stasis and colonization of the intestinal villi can occur with similar effects to those seen in the young neonatal piglets[60] (*Figures 8.4 and 8.5*).

A rather different case of interaction between microbe and host is demonstrated by *Cl. perfringens* food poisoning. In cases of *Cl. perfringens* food poisoning heat resistant spores ingested in contaminated food germinate in the intestine followed by phases of growth and sporulation[9, 21]. During sporulation a sporulation associated product, the enterotoxin, is produced in the cytoplasm of the cells and this is released during lysis of the cell[9, 10, 11, 12, 18, 28, 48, 52]. Unlike the enterotoxin of *V. cholerae* the enterotoxin of *Cl. perfringens* causes some damage to the epithelium at the tip of the ileal villi in rabbits. In addition, cyclic AMP has not been found to be involved in the clostridial model and the biochemical changes suggest a general pattern of cell degeneration and metabolic inhibition[34, 35]. Presumably the initial germination of spores occurs in the lumen followed by attachment of the organisms and production of toxins.

POSSIBLE CONTROLLING MECHANISMS

There is some evidence for the control of the normal microbial population by antibodies produced in response to organisms grown in the intestine. This subject is thoroughly reviewed by Savage[54] and in this section attention will be focused on more recent developments of the importance of cellular immunity as a possible mechanism of controlling populations.

Rather more light on possible controlling mechanisms has been found from studies on Thiry-Vella loops in pigs[4,5]. Thiry-Vella loops have been prepared from the duodenum by sectioning the gut at two places, the first approximately 90 cm and again at 12 cm posterior to the pylorus. The section of gut between the two cuts, having an intact blood supply, can be converted into a Thiry-Vella loop by bringing out the ends of the gut via stab wounds through the flank and stitching them to the skin, thus allowing ready access to the lumen of the loop. The continuity of the intestine can then be re-established. Closing of the loop is achieved by the use of Foley catheters. There is considerable evidence that for the period of experimentation the loops can be regarded as representative of the small intestine[27] although clearly there are differences, notably the lack of continuity with the small intestine.

It has been shown that following the introduction of *E. coli* serotype 0149 into the loop, elimination of the organism takes place over a period of 24 hours[5,6] (*Table 8.3*). On first exposure no drop in viable count was observed during the first 4–8 hours after incubation. However, after this period elimination of *E. coli* occurred in all loops and by 24 hours there was a 75–85 per cent decrease in recovery of viable *E. coli* from the loop[5,6]. If the loop was frequently stimulated in this way the rate of elimination of *E. coli* organisms was considerably increased up to a period of five exposures. By 24 hours the viability of the challenge organism had dropped by a factor of 10^3. This elimination pattern was evident whether the results were presented as numbers of colony-forming units of *E. coli*/ml of loop secretion or as total numbers of the challenge organism in the loop secretion.

Table 8.3 Elimination of *E. coli* 0149 from Thiry-Vella loops following repeated stimulation. (Reproduced by courtesy of Dr Bhogal[5])

Pig no.	*Exposure no.*	*Inoculum* E. coli *0149* $\times 10^6$ *per ml*	*Viable* E. coli *0149 (*$\times 10^6$ *per ml) recovered from the loop* *Hours following exposure* 1	2	4	6	8	12	24
	1	2.6	3.8	2.3	2.9	0.79	0.67	0.78	0.56
	2(10)	2.8	0.76	0.74	0.68	0.67	0.54	0.40	0.51
	3(3)	2.7	0.40	0.38	0.071	0.039	0.04	0.026	0.007
1	4(6)	3.1	0.58	0.42	0.084	0.050	0.031	0.020	0.006
	5(2)	3.1	0.64	0.57	0.063	0.029	0.0078	0.0061	0.00052
	6(2)	2.4	0.36	0.20	0.021	0.018	0.0038	0.0029	0.0004
	7(4)	2.6	0.49	0.38	0.041	0.031	0.0027	0.0021	0.0002
	8(1)	3.0	0.59	0.41	0.037	0.038	0.0019	0.0010	0.0002
	9(1)	2.9	0.26	0.24	0.043	0.0079	0.0040	0.0020	0.0001

Figures in parentheses indicate the interval (days) between two consecutive exposures of the loop to *E. coli* 0149.

Thereafter the rate of elimination remained constant. When repeatedly challenged loops were rested for varying periods of time and re-exposed to the same challenge organism the elimination pattern of the loops changed (*Table 8.4*). The rate of elimination did not alter appreciably up to 1½ months of resting. However, after 3 or 4 months the rate of elimination of *E. coli* decreased substantially and by 5–7 months the loops exhibited the same elimination pattern as a virgin loop and the process has to be repeated in order to stimulate effective elimination. Furthermore, if during the period of maximum elimination of a particular serotype from the loop, the loop is challenged with a non-related serotype, then the rate of elimination of the new serotype is that of a virgin loop (*Table 8.5*). The loop failed to eliminate either a calf or human strain of *E. coli* which had been introduced. There is, thus, considerable specificity in the mechanisms involved in elimination of various serotypes of *E. coli*.

Further light on the mechanisms involved are highlighted by studying the pattern of cellular infiltration into the loops following varying periods of stimulation and analysing the basic protein and lactoferrin content of the secretions[5,6]. Pre-exposure loop fluid had very few intact leucocytes and of these the overwhelming majority were mononuclear cells. Viability of the cellular population, as judged by staining with toluidine blue, was less than 30 per cent. In a maximum eliminating loop following stimulation considerable numbers of polymorphonuclear leucocytes (neutrophils) appeared in the loop secretions as early as 15 min after stimulation. The viability of the leucocytes in these samples was more than 80 per cent and contained large numbers of bacteria in varying stages of degradation. The vacuoles contained in addition to phagocytoed bacteria small particles resembling secondary or specific granules of neutrophils (*Figure 8.6*). Many dense primary granules were seen in the cytoplasm but few secondary granules. Some of the phagocytic granules were not closed and the contents of the vacuoles could be seen escaping (*Figure*

Table 8.4 Elimination of *E. coli* 0149 from maximally stimulated Thiry-Vella loops rested for varying intervals of time. (Reproduced by courtesy of Dr. Bhogal[5])

Pig no.	*Interval between two consecutive exposures of the loop to* E. coli *0149*	*Viable counts* of* E. coli *0149 per ml recovered from the loop — Hours following exposure*							
		0	*1*	*2*	*4*	*6*	*8*	*12*	*24*
	–	3.3	0.40	0.39	0.028	0.0076	0.0034	0.001	0.00023
1	1 month	2.3	0.21	0.26	0.014	0.0048	0.0021	ND	0.00020
	3 months	2.5	4.5	4.5	0.67	0.62	ND	ND	0.087
	5 months	3.5	4.6	3.9	0.91	0.87	ND	ND	0.76
	–	2.9	0.26	0.24	0.043	0.0079	0.0040	0.0020	0.0001
2	1½ months	3.8	0.56	0.42	0.087	0.0047	ND	ND	0.00072
	3 months	2.8	3.2	2.9	0.89	0.87	0.68	ND	0.064
	7 months	3.0	4.1	4.9	3.9	2.9	0.97	ND	0.91

* All counts are given as $\times 10^6$ colony forming units per ml.

Table 8.5 Elimination of different strains of *E. coli* from porcine duodenal Thiry-Vella loops immunized with *E. coli* 0149. (Reproduced by courtesy of Dr. Bhogal[5])

Pig no.	*Strain of* E. coli	*Viable* E. coli *recovered* ($\times 10^6$ *per ml) from the loop* *Hours following exposure*					
		0	*1*	*2*	*4*	*6*	*24*
	0149	2.7	0.64	0.26	0.074	0.0046	0.00032
1	3206*(2)	4.9	6.4	4.6	3.8	3.5	0.65
	0149(2)	3.0	0.49	0.39	0.067	0.0052	0.00029
	0149	1.8	0.40	0.34	0.071	0.0048	0.00030
2	026†(2)	2.5	2.9	3.0	2.8	2.4	0.80
	0149(2)	2.7	0.39	0.27	0.058	0.0060	0.00012

* 3206 *E. coli* isolated from calf diarrhoea.
† 026 *E. coli* isolated from human diarrhoea.
Figures in parentheses indicate the interval (days) between the two consecutive exposures of the loop to *E. coli* serotypes

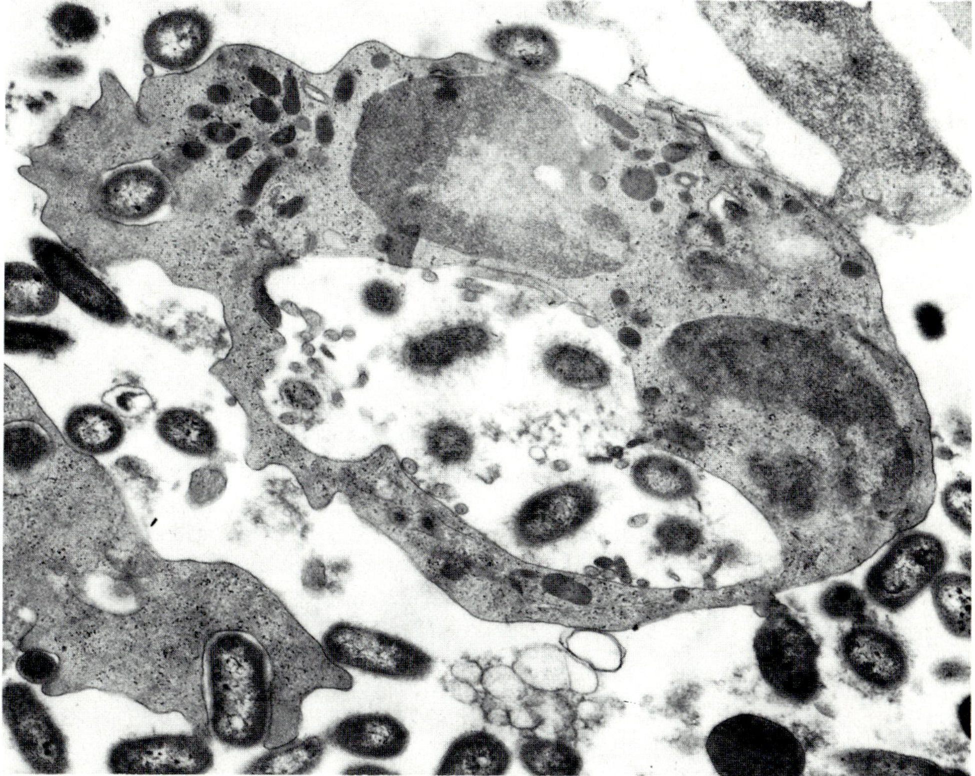

Figure 8.6 Ultrathin section of loop fluid collected 15 minutes after exposure showing a neutrophil with phagocytosed bacteria undergoing lysis. Note dense intact primary granules in the cytoplasm and smaller secondary granules in the vacuoles. (× 19 800)

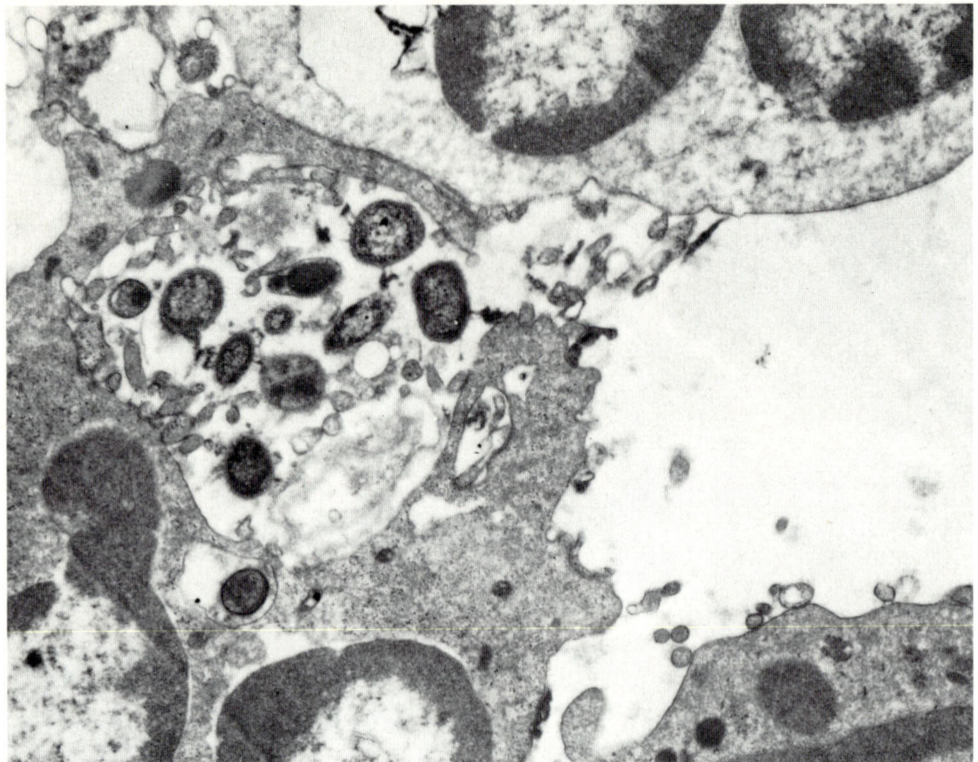

Figure 8.7 Ultrathin section of loop fluid collected 15 minutes after exposure showing an incompletely closed phagocytic vacuole with contents escaping. (×18 225)

8.7). Bacteria were also seen lysing in close proximity to the incompletely closed phagocytic vacuoles. Samples taken at further intervals up to 4 hours revealed a similar picture with further infiltrations of leucocytes, phagocytosed, disintegrating bacteria and an accumulation of debris. After 6 hours the picture changed into one of fewer leucocytic cells with decreased viability (40–50 per cent) and accumulation of cellular debris and cytoplasmic granules. Disintegrating bacteria were seen in close proximity to the granules which may have been released due to disruption of neutrophils (*Figure 8.8*). By 24 hours the appearance of the loop was similar to that of the pre-exposure samples.

Addition of iron (0.015 per cent ferric iron/ml) to the loop at the time of challenge significantly reduced the rate of elimination. The presence of iron did not affect phagocytosis or degranulation but the bacteria in the phagocytic granules appeared to be intact (*Figures 8.9 and 8.10*).

At the time of exposure very little lactoferrin was present in loop secretions but this increased appreciably after stimulation and by 6 hours increased 50–100 fold.

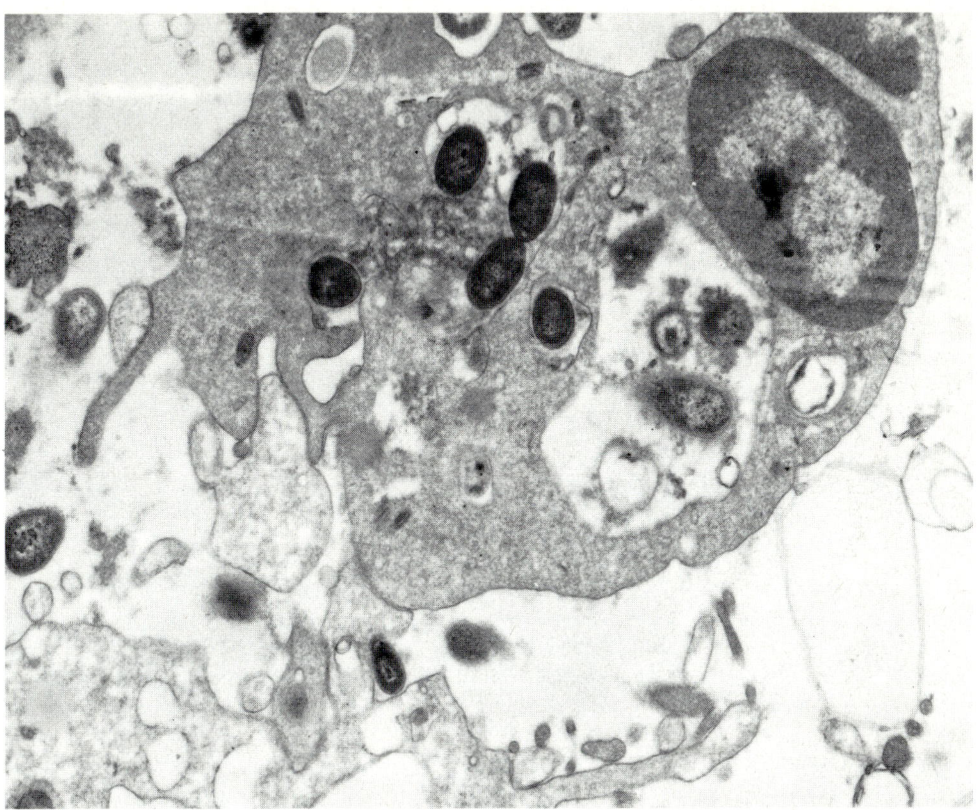

Figure 8.8 Ultrathin section of loop fluid collected 4 hours after exposure. Phagocytic cells with bacteria in their vacuoles are in various stages of disintegration and lysed bacteria and some granular-like contents can be seen outside the cells. (Reproduced by courtesy of Dr Bhogal[5]) (× 18 225)

Thereafter, the concentration of lactoferrin decreased. There was also a significant increase in the basic amino acid content of the secretions at 1 and 6 hours exposure but no change in the neutral or acid amino acid content.

These studies appear to show that there exists in the loop a specific immunological stimulation of polymorphs causing them to enter the loop and phagocytose invading bacteria. These organisms are killed by products released from the secondary granules and, in addition, granules are discharged extracellularly where they can also kill invading bacteria. It has been reported that disrupted granulocytes are as rapidly bactericidal for *E. coli* as intact granulocytes[13]. The fact that some of these effects can be reversed by the presence of additional iron suggests the role of secondary granules and particularly lactoferrin in this mechanism. The possibility that such mechanisms may operate in the intact small intestine leading to elimination of pathogens and possibly as a general control mechanism should be considered.

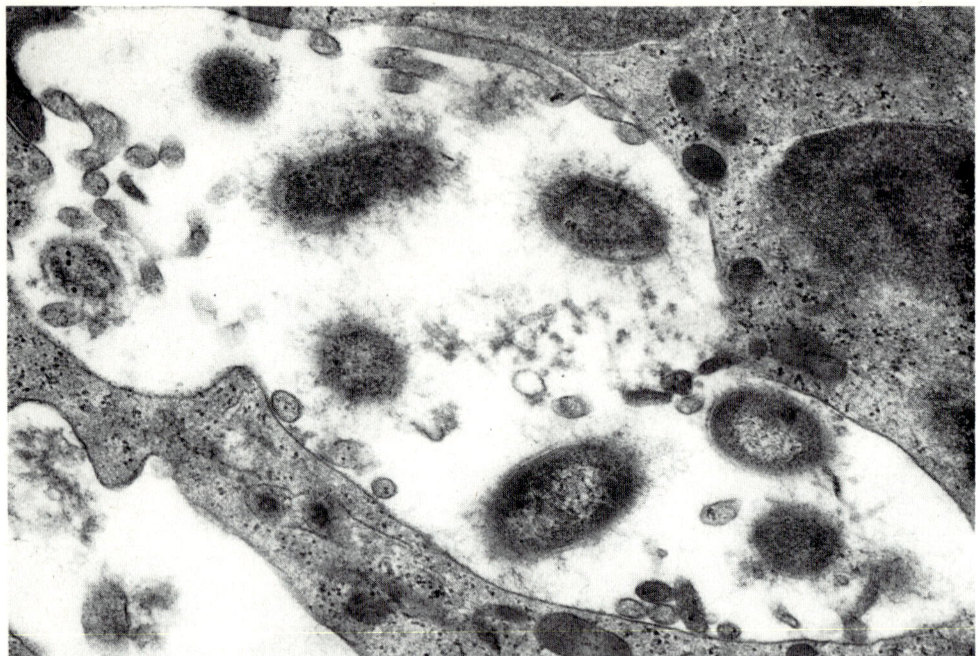

Figure 8.9 Ultrathin section of loop fluid without iron treatment 15 minutes after exposure showing a phagocytic vacuole containing bacteria in various stages of distintegration. (Reproduced by courtesy of Dr Bhogal[5]) (× 30 442)

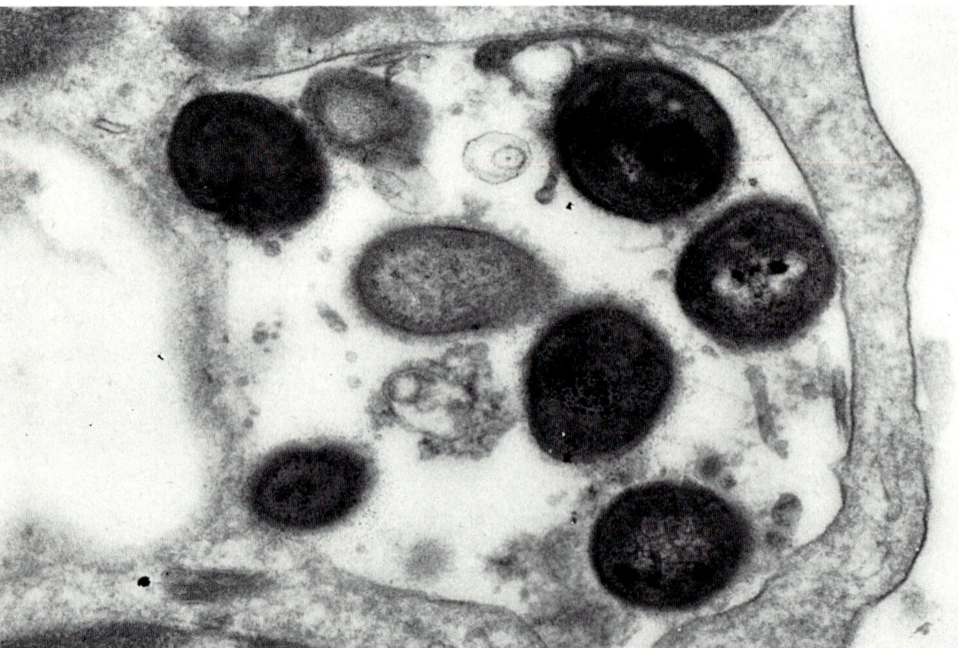

Figure 8.10 Ultrathin section of loop fluid from a loop treated with iron collected 15 minutes after exposure. Most of the bacteria in the phagocytic vacuole are seen intact. (Reproduced by courtesy of Dr Bhogal[5]) (× 47 512)

GENERAL DISCUSSION

The importance of attachment as a first stage in colonization is shown by the work on *E. coli*. Specific attachment mechanisms have been developed by the organisms. However, as has been discussed the possession of specific adhesive antigens may only provide a selective advantage for a limited period. Certainly there is evidence in mice, reviewed by Savage[54], for the colonization of the small intestine by segmented, filamentous bacteria that can attach end-on to the special membranes of epithelial cells in their habitat beginning in the upper third of the small intestine. In the case of pathogenic bacteria, secondary symptoms are caused by toxins elaborated from the cell. The increased release of fluid due to enterotoxin production is probably a factor in limiting infections of this type due to flushing out of the organisms. On the other hand, it is clear that in addition to antibody specific immune mechanisms involving leucocytes may be involved. There is strong evidence to suggest the importance of phagocytic cells in the antibacterial defence mechanisms of the lung as well as the bovine mammary gland[47] and the importance of such cells in the gastrointestinal tract should be considered. Following recovery from cholera, patients have been shown to be refractory to challenge with the organism. Whilst this may be the result of production of antibodies interfering with adhesion which has been shown to be an important factor[16, 17, 29, 46, 55] in infection, it could equally result from killing due to a sensitized leucocytic system as involved in Thiry-Vella loops. In endemic areas continuous stimulation of sensitized individuals could be provided from organisms present in the environment. Although some studies have indicated poor functional capabilities of neutrophils on mucosal surfaces[53], these *in vitro* studies may not be comparable to the *in vivo* situation where a continual replenishment of healthy neutrophils occurs in the presence of antigen. The observations on the presence of structures similar to secondary granules in the phagocytic vacuoles and the observation that in some cases the latter were incompletely closed and the contents extruding are consistent with *in vitro* studies[33] which showed that during phagocytosis the secondary granules are discharged first into the phagocytic vacuoles followed by the primary granules and that more than 85 per cent of the lactoferrin content of the secondary granules was released extracellularly.

While the increase of lactoferrin and basic amino acid in the loop secretion is not itself proof that these substances participate in the bactericidal section observed in the loop, *in vitro* studies indicate that lactoferrin in human[7] and porcine[45] colostrum and milk could inhibit growth of *E. coli* involved in neonatal diarrhoea and addition of iron reversed the inhibition. Gladstone and Walton[19] showed that the *in vitro* antibacterial effect of neutrophils was due to cationic proteins and addition of iron abolished the antibacterial effect.

It is clear that a specific immunological mechanism such as described above could not only eliminate pathogens but could, if it was stimulated when the numbers of an individual organism in a population reached threshold levels, regulate its numbers.

Acknowledgements

I should like to thank Dr. B. S. Bhogal for his kindness in allowing me to quote from his Thesis and to reproduce *Figures 8.8–8.10*.

References

1 ARBUCKLE, J. B. R. The attachment of *Clostridium welchii* (*Cl. perfringens*) type C to intestinal villi of pigs. *Journal of Pathology*, **106,** 65–72 (1972)

2 ALEXANDER, M. In *Microbial Ecology*. New York, John Wiley & Sons (1971)

3 BERGELAND, M. E. Pathogenesis and immunity of *Clostridium perfringens* type C enteritis in swine. *Journal of the American Veterinary Medical Association*, **160,** 568–571 (1972)

4 BENNETTS, H. W. Infectious enterotoxaemia of sheep in Western Australia. *Bulletin of the Council for Scientific Industrial Research (Australia),* **57** (1932)

5 BHOGAL, B. S. A study of some of the immunological mechanisms involved in the protection of the gastrointestinal tract of the pig against *Escherichia coli* infection. *Doctor of Philosophy Thesis*, National Council for Academic Awards (1978)

6 BHOGAL, B. S., NAGY, L. K. and WALKER, P. D. (unpublished observations)

7 BULLEN, J., ROGERS, H. J. and LEIGH, L. Iron bonding proteins in milk and resistance to *Escherichia coli* infection in infants. *British Medical Journal*, **1,** 69–75 (1972)

8 BULLEN, J. J. and SCARISBRICK, R. Enterotoxaemia of sheep: experimental reproduction of diseases. *Journal of Pathology and Bacteriology*, **73,** 495–509 (1957)

9 DUNCAN, C. L. Time of enterotoxin formation and release during sporulation of *Clostridium perfringens* type A. *Journal of Bacteriology*, **113,** 932–936 (1973)

10 DUNCAN, C. L., KING, G. J. and FRIEBEN, W. R. A paracrystalline inclusion formed during sporulation of enterotoxin producing strains of *Clostridium perfringens* type A. *Journal of Bacteriology*, **114,** 845–859 (1973)

11 DUNCAN, C. L. and STRONG, D. H. Sporulation and enterotoxin production by mutants of *Clostridium perfringens. Journal of Bacteriology*, **110,** 378–391 (1972)

12 DUNCAN, C. L., SUGIYAMA, J. and STRONG, D. H. Rabbit ileal loop response to strains of *Clostridium perfringens. Journal of Bacteriology*, **95,** 1560–1566 (1968)

13 ELSBACH, P., BECKERDITE, S., PETTIS, P. and FRANSON, R. Persistence of regulation of macromolecular synthesis by *Escherichia coli* during killing by disrupted rabbit granulocytes. *Infection and Immunity*, **9,** 663–668 (1974)

14 FIELD, H. I. and GIBSON, E. A. Studies on piglet mortality. II. *Clostridium welchii* infection. *Veterinary Record*, **67,** 31–35 (1955)

15 FLOCK, M. H., GERSHENGOREN, W. and FREEDMAN, L. R. Methods for the quantitative study of the aerobic and anaerobic intestinal bacterial flora of man. *Yale Journal of Biological Medicine*, **41,** 50–61 (1968)

16 FRETER, R. Studies on the mechanism of action of intestinal antibody in experimental cholera. *Texas Reports on Biology and Medicine*, **27,** 299–316 (1969)

17 FRETER, R., SMITH, H. L. and SWEENEY, F. J. Jr. An evaluation of intestinal fluids in the pathogenesis of cholera. *Journal of Infectious Diseases*, **109,** 35–42 (1961)

18 FRIEBEN, W. R. and DUNCAN, C. L. Heterogeneity of enterotoxin-like protein extracted from spores of *Clostridium perfringens* type A. *European Journal of Biochemistry*, **55,** 455–463 (1975)

19 GLADSTONE, G. P. and WALTON, E. The effect of iron and haematin on the killing of staphylococci by rabbit polymorphs. *British Journal of Experimental Pathology*, **52,** 452–464 (1971)

20 GORBACH, S. L. Intestinal flora. *Progress in Gastroenterology*, **60,** 1110–1129 (1971)

21 HAUSCHILD, A. H. W. and HILSHEIMER, R. Purification and characteristics of the enterotoxin of *Clostridium perfringens* type A. *Canadian Journal of Microbiology*, **17,** 1425–1433 (1971)

22 HOGH, P. Porcine infectious necrotising enteritis caused by *Clostridium perfringens. PhD. Dissertation*, Royal Veterinary Agricultural University, Copenhagen (1974)

23 HOWARD, F. M., FLYNN, D. M., BRADLEY, J. M., NOONE, P. and SZAWATKOWSKI, M. Outbreak of necrotising enterocolitis caused by *Clostridium butyricum. Lancet*, **2,** 1099–1102 (1977)

24 ISAACSON, R. E., NAGY, B. and MOON, H. W. Colonisation of porcine small intestine by *Escherichia coli*: colonisation and adhesion of piglet enteropathogens that lack K88. *Journal of Infectious Diseases*, **135,** 531–538 (1977)

25 JONES, G. W. and RUTTER, J. M. Role of the K88 antigen in the pathogenesis of neonatal diarrhoea caused by *Escherichia coli* in piglets. *Infection and Immunity*, **6,** 918–927 (1972)

26 KALLENIUS, G., SVENSON, S. B., HULTBERG, H., MOLBY, R., HELIN, I., CEDERGREN, B. and WINBERG, J. Occurrence of 'P' fimbriated *Escherichia coli* in urinary tract infections. *Lancet*, **2,** 1369–1372 (1981)

27 KEREN, D. F., ELLIOT, H. L., BROWN, G. D. and YARDLEY, J. G. Atrophy of villi with hypertrophy and hyperphasia of Paneth cells in isolated (Thiry-Vella) ileal loops in rabbits. *Gastroenterology*, **68,** 83–93 (1975)

28 LABBE, R. G. and DUNCAN, C. L. Sporecoat protein and enterotoxin synthesis in *Clostridium perfringens. Journal of Bacteriology*, **131,** 713–715 (1977)

29 LABREC, C. H., SPRINZ, H., SCHNEIDER, H. and FORMAL, S. R. Localisation of vibrios in experimental cholera: a fluorescent antibody study in guinea pigs. In *Proceedings of the Cholera Research Symposium* (Honolulu, Hawaii) US Public Health Service, Publication No. **1328,** 262–276. Washington DC., US Government Printing Office (1965)

30 LAWRENCE, G. and COOKE, R. Experimental pig-bel: the production and pathology of necrotising enteritis due to *Clostridium welchii* type C in the guinea pig. *British Journal of Experimental Pathology*, **61,** 261–271 (1981)

31 LAWRENCE, G. and WALKER, P. D. Pathogenesis of enteritis necroticans in Papua New Guinea. *Lancet*, **1,** 125 (1976)

32 LAWRENCE, G., WALKER, P. D., GARAP, J. and AVUSI, M. The occurrence of *Clostridium welchii* type C in Papua New Guinea. *Papua New Guinea Medical Journal*, **22,** 69–73 (1979)

33 LEFFELL, M. S. and SPIZNAGEL, J. K. Intracellular extracellular degranulation of human polymorphonuclear azurophil and specific granules induced by immune complexes. *Infection and Immunity*, **10,** 1241–1249 (1974)

34 McDONEL, J. L. and DUNCAN, C. L. Effects of *Clostridium perfringens* enterotoxin on metabolic indexes of everted rat ileal sacs. *Infection and Immunity*, **12,** 274–280 (1975a)

35 McDONEL, J. L. and DUNCAN, C. L. Histopathological effect of *Clostridium perfringens* enterotoxin in the rabbit ileum. *Infection and Immunity*, **12,** 1214–1218 (1975b)

36 MCDONEL, J. L. and DUNCAN, C. L. Effect of *Clostridium perfringens* enterotoxin on mitochondrial respiration. *Infection and Immunity*, **15,** 999–1001 (1977)

37 MOON, H. W. and BERGELAND, M. E. *Clostridium perfringens* type C enterotoxaemia of the newborn pig. *Canadian Veterinary Journal*, **6,** 159–161 (1965)

38 MOON, H. W. and DILLMAN, R. C. Comments on clostridia and enteric disease in swine. *Journal of the American Veterinary Medical Association*, **160,** 572–583 (1972)

39 MOON, H. W., NAGY, B., ISAACSON, R. E. and ORSKOV, I. Occurrence of K99 antigen on *Escherichia coli* isolated from pigs and colonisation of pig ileum by K99+ enterotoxigenic *E. coli* from calves and pigs. *Infection and Immunity*, **15,** 614–620 (1977)

40 MURRELL, T. G. C., EGERTON, J. R., RAMPLING, A., SAMELS, J. and WALKER, P. D. The ecology and epidemiology of the pig-bel syndrome in man in New Guinea. *Journal of Hygiene* (*Cambridge*), **64,** 375–396 (1966)

41 MURRELL, T. G. C., EGERTON, J. R., ROTH, L., SAMELS, J. and WALKER, P. D. Pig-bel enteritis necroticans: A study in diagnosis and management. *Lancet*, **1,** 217–222 (1966)

42 NAGY, L. K., BHOGAL, B. S., WALKER, P. D. and MACKENZIE, T. Mode of action of *Escherichia coli* bacterins with or without K88 antigens in passive protection of piglets against experimental enteric colibacillosis. In *Proceedings of the Second International Symposium on Neonatal Diarrhoea*, edited by D. S. Acres, 414–426. Canada, Veterinary Infection Disease Association (1978)

43 NAGY, B., MOON, H. W. and ISAACSON, R. Colonisation of porcine small intestine by *Escherichia coli*: ileal colonisation and adhesion of pig enteropathogens that lack K88 antigen and by some acapsular mutants. *Infection and Immunity*, **13,** 1214–1220 (1976)

44 NAGY, B., MOON, H. W. and ISAACSON, R. W. Colonisation of porcine intestine by enterotoxigenic *Escherichia coli*: selection of piliated forms *in vivo* adhesion of piliated forms to epithelial cells *in vitro* and incidence of a pilus antigen among porcine enteropathogenic *E. coli. Infection and Immunity*, **16,** 344–352 (1977)

45 NAGY, L. K., PENN, C. W. and MacKENZIE, T. Studies of immunity of colienteritis in the pig. *Research in Veterinary Science*, **17,** 215–221 (1974)

46 NELSON, E. T., CLEMENTS, J. D. and FINKELSTEIN, R. A. *Vibrio cholerae* adherence and colonisation in experimental cholera: electron microscopic studies. *Infection and Immunity*, **14,** 527–547 (1976)

47 NEWBOULD, F. H. A. and NEAVE, F. K. The response of the bovine mammary gland to invasion of *Staphylococcus aureus. Journal of Dairy Research*, **32,** 163–167 (1965)

48 NILO, L. Enterotoxin formation by *Clostridium perfringens* type A studied by the use of fluorescent antibody. *Canadian Journal of Microbiology*, **23,** 908–915 (1977)

49 ORSKOV, I., ORSKOV, F., SMITH, H. W. and SOJKA, W. J. The establishment of K99 a thermolabile transmissible *Escherichia coli* K antigen previously called 'KCO' possessed by calf and lamb enteropathogenic strains. *Acta pathologica et Microbiologica Scandinavica*, Section B, **83,** 31–36 (1975)

50 PARNAS, J. The effects of *Clostridium perfringens* beta toxin (type C) on the motility of intestinal segments *in vitro*. (abstract) *Zentralblatt fur Bakteriologie, Parasitenkunde, Infektionskrankheiten und Hygiene*, **234,** 243–246 (1976)

51 PLAUT, A. G., SHERWOOD, L., GORBACH, M. D. Studies of intestinal microflora. III. The microbial flora of human small intestinal mucosa and fluids. *Gastroenterology*, **53,** 868–873 (1967)

52 RIEBEN, W. R. and DUNCAN, C. L. Homology between enterotoxin protein and spore structural protein in *Clostridium perfringens* type A. *European Journal of Biochemistry*, **39,** 393–401 (1973)

53 RUSSELL, M. W. and REITER, B. Phagocytic deficiency of bovine milk leucocytes: an effect of casein. *Journal of the Reticuloendothelial Society*, **18,** 1–13 (1975)

54 SAVAGE, D. C. Interactions between the host and its microbes. In *Microbial Ecology of the Gut*, edited by R. T. J. Clark and T. Bauchop, 277–310. London, Academic Press (1977)

55 SCHRANK, G. D. and VERWEY, W. F. Distribution of cholera organisms in experimental *Vibrio cholerae* infections: proposed mechanisms of pathogenesis and antibacterial immunity. *Infection and Immunity*, **13,** 195–213 (1976)

56 SMITH, H. W. and HUGGINS, M. B. The influence of plasmid determined and other characteristics of enteropathogenic *Escherichia coli* on their ability to proliferate on the alimentary tracts of piglets, calves and lambs. *Journal of Medical Microbiology*, **11,** 471–492 (1978)

57 SMITH, H. W. and LINGGOOD, M. A. Observations on the pathogenic properties of the K88 and ENT plasmids of *Escherichia coli* with particular reference to porcine diarrhoea. *Journal of Medical Microbiology*, **4,** 467–485 (1971)

58 SMITH, H. W. and LINGGOOD, M. A. Further observations on *Escherichia coli* enterotoxins with particular regard to those produced by atypical piglet strains and by calf and lamb strains. The transmissible nature of these enterotoxins and of a K antigen possessed by calf and lamb strains. *Journal of Medical Microbiology*, **5,** 243–250 (1972)

59 WALKER, P. D. and NAGY, L. K. Adhesion of organisms to animal tissues. In *Microbial Adhesion to Surfaces*, edited by R. C. W. Berkeley, J. M. Lynch, J. Melling, P. R. Rutter and B. Vincent, 473–494. London, Society for Chemical Industry (1980)

60 WALKER, P. D., NAGY, L. K. and MURRELL, T. G. C. Scanning electron microscopy of the jejunum in enteritis necroticans. *Journal of Medical Microbiology*, **13,** 445–450 (1980)

9
Intestinal parasites

H. R. P. Miller

INTRODUCTION

The clinical picture of enteric parasitism, characterized by inappetence, failure to thrive, hypoproteinaemia and, in severe cases, diarrhoea, is surprisingly mild in view of the extensive and severe pathological and physiological changes occurring in the gut. These include flattening of the mucosa with loss of brush border enzymes, oedema and inflammation of the lamina propria, altered levels of gastrointestinal peptide hormones, smooth muscle hypertrophy and altered intestinal motility (reviewed by Castro[10]).

It is important to distinguish which, if any, of these pathophysiological changes protect the host either by eliminating the established parasite, or by preventing further infection. Enteric parasites occupy well-defined sites within the gut and it is appropriate to examine the immunologically mediated effector mechanisms which might operate at these sites. Since limitation of space precludes a comprehensive review of the subject, an attempt will be made to discuss recent advances in our understanding of intestinal immunity to parasites and to comment on the likely direction of future developments in this field.

PARASITES AND PARASITE ANTIGENS

Helminths provide stable, non-replicating populations which are readily visualized and quantitated and which survive in the intestine for defined periods of time. Protozoa, on the other hand, are more difficult to detect and enteric infection is usually monitored by faecal counts of oocysts and by histological examination of the intestine[41]. Recently however, it has proved possible to recover trophozoites of *Giardia muris* quantitatively from the small intestine[19]. Certain protozoa persist in the intestine for many months, others remain only for the duration of their life cycle[41].

The host specificity and intestinal localization of some representative examples of the parasites to be discussed in this chapter are summarized in *Table 9.1* which

Table 9.1 Intestinal localization of some enteric helminths and protozoa

Parasite	*Distribution*	*Site*	*Host(s)*
Nippostrongylus brasiliensis	Proximal jejunum	Luminal between villi	Rat
Giardia muris	Jejunum	Surface of brush border	Mouse
Trichinella spiralis	Varies	Intraepithelial lamina propria and lumen	Various
Trichostrongylus colubriformis	Proximal intestine	Intraepithelial lamina propria and lumen	Sheep Guinea pig
Eimeria spp.	Varies according to spp.	Intraepithelial	Various
Taenia taeniaformis (larval stage)	Not known (transitory)	Migratory	Various

also shows that the intestine is a portal of entry for some of the tissue-migrating parasites.

The extent to which the battery of enzymes, cuticular antigens, protease inhibitors and so on, produced by enteric parasites alter the pathophysiology of the intestine has yet to be fully assessed. For example, the nematode *Trichinella spiralis* exerts an immunosuppressive and antiphlogistic effect in the host[10]. Phospholipids extracted from *Ascaris* spp. induce mast cell granule lysis and eosinophilia[3], and it has been postulated that nematode cholinesterases could favour parasite survival by altering intestinal motility[40].

Analysis of serum antibodies to parasites has permitted the characterization of cuticular as well as secretory antigens[47]. Furthermore, the cuticular antigens and the antibodies directed against them are specific for different stages in the life cycles of certain nematodes[38]. Similar studies should be extended to other species of helminths in order to determine the extent to which the immune system can recognise and respond to antigens on the surface of parasites. The presence of immunogenic surface antigens is clearly relevant to the nature of the enteric protective response.

The elicitation of a sterilizing and lasting immunity to enteric parasites by vaccination with parasite antigens is the ultimate goal for all immunoparasitologists. Recent progress in this area has been reviewed[25], as have the difficulties of identifying and purifying protective antigens from helminths. As yet, there has been no concerted effort to standardize the type of antigen and route of vaccination, nor is it generally known whether adjuvants help or hinder the protective immune response. Soluble antigens prepared from cestodes, nematodes, and flukes often confer substantial protection[44] although they tend to be less effective than attenuated or natural infections with living parasites[25]. The reasons for this may become more fully apparent when the nature of the intestinal protective response is discussed later in this review.

THE EXPRESSION OF RESISTANCE AGAINST ENTERIC PARASITES

The kinetics of establishment and expulsion of enteric nematodes is exemplified by infection of rats with *Nippostrongylus brasiliensis*. This parasite persists in the jejunum for 7–10 days (plateau phase) before being expelled in an exponential fashion over a period of 2–3 days[20]. Following a secondary challenge of immune rats the duration of the plateau phase is reduced, and the loss phase is accelerated[20]. Expulsion of both *N. brasiliensis*[32] and *T. spiralis*[10] from immune rats and mice can occur extremely rapidly, being complete within a few hours of experimental intraduodenal challenge and this process is normally referred to as rapid expulsion. The worms are, however, viable and will, after rapid expulsion, establish normally in non-immune intestine[17].

Other manifestations of the protective response against helminths include structural damage to their internal organs; reduced fecundity and stunted growth may also occur and a more subtle effect of the immune response is reflected by the redistribution of the parasites to sites proximal to and distal from their normal predilection site[40,47].

The immune expulsion of protozoa is more difficult to monitor and for certain species, such as *Eimeria*, measurement is complicated by the relatively short duration of their life cycles. Trophozoites of *Giardia muris* are detectable in the bowel even when no oocysts are found in the faeces[19] and it is possible that the partial immunity measured by suppression of oocyst formation differs from the sterilizing immunity where trophozoites are completely eliminated from the gut.

Probably the best measure of the immune status of the gut to *Eimeria* spp. is achieved by challenge experiments where it has been shown that the sporozoites can establish within the epithelium of immune gut but that their development is inhibited and, after a short space of time, they lose infectivity when transferred to naive recipients[41].

It must be stressed that the examples cited here take no account of the many factors which influence the expression of resistance. For example the level of infection, the sex and hormonal status of the host and, above all, its genetic background are crucial elements in the determination of the response to enteric parasites. The exploitation of genetic differences in the host to determine the genetically controlled protective responses is already a rapidly developing branch of immunoparasitology[48].

ENTERIC IMMUNE RESPONSES TO PARASITES

Considerable advances in the understanding of enteric immune responses to parasites have been achieved by techniques originally used to study the homograft reaction. These include thymus deprivation, drug–induced immunosuppression, lymphocyte depletion, adoptive immunization with lymphocytes, passive transfer of immune serum and *in vitro* assessment of cell mediated responses and humoral antibodies. For a comprehensive coverage of these techniques, the reviews by Ogilvie and Jones[40], Wakelin[47], and Befus and Bienenstock[8] are recommended.

There is little doubt that the thymus plays a central role in the expression of resistance against enteric parasites (*Table 9.2*) although there are exceptions to this general rule (e.g. the expulsion of adult cestodes from athymic mice[1]). This does not, however, mean that T-cells are necessarily involved in the final effector mechanism. They may, for example, provide help for systemic or local antibody production and/or they may influence the functions of accessory cells as well as the extensive remodelling of the mucosal architecture which occurs during parasite infections (*Table 9.2*). For convenience, antibody and cellular responses will be discussed separately.

Table 9.2 Influence of the thymus* on intestinal responses to parasites

Response	*Host*	*Parasite*	*Reference*
Parasite expulsion and/or resistance to rechallenge	Mouse, rat	*N. brasiliensis*	8, 39, 40
	Mouse	*T. spiralis*	8
	Guinea pig	*T. colubriformis*	43
	Mouse	*G. muris*	8
Villous atrophy/ crypt hyperplasia	Rat	*N. brasiliensis*	8
	Mouse	*T. spiralis*	8, 26
Mastocytosis	Rat	*N. brasiliensis*	28, 30
	Mouse	*T. spiralis*	5, 8, 30
Basophil infiltration	Guinea pig	*T. colubriformis*	43
Eosinophil infiltration	Guinea pig	*T. colubriformis*	43

* The responses listed are either absent or reduced in neonatally thymectomised or athymic hosts.

Antibodies to enteric parasites

IgA

Specific antiworm antibodies have been detected both in luminal secretions and on the teguments of cestodes[8] and the cuticles of nematodes[45]. IgA is the predominant antibody in the intestines of *Nippostrongylus*-infected rats whereas parasite-specific IgG predominates in the serum[45]. Studies of the effects of colostral IgA against infection with larval cestodes[8] or with *Giardia muris*[2], in rats and mice respectively, suggest that this immunoglobulin isotype serves a protective role in the intestine. Several mechanisms may be postulated for the action of IgA. These include:

(1) immune exclusion of soluble antigens essential for the survival of the parasite;
(2) binding of IgA to the surface of the parasite and impairment of its ability to maintain contact with or penetrate into the mucosa;
(3) promotion of mucus trapping (*see later*);
(4) modulation of accessory cell function following the binding, via IgA Fc receptors or immune complexes, to the cell surface.

IgE

Potent parasite-specific IgE responses occur following enteric helminthiasis[21] whereas there is less evidence to suggest that protozoa induce IgE antibody synthesis even though sensitization for intestinal anaphylaxis is a feature of *Eimeria* spp. infections[41]. It is characteristic of almost all heminth infections that parasite-specific and non-specific IgE are produced together with hyperplasia of mast cells and infiltration of basophils and eosinophils, and that these events are associated with the occurrence of immediate hypersensitivity reactions[21]. Enteric helminthiasis is no exception to this generalization and immediate hypersensitivity reactions in the immune gut to systemically administered parasite allergen are characterized by release of mucus, increased fluidity in the gut lumen, and hyperaemia and oedema of the mucosa[21].

The view that such reactions are, in part, responsible for the immune elimination of enteric nematodes is disputed,[5, 30, 34] especially with regard to the expulsion of primary nematode infections. In such instances worm expulsion usually precedes the detection of circulating parasite-specific IgE by several days[5, 30, 34]. However, intestinal hypersensitivity, local cutaneous anaphylaxis, and sensitization of peritoneal mast cells occur much earlier in infection which would suggest that specific IgE is present and is bound to the tissues[21]. Furthermore, experimental studies have shown that hypersensitivity reactions induced by heterologous anaphylactic shock are detrimental to parasite survival[6], possibly as a result of the pathotopic transfer of serum antibodies into the gut lumen[6, 34].

The effector functions of both macrophages and eosinophils, especially against tissue-dwelling helminths, are altered and augmented by the presence of IgE on the cell surface. Whilst it is difficult to determine what influence these cells might have on lumen-dwelling helminths, the selective suppression of IgE synthesis in *T. spiralis* infected rats not only reduces resistance to the migration of newborn larvae from the gut to the skeletal tissues but also suppresses the eosinophil response[14]. These findings suggest that IgE has several biological functions in the gastrointestinal tract, which have yet to be thoroughly characterised.

IgG

The passive transfer of immune rat serum IgG into non-immune recipients confers substantial protection against *N. brasiliensis*[18]. It is tempting to conclude that IgG *per se* mediates worm expulsion, however, careful examination of the kinetics of protection in passively immunized rats suggests the mechanisms are complex[31] and involves extensive alterations of the cell populations in the mucosa[29, 33]. Passive transfer of immune serum confers some protection against *Eimeria* spp. although the site at which antibody acts in the gut is not known[41]. This is also true of the migratory parasites such as larval cestodes[8] where it is not clear whether the oncospheres are inhibited either at the mucous surface or soon after they have penetrated into the lamina propria.

Active transport of IgG to mucous surfaces occurs in ruminants whereas this class of immunoglobulin, although present in the lamina propria of other species, normally reaches the intestinal lumen by passive diffusion[34]. This process is augmented by the occurrence of hypersensitivity reactions in the mucosa[34, 35] and, once it reaches the lumen, parasite-specific IgG may have similar functions to those described for IgA. In addition, IgG immune complexes are reported to trigger the release of mucin glycoproteins from goblet cells in the rat[23]. This may be an important part of the mucus-trapping mechanism to be described later in this review.

Some tissue-migrating enteric nematodes, such as the larval stages of *Nematospiroides dubius* in mice, stimulate massive increases in circulating IgG[22]. Parasite-specific IgG antibodies are thought to promote eosinophil-mediated killing of helminths in the tissues[9] and these mechanisms presumably operate with the intestinal mucosa.

In summary, IgA and IgG are effective both within the lumen and tissues of the intestinal tract. These two isotypes apparently interact with soluble antigens and with complex parasite surface antigens and, via their heavy-chain Fc regions, bind to and promote the functions of various effector cells. By contrast IgE seems to have little biological function in the gut lumen, presumably because it is so rapidly and effectively bound to the surfaces of cells bearing IgE Fc receptors. It may, however, promote the translocation of serum IgG into the gut lumen. In the future, identification of *relevant* parasite antigens, together with the development of appropriate methods of quantitating parasite-specific antibodies in the small intestine will be essential not only for a better understanding of enteric protective responses but also for the development of effective vaccines.

Cellular responses to enteric parasites

Lymphoid cells

The intestine is richly populated with lymphoid cells dispersed in the lamina propria and epithelium, and, aggregated in the Peyer's patches[8]. It is also the major source of recirculating lymphocytes which traverse the mesenteric lymph nodes en route to the thoracic duct. Whether Peyer's patches are involved in recognition of parasite antigens and the dissemination of responding lymphocytes to other regions of the gut has not yet been clarified[8]. Nevertheless, enteric nematodiasis has been particularly useful as a system for studying the localization of recirculating lymphoid cells[26].

Lymphoid cells derived from gut-associated lymphoid tissue will adoptively confer resistance against a variety of nematode and protozoal infections[8]. The mechanism by which they do this has not been established and some of the consequences of passive immunization with either lymphocytes or immune serum are summarized in *Table 9.3*. Adoptive immunization with either T cells[37] or B cells[13,37] may confer resistance, depending on the immune status of the cell donor. The same is true of the passive transfer of immune serum[31]. Both manipulations may have a final common pathway in promoting the mucosal changes responsible for worm expulsion (*Table 9.3*). Clearly, it is now essential to further characterize the local intestinal antibody and cellular responses in order to define the roles of adoptively transferred B cell and T cell subpopulations.

Table 9.3 Intestinal responses to enteric parasites which can be passively transferred with either immune lymphoid cells or immune serum

Response	*Host*	*Parasite*	*Mechanism(s)*	*Reference*
Parasite expulsion	Rat, mouse	*T. spiralis*	Cells	13, 49
	Rat	*N. brasiliensis*	Cells or serum	31, 36, 37
	Guinea pig	*T. colubriformis*	Cells	42, 43
	Rat	*Eimeria* spp.	Cells	41
Villous atrophy/crypt hyperplasia	Mouse	*T. spiralis*	Cells	26
Mastocytosis	Rat	*N. brasiliensis*	Cells or serum	7, 29, 36
Basophil infiltration	Guinea pig	*T. colubriformis*	Cells	42
Eosinophil infiltration	Guinea pig	*T. colubriformis*	Cells	42
Goblet cell hyperplasia	Rat	*N. brasiliensis*	Cells or serum	33

Whether lymphoid cells in the mucosa act directly against the parasites is not yet known but, with recent developments in the isolation of functional lymphoid cells from the intestinal mucosa[8], studies of *in vitro* interactions between enteric parasites and mucosal lymphocytes should now be feasible.

Accessory cells

Histological assessment of the cell kinetics in parasitized intestinal mucosae have shown that basophils[42], eosinophils[42], and mast cells[30] increase in number at about the time of nematode expulsion and that the principal infiltrating cells in *Eimeria*-infected gut are neutrophils[41]. Granulocytes arise in bone marrow, and it seems likely that the requirement for bone marrow cells as well as sensitized lymphocytes for the successful transfer of resistance against nematodes in irradiated rats[15] and mice[49] is related to the presence and function of these accessory cells in the mucosa.

The participation of the immune system in the generation of basophils and eosinophils and in the release of these cells into the peripheral circulation is well established[4,5], and it is clear from *Table 9.3* that the infiltration of these cells into parasitized mucosa is under immunological control. The precursors of mast cells also arise in bone marrow but are seeded out to the tissues where they differentiate[5]. It is likely, but as yet unproven, that the precursors of mucosal mast cells in the intestinal lamina propria also arise in bone marrow[5,30], however, the differentiation and proliferation of this subpopulation of cells within parasitized intestine is influenced not only by the thymus and/or T cells but also by factors in serum (*Table 9.3*).

There is no reason to suspect that eosinophils within the gut function differently from those elsewhere in the body and on this basis it must be assumed that they are active against parasites in the mucosa via the antibody dependent (IgE[21] and IgG – *see preceding section*) helminthotoxic mechanisms which have been intensively studied in the last few years (reviewed by Butterworth[9]). It remains to be shown, however, whether eosinophils are helminthotoxic against luminal parasites.

Studies by Rothwell[42,43] indicate that basophils participate in the rejection of *Trichostrongylus colubriformis* from guinea pig intestine. The numbers of these cells increase at the time of worm expulsion and, in parallel, the levels of histamine and 5HT are also increased[4]. Infusion of these amines directly into the intestinal lumen effects expulsion of fourth stage *T. colubriformis* larvae[4]. Evidence that mucosal mast cells participate in similar reactions against *T. spiralis* and *N. brasiliensis* is more controversial not only because of the kinetics of appearance of parasite-specific IgE, but also because primary worm expulsion can occur in the absence of mast cells[21]. However, since mucosal mast cells[16,46] and basophils[4] in many species, including man, require special fixation and histochemical techniques for their adequate demonstration in the gut, they may not be detected if routine methods of histological assessment are made. This is true of *N. brasiliensis*-infected rat intestine where basophil infiltration, which precedes mucosal mastocytosis, is only detectable in plastic-embedded tissues[30].

Befus and Bienenstock[8] have emphasized the dangers of assuming that monoamines are involved only in local hypersensitivity reactions, and have listed the variety of ways in which, for example, histamine can modulate cell function via H_1 and H_2 receptors. Nevertheless, recent studies indicate that mucosal mast cells in immune rat gut release serine protease from their granules during the rapid expulsion of *N. brasiliensis* (Miller, Woodbury and Huntley, unpublished observations). Since this protease is specific to rat mucosal mast granules[51] it provides an excellent system for monitoring the secretory function of these cells during parasitic infection[50].

The following functions have been proposed for mucosal mast cell or basophil mediated intestinal hypersensitivity rections[32]:

(1) IgE-mediated release of monoamines from mucosal mast cells/basophils;
(2) the direct effects of monoamines against the parasites[4];
(3) monoamine-induced release of mucins from goblet cells[23];
(4) increased mucosal permeability and transfer of immunoglobulin into the gut lumen[34,35];
(5) altered intestinal motility[10,21].

The participation of all, or some, of these effector mechanisms would seem likely to promote the rapid expulsion of a challenge infection and further, more detailed, analysis of the mechanisms of rapid expulsion is urgently required.

THE PROTECTIVE FUNCTION OF INTESTINAL EPITHELIUM

The primary line of defence in the gut is the epithelial surface and there is increasing interest in its protective role. Whilst it is not yet certain that local cell-mediated responses are the sole cause of villous atrophy and crypt hyperplasia in parasitized gut[8], there is good evidence to support the contention that they are in part caused by T cells (*Table 9.3*). There is also a correlation between the appearance of these changes and the immune expulsion of *T. spiralis*[26] but the significance of this correlation is not known.

More direct evidence of the involvement of mucosal epithelia in nematode expulsion has arisen from *in vivo* and *in vitro* studies on the trapping of the nematodes *N. brasiliensis* and *T. spiralis* in rat intestinal mucus[23, 32]. It would appear that the superficial mucus in immune intestine excludes the parasites from their predilection sites close to the mucosa[24, 32]. Immunologically mediated hyperplasia of the goblet cell population[33], discharge of mucin[32], and increased intestinal motility may also promote the inhibitory effects of superficial mucus. *In vitro* studies suggest that specific antibody and heat-labile non-specific factors (e.g. complement) promote the trapping of infective *T. spiralis* in intestinal mucus[26]. Since immediate hypersensitivity reactions promote mucus release[23] as well as the translocation of serum macromolecules into the gut lumen[23, 34] it is possible that such mechanisms facilitate co-operative interaction between mucin glycoproteins and parasite specific antibodies. Those antibodies recognising cuticular antigens[8, 38, 45] may thus be ideally suited to promote mucus trapping.

Recent studies indicate that intestinal epithelia in immune rats not only mount a net secretory response within minutes of challenge with *T. spiralis*[12] but also that the carbohydrate composition of their brush borders is altered by infection with this parasite[11]. The fact that the expression of serologically defined Ia antigens on intestinal epithelia is greatly increased in response to immunological stimuli[27] adds further impact to the exciting prospect that profound biochemical and functional changes occur within immunologically compromised mucosal epithelia. The significance of these changes for intestinal parasites has yet to be fully explored.

References

1 ANDREASSON, I., HINSBO, O. and RUITENBERG, E. J. *Hymenolepis diminuta* infections in congenitally athymic (nude) mice: worm kinetics and intestinal histopathology. *Immunology*, **34,** 105–113 (1978)

2 ANDREWS, J. S. and HEWLETT, E. L. Protection against infection with *Giardia muris* by milk containing antibody to *Giardia*. *Journal of Infectious Diseases*, **143,** 242–246 (1981)

3 ARCHER, G T., ROBSON, J. E. and THOMPSON, A. R. Eosinophilia and mast cell hyperplasia induced by parasite phospholipid. *Pathology*, **9,** 137–153 (1977)

4 ASKENASE, P. W. Role of basophils, mast cells and vasoamines in hypersensitivity reactions with a delayed time course. *Progress in Allergy*, **23,** 199–320 (1977)

5 ASKENASE, P. W. Immunopathology of parasitic diseases: involvement of basophils and mast cells. *Springer Seminars in Immunopathology*, **2,** 417–442 (1980)

6 BARTH, E. E. E., JARRETT, W. F. H. and URQUHART, G. M. Studies on the mechanism of the self-cure reaction in rats infected with *Nippostrongylus brasiliensis*. *Immunology*, **10,** 459–464 (1966)

7 BEFUS, A. D. and BIENENSTOCK, J. Immunologically-mediated mastocytosis in *Nippostrongylus brasiliensis* infected rats. *Immunology*, **38,** 95–101 (1979)

8 BEFUS, A. D. and BIENENSTOCK, J. Factors involved in symbiosis and host resistance at the mucosa-parasite interface. *Progress in Allergy*, **31,** 76–177 (1982)

9 BUTTERWORTH, A. E. Eosinophils and immunity to parasites. *Transactions of the Royal Society of Tropical Medicine and Hygiene.* **74** (Suppl.) 38–43 (1980)

10 CASTRO, G. A. Physiology of the gastrointestinal tract in the parasitized host. In *Physiology of the Gastrointestinal Tract*, edited by L. R. Johnson, 1381–1406, Raven Press, New York (1981)

11 CASTRO, G. A. and HARARI, Y. Intestinal epithelial membrane changes in rats immune to *Trichinella spiralis*. Abstract: *Proceedings of the American Society for Parasitology*, Montreal, Canada (1981)

12 CASTRO, G. A., HESSEL, J. J. and WHALEN, G. Altered intestinal fluid movement in response to *Trichinella spiralis* in immunized rats. *Parasite Immunology*, **1,** 259–265 (1979)

13 CRUM, E. D., DESPOMMIER, D. D. and McGREGOR, D. D. Immunity to *Trichinella spiralis*. I. Transfer of resistance by two classes of lymphocytes. *Immunology*, **33,** 787–795 (1977)

14 DESSEIN, A. J., PARKER, W. L., JAMES, S. L. and DAVID, J. R. IgE antibody and resistance to infection. 1 Selective suppression of the IgE antibody response in rats diminishes the resistance and eosinophil response to *Trichinella spiralis* infection. *Journal of Experimental Medicine*, **153,** 423–436 (1981)

15 DINEEN, J. K. and KELLY, J. D. Expulsion of *Nippostrongylus brasiliensis* from the intestine of rats: the role of a cellular component derived from bone marrow. *International Archives of Allergy*, **45,** 759–766 (1973)

16 ENERBACK, L. Mast cells in rat gastrointestinal mucosa. 2. Dyebinding and metachromatic properties. *Acta Pathologica et Microbiologica Scandinavica*, **66,** 303–312 (1966)

17 HESSELL, J. J., RAMASWAMY, K. and CASTRO, G. A. Reduced hexose transport by enterocytes associated with rapid, noninjurious rejection of *Trichinella spiralis* from immune rats. *Journal of Parasitology*, **68,** 202–207 (1982)

18 JONES, V. E., EDWARDS, A. J. and OGILVIE, B. M. The circulating immunoglobulins involved in protective immunity to the intestinal stage of *Nippostrongylus brasiliensis* in the rat. *Immunology*, **18,** 621–633 (1970)

19 GILLON, J., Al THAMERY, D. and FERGUSON, A. Features of small intestinal pathology (epithelial cell kinetics, intraepithelial lymphocytes, disaccharidases) in a primary *Giardia muris* infection. *Gut*, **23,** 498–506 (1982)

20 JARRETT, E. E. E., JARRETT, W. F. H. and URQUHART, G. M. Quantitative studies on the kinetics of establishment and expulsion of intestinal nematode populations in susceptible and immune hosts. *Nippostrongylus brasiliensis* in the rat. *Parasitology*, **58,** 625–639 (1968)

21 JARRETT, E. E. E. and MILLER, H. R. P. The production and activities of IgE in helminth infections. *Progress in Allergy*, **31,** 178–233 (1982)

22 KNOPF, P. M., CHAPMAN, C. B., HICKS, J. D., MANDEL, T. E. and MITCHELL, G. F. Localization of IgG_1-producing cells within a hyperstimulated lymph node of mice infected with an intestinal nematode parasite. *Immunology Letters*, **1,** 137–140 (1979)

23 LAKE, A. M., BLOCH, K. J., SINCLAIR, K. J. and WALKER, W. A. Anaphylactic release of intestinal goblet cell mucus. *Immunology*, **39,** 173–178 (1980)

24 LEE, G. B. and OGILVIE, B. M. The mucous layer in intestinal nematode infections. In *The Mucosal Immune System in Health and Disease* (Proceedings of the 81st Ross Conference on Pediatric Research), edited by P. L. Ogra and J. Bienenstock, 175–187. Columbus, Ohio, Ross Laboratories (1981)

25 LLOYD, S. Progress in immunization against parasitic helminths. *Parasitology*, **83,** 225–242 (1981)

26 MANSON-SMITH, D. F., BRUCE, R. G. and PARROTT, D. M. V. Villous atrophy and expulsion of intestinal *Trichinella spiralis* are mediated by T cells. *Cellular Immunology*, **47,** 285–292 (1979)

27 MASON, D. W., DALLMAN, M. and BARCLAY, A. N. Graft-versus-host disease induces expression of Ia antigen in rat epidermal cells and gut epithelium. *Nature*, **293,** 150–151 (1981)

28 MAYRHOFER, G. and FISHER, R. Mast cells in severely T-cell depleted rats and the response to infestation with *Nippostrongylus brasiliensis*. *Immunology*, **37,** 145–155 (1979)

29 MILLER, H. R. P. Passive transfer of the mucosal mast cell response its relationship to goblet cell differentiation. In *The Mast Cell, its Role in Health and Disease* edited by J. Pepys and A. M. Edwards, 738–742. Pitman Medical, Tunbridge Wells (1979)

30 MILLER, H. R. P. The structure, origin and function of mucosal mast cells: a brief review. *Biologie Cellulaire*, **39,** 229–232 (1980)

31 MILLER, H. R. P. Expulsion of *Nippostrongylus brasiliensis* from rats protected with serum. I The efficacy of sera from singly and multiply infected donors related to time of administration and volume of serum injected. *Immunology*, **40,** 325–334 (1980)

32 MILLER, H. R. P., HUNTLEY, J. F. and WALLACE, G. R. Immune exclusion and mucus trapping during the rapid expulsion of *Nippostrongylus brasiliensis* from primed rats. *Immunology*, **44,** 419–429 (1981)

33 MILLER, H. R. P. and NAWA, Y. Immune regulation of intestinal goblet cell differentiation. Specific induction of nonspecific protection against helminths? *Nouvelle Revue Francaise d'Hematologie*, **21,** 31–45 (1979)

34 MURRAY, M. Immediate hypersensitivity effector mechanisms. II *In vivo* reactions. In *Immunity to Animal Parasites*, edited by E. J. L. Soulsby, 155–190, New York, Academic Press (1972)

35 NAWA, Y. Increased permeability of gut mucosa in rats infected with *Nippostrongylus brasiliensis*. *International Journal for Parasitology*, **9,** 251–256 (1979)

36 NAWA, Y. and MILLER, H. R. P. Adoptive transfer of the intestinal mast cell response in rats infected with *Nippostrongylus brasiliensis*. *Cellular Immunology*, **42,** 225–239 (1979)

37 NAWA, Y., PARISH, C. R. and MILLER, H. R. P. The protective capacities of fractionated immune thoracic duct lymphocytes against *Nippostrongylus* brasiliensis. *Cellular Immunology*, **37,** 41–50 (1978)

38 PHILIPP, M., TAYLOR, P. M., PARKHOUSE, R. M. E. and OGILVIE, B. M. Immune response to stage-specific surface antigens of the parasitic nematode *Trichinella spiralis. Journal of Experimental Medicine*, **154,** 210–215 (1981)

39 OGILVIE, B. M. and JONES, V. E. Reaginic antibodies and immunity to *Nippostrongylus brasiliensis* in the rat. *Parasitology*, **57,** 335–349 (1967)

40 OGILVIE, B. M. and JONES, V. E. *Nippostrongylus brasiliensis*: a review of immunity and the host/parasite relationship in the rat. *Experimental Parasitology*, **29,** 138–177 (1971)

41 OGILVIE, B. M. and ROSE, M. E. The response of the host to some parasites of the small intestine: *coccidia* and nematodes. *Les Colloques de L'Institut National de la Sante et de la Recherche Medicale*, INSERM **72,** 237–248 (1977)

42 ROTHWELL, T. L. W. and DINEEN, J. K. Cellular reactions in guinea-pigs following primary and challenge infection with *Trichostrongylus colubriformis* with special reference to the roles played by eosinophils and basophils in rejection of the parasite. *Immunology*, **22,** 733–745 (1972)

43 ROTHWELL, T. L. W. and LOVE, R. J. Studies of the responses of basophils and eosinophil leucocytes and mast cells to the nematode *Trichostrongylus colubriformis*. II Changes in cell numbers following infection of thymectomised and adoptively or passively immunised guinea-pigs. *Journal of Pathology*, **116,** 183–194 (1975)

44 ROTHWELL, T. L. W. and LOVE, R. J. Vaccination against the nematode *Trichostrongylus colubriformis.* 1 Vaccination of guinea-pigs with worm homogenates and soluble products released during *in vitro* maintenance. *International Journal for Parasitology*, **4,** 293–299 (1974)

45 SINSKI, E. and HOLMES, P. H. *In vitro* binding of IgG and IgA to *Nippostrongylus brasiliensis* measured by radio-immunoassay. *Journal of Parasitology*, **64,** 189–191 (1978)

46 STROBEL, S., MILLER, H. R. P. and FERGUSON, A. Human intestinal mucosal mast cells: evaluation of fixation and staining techniques. *Journal of Clinical Pathology*, **34,** 851–858 (1981)

47 WAKELIN, D. Immunity to intestinal parasites. *Nature*, **273,** 617–620 (1978)

48 WAKELIN, D. and DONACHIE, A. M. Genetic control of immunity to parasites: adoptive transfer of immunity between inbred strains of mice characterised by rapid and slow immune expulsion of *Trichinella spiralis. Parasite Immunology*, **2,** 249–260 (1980)

49 WAKELIN, D. and WILSON, M. M. Immunity to *Trichinella spiralis* in irradiated mice. *International Journal for Parasitology*, **10,** 37–41 (1980)

50 WOODBURY, R. G. and MILLER, H. R. P. Quantitative analysis of mucosal mast cell protease in the intestines of *Nippostrongylus*-infected rats. *Immunology*, **46,** 487–496 (1982)

51 WOODBURY, R. G. and NEURATH, H. Purification of an atypical mast cell protease and its levels in developing rats. *Biochemistry*, **17,** 4298–4304 (1978)

10
Alpha chain disease and intestinal lymphoma

C. Hocine Asselah and Fatima Asselah

INTRODUCTION AND HISTORICAL BACKGROUND

Alpha chain disease is a fascinating disorder which has attracted great interest among gastroenterologists and immunologists, for the last thirteen years. However, even though more than 200 cases have been reported, the aetiology remains unknown, the pathogenesis obscure and the management still controversial. Alpha chain disease belongs to a group of disorders known as heavy chain diseases. These are lymphoproliferative disorders characterized by the production of an incomplete immunoglobulin devoid of light chains and comprising defective heavy chains with an intact Fc portion, a major deletion in the Fd portion and/or a deletion in the hinge region. In 1964 Franklin *et al.*[44] opened the chapter of heavy chain diseases by describing the first case of α-chain disease. They then foresaw the discovery of similar disorders related to other classes of immunoglobulins. Within a few years, α-chain disease[92, 116], in 1968, μ-chain disease[40], in 1970, and recently δ-chain disease[133], in 1978, have been subsequently identified.

Alpha chain disease appears now to be the most common form of the heavy chain diseases. It was initially recognized in a serum of a young female Syrian patient suffering from a primary diffuse intestinal lymphoma associated with malabsorption[92, 116]. This type of lymphoma was known, for many years, as 'Mediterranean abdominal lymphoma'[114] because of its high incidence and initial confinement in the Mediterranean region[8, 36, 100], but now appears to exist in other parts of the world as well. It is distinct from other primary intestinal lymphomas occurring in western countries among older patients who present either signs of neoplasm or malabsorption in association with adult coeliac disease. Although α-chain disease and Mediterranean type lymphoma share the same clinicopathological features, the only distinction being the evidence of α-chain disease protein secretion in the former disease, the question of their relationship is still in controversy. A number of synonyms such as primary upper small intestinal lymphoma[56, 78], Middle Eastern lymphoma[63, 138], or immunoproliferative small intestinal disease[135] are used, adding even more to the confusion. None of these terms seem appropriate. The term 'Mediterranean type lymphoma' has been sanctioned by usage.

Alpha chain disease has now been described in nearly all parts of the world. Characterized by a diffuse and massive plasmacytic infiltration of the lamina propria of the intestine and the mesenteric lymph nodes, the disease affects mainly young adults in whom diarrhoea, severe malabsorption, weight loss and abdominal pain are the major clinical features. The disease is usually progressive and fatal although a few remissions have been reported. It is our purpose to provide a review of the pathological features, the clinical aspects, the pathogenesis, the management of α-chain disease and its relationship to intestinal lymphoma of Mediterranean type. At the time of writing, we are aware of 42 cases of α-chain disease which have been diagnosed in Algeria since 1968. The study is based on our experience and on the relevant data found in the available literature. All the cases of α-chain disease have involved the gastrointestinal tract, except for three cases[37, 39, 126] so far reported, which affected the respiratory tract and showed that α-chain disease may affect the whole IgA secretory system.

PATHOLOGY

The pathological features of the gastrointestinal form of α-chain disease have been repeatedly reported as fairly uniform. A diffuse infiltration of both the mesenteric lymph nodes and the small intestinal mucosa along the whole length of the bowel with plasmacytes secreting abnormal immunoglobulin are the main features of the disease. Although the initial cell proliferation usually appears benign and confined to the enteromesenteric area, overt malignant lymphomas arise in the small intestine and/or the mesenteric lymph nodes with, in most cases, little evidence of distant spread. Recent biosynthetic and immunohistochemical studies[14, 16, 85, 102, 121] strongly suggest that the obviously malignant lymphomas may derive from the same cell populations as the benign appearing plasmocytes secreting the α-chain disease protein. Alpha chain disease presents similar pathological features to the so-called Mediterranean type lymphoma. This will be discussed in more detail in the following paragraph.

Macroscopic appearances

The main macroscopic features of the disease are a diffuse thickening of the small intestine along its whole length caused by a mucosal lesion and a constant involvement of the mesenteric lymph nodes. In most patients seen at laparotomy, the serosal aspect of the small bowel appears normal, although, on palpation, the intestinal loops are felt heavier and more rigid. In resected specimens the mucosal folds are uniformly thickened. The mesenteric nodes are moderately and irregularly enlarged and appear reactive (*Figure 10.1*). Only a small number of patients present para-ortic lymphadenopathy[4, 11, 66, 87]. But, with most of them, the enteromesenteric involvement remains isolated. The peripheral nodes are not

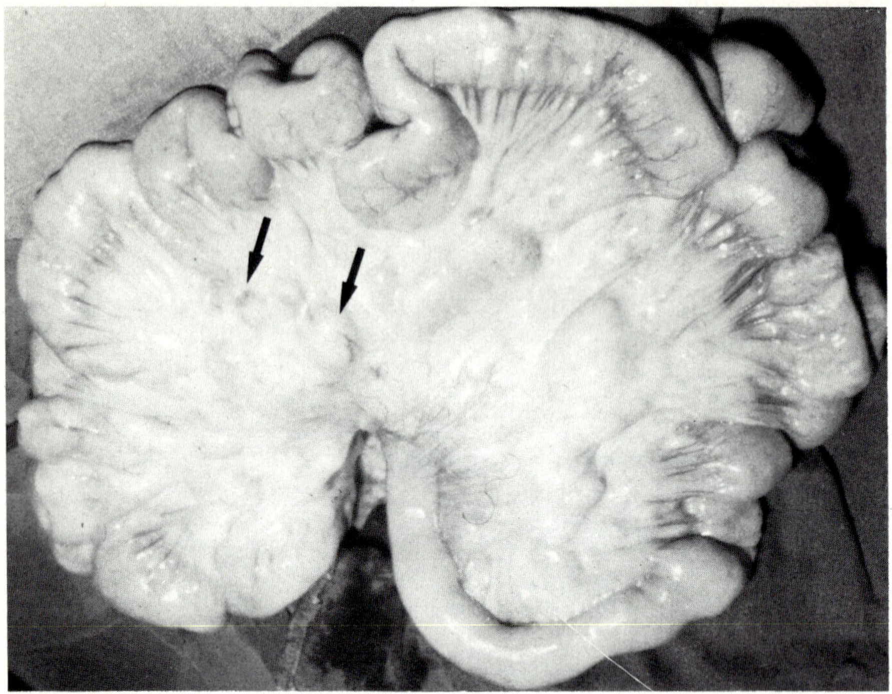

Figure 10.1 Gross findings at an early stage of α-chain disease. At laparotomy a slight and diffuse thickening of the small bowel wall is associated with an irregular enlargement of the mesenteric lymph nodes (arrows)

enlarged, the liver and the spleen are unremarkable – except in one case only where splenic atrophy was reported[58].

However, when the patient has reached a more advanced phase, he develops severe lesions: large tumours in the mesentery and a more marked intestinal thickening (*Figure 10.2*) generally associated with isolated[4, 79, 80] or multiple[14, 21, 35, 56, 71, 131] circumscribed and obviously malignant changes in the bowel. These areas appear to be thickened, stenotic, ulcerated and/or perforated with cobblestone or polypoid changes in the mucosa. Extrinsic involvement of the intestinal wall caused by mesenteric masses may lead to subacute obstruction[1, 12, 56, 73, 78, 79]. Although intussusception[14, 31] and perforation[12, 35, 70] with peritonitis have been reported, fissuring and fistula remain rare. Extensive lymphomatous involvement in the whole gastrointestinal tract, characterized by multiple nodules is found in few patients at a final stage[4] and a case of multiple lymphoid polyposis has been reported[23]. Generally, signs of gross neoplastic dissemination are unseen at an early stage. They become more apparent when the disease has progressed, but remain relatively discrete with involvement of the intra-abdominal lymph nodes. However, at a terminal stage, the stomach, the large bowel and many other organs may be involved[1, 4, 67, 128].

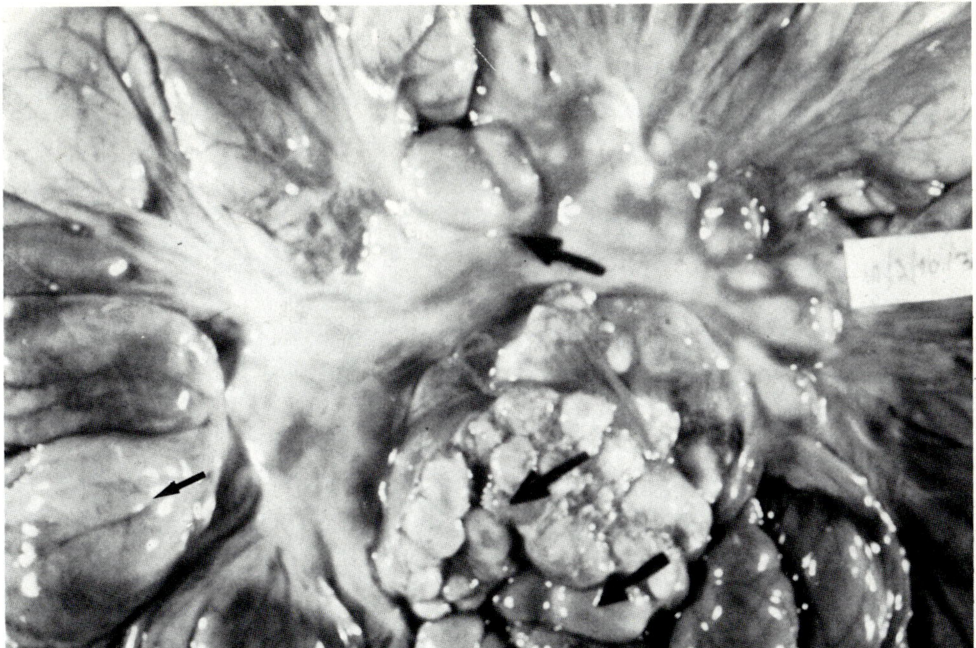

Figure 10.2 At necropsy, large lymphomatous masses are found in the mesentery (large arrows); the small intestine is diffusely and evenly thickened (small arrows)

Light microscopy

The main histological feature is a diffuse, massive mononuclear cell infiltrate located within the lamina propria at any level of the small intestine, associated with characteristic distortion of the mucosal architecture. The cell proliferation thickens the mucosa and obliterates the core of the villi. As a result, the mucosa becomes more or less flat (*Figure 10.3*). However, the surface epithelium is relatively well preserved and presents a regular brush border (*Figure 10.4*). The intraepithelial lymphocyte count is within the normal limits[4, 32] and crypts are sparse and widely spaced. These features clearly distinguish α-chain disease and Mediterranean type lymphoma from coeliac disease. In the early stage, the cell infiltrate is moderately dense, limited within the lamina propria and shows no sign of atypia (*Figure 10.4*). It is composed of mature appearing plasmacytes with eccentric clock-face nuclei and prominent nucleoli. Their cytoplasm is abundant, vacuolated, basophilic and slightly PAS positive. Occasional PAS positive intranuclear vacuoles may be found. Few lymphocytes, macrophages and a larger number of mast cells and eosinophils are found within this infiltrate. Lymphangiectasia is inconstant. Special histochemical stains fail to reveal amyloid. In some cases, the cell proliferation is more massive and infiltrates the submucosa. The cells appear less mature with larger, clearer nuclei and enlarged nucleoli. Atypical cells are seen scattered in the lamina

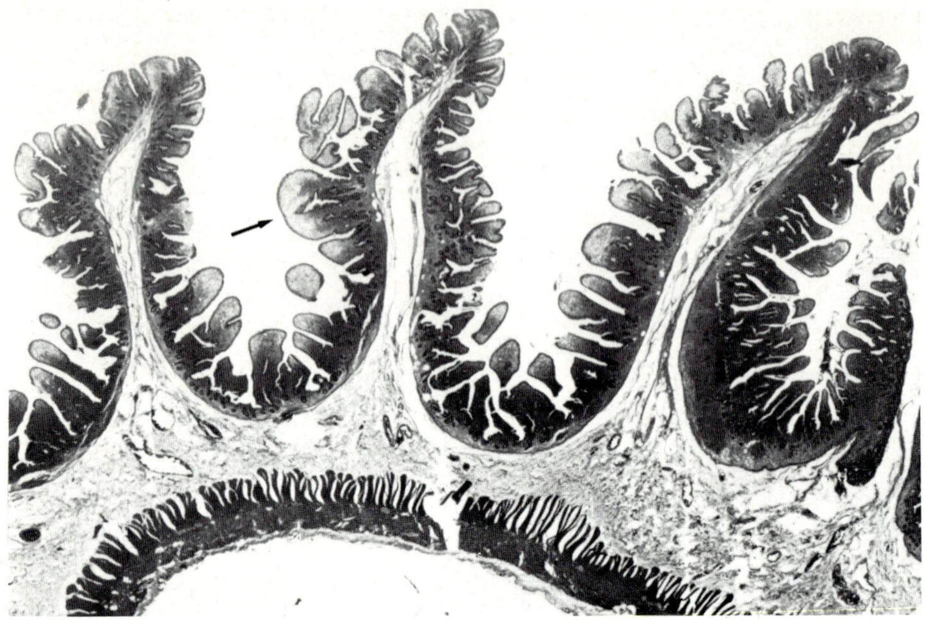

Figure 10.3 Low power view showing a severe thickening of the mucosa; the villi are blunted (arrows), the crypts widely spaced; the distorsion of the villous architecture may be more severe, resulting in a flat mucosa (H & E × 14)

propria, assembled in nodules located deep in the mucosa or infiltrating and destroying crypts (*Figure 10.5*). These features are widely accepted signs of incipient malignancy[4, 36, 51, 63, 103]. Malignant lymphomas seen at advanced stages are diffuse, or constitute multiple foci adjacent to the benign appearing cell population. The mesenteric lymph nodes usually show a well preserved architecture and a diffuse plasma cell infiltrate within the sinusoids and medullary cords. Lymphomas are associated with complete or partial loss of the lymph node architecture. Necrosis, haemorrhage, sclerosis, hyaline deposits and granulomas can all be observed but there is no evidence of amyloid.

A spectrum of lymphomas has been described in association with α-chain disease: reticulum cell sarcoma and Hodgkin's disease[75, 89, 103], plasma cell tumours[59, 124], immunocytoma[4, 69, 121], immunoblastic sarcoma[4, 135] and follicular lymphoma[4, 65]. They appear as B lymphomas with, in most cases, a high plasma cell differentiation. However, these lymphomas do not resemble soft tissue plasmocytomas morphologically, nor do they behave like them[4, 5, 32, 70]. None of them had the features of primary malignant histiocytosis of the small intestine[62]. Spread of the abnormal cells to the stomach[4, 6], rectum[4, 12, 66], caecum[4, 6], bone marrow[11, 32, 35, 92], peripheral nodes[3, 4, 20, 73, 107, 121, 128], nasopharyngeal tissue[32], tonsils[7], and peripheral blood[6, 32] has been demonstrated. In the liver, slight or moderate, portal or intralobular mononuclear cell infiltrate may be found[4, 35, 56, 107]. In contrast to malignant histiocytosis[62] there is no sign of phagocytosis in the neoplastic cells or isolated malignant cells in the sinusoids[4]. The spleen may be partly[128] or diffusely[6] involved with lymphoma, however, this remains exceptional. The presence of

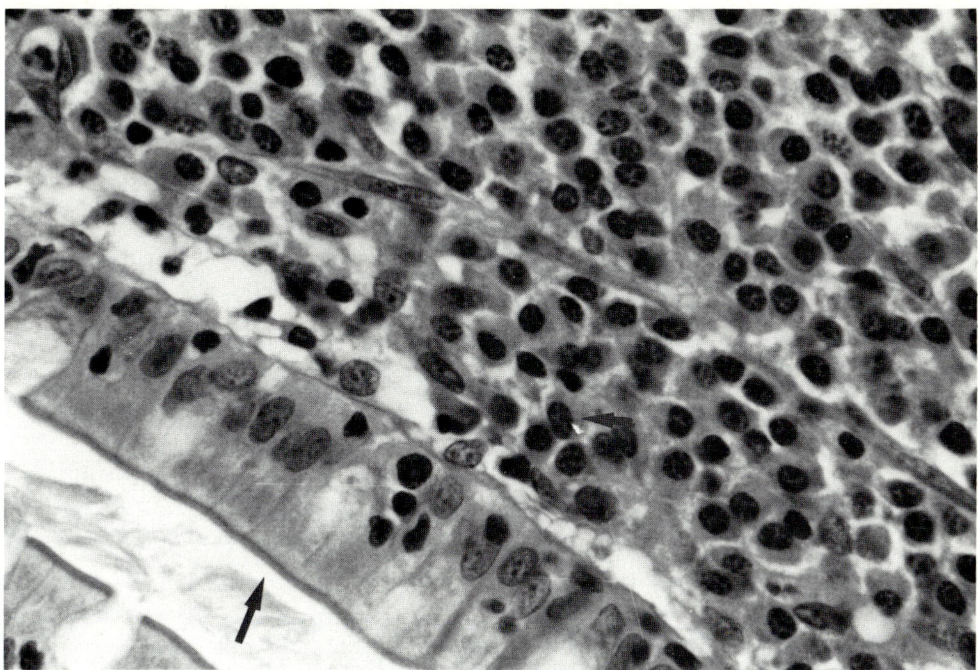

Figure 10.4 High power photomicrograph showing a relatively well preserved surface epithelium with a regular brush border; the intraepithelial lymphocyte count is moderately increased; the massive cell proliferation in the lamina propria is mainly composed of mature-looking plasma cells (H & E × 640)

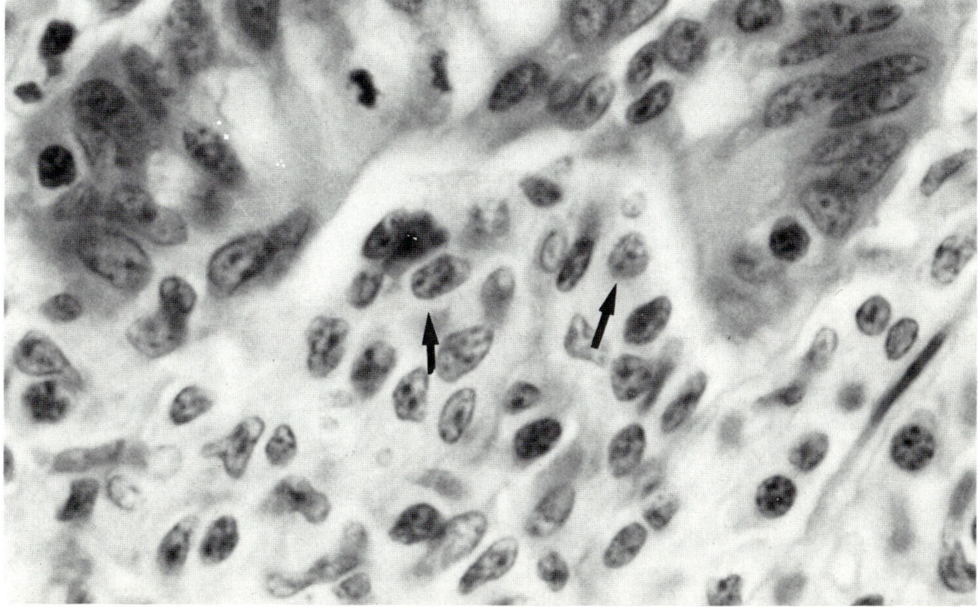

Figure 10.5 Atypical cells infiltrating and destroying crypts is a useful criterion for malignancy (H & E × 1000)

cellular proliferation of both benign and malignant appearances at different places of the small intestine and/or the mesenteric nodes is frequent. The progression of the disease, from a limited apparently benign cell proliferation to a more extensive and malignant one has been followed by sequential histological examinations[4, 12, 22, 32, 52].

Electron microscopy

Ultrastructural studies of a few cases of α-chain disease[32, 49, 80, 87, 113, 123] confirm the plasmacytoid features of the proliferating cells. The latter appear either like mature and actively-secreting plasma cells, or malignant with pale and enlarged nuclei, enlarged nucleoli, signs of nuclear cytoplastic asynchrony and mitochondrial abnormalities. A moderately dense amorphous or less often crystalline material is found in the distended cysternae of the rough endoplasmic reticulum (*Figure 10.6*).

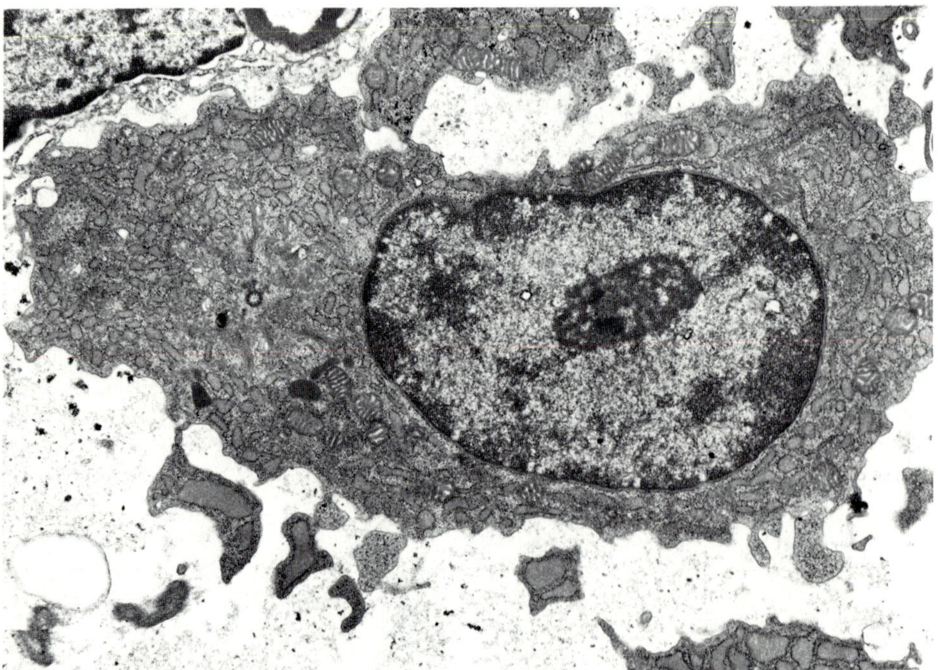

Figure 10.6 Electron micrograph of a mature-looking plasma cell found in α-chain disease in the small intestinal mucosa; the eccentric located nucleus shows the characteristic peripheral condensation of the chromatin into coarse clumps; the nucleolus is prominent; a moderately dense, granular material is present within the distended cysternae of the rough endoplasmic reticulum (× 10 000); the rather large Golgi region contains a centrosome: a few mitochondria are seen

Occasional intranuclear inclusions are seen. Besides these abnormal plasma cells[9], few lymphocytes, eosinophils, neutrophils, mast cells and macrophages are found. The surface epithelium is usually normal[81, 123] (Asselah: unpublished observations), in some cases mildly and patchily[113] or more severely altered[87]. Intraepithelial coccidian microorganisms of the subphylum Sporozoa, class Teleosporea, have been identified in one patient[58]. The few α-chain disease cases studied showed once more how difficult it is to recognize cell malignancy. Although, both electron microscopy and light microscopy showed similar aspects of plasma cell proliferation, either mature and highly secreting or more malignant, the true nature of the initial benign appearance remains difficult to determine.

Immunohistochemistry

Immunofluorescent studies have been used to demonstrate α-chain disease protein secretion by the abnormal cells and for the evaluation of the progression of the disease[12, 32, 52, 71, 92, 93, 116, 117, 131].

Where fluorescent monospecific antisera were used, the proliferating cells did not show any κ or λ light chain secretion. The cytoplasm of a few of them fluoresced slightly with anti-IgA antisera. Malignant cells showed surface immunoglobulins[16], but no cytoplasmic immunoglobulins[12, 52].

Immunoperoxidase

Although this technique[130] offers numerous advantages, it has only been used in a few cases[4, 57, 63, 121, 124]. The abnormal cells showed heavy and specific staining with both anti-IgA and anti-J chain antisera, but not with anti-κ and anti-λ light chains antisera (*Figures 10.7, 10.8 and 10.9*). Occasional cells exhibited IgG, IgM, κ and λ light chains secretion. Malignant cells showed no evidence at all[63], or mild and variable immunoglobulin secretion[4, 57, 121]. Using immunoperoxidase, a monotypic complete immunoglobulin secretion has been recognised in very few plasma cell tumours associated with α-chain disease[4, 90, 124]. Immunohistochemistry has been especially useful in the recognition of non-secretory forms of the disease[69, 97], and of other types of protein abnormalities[9, 10, 21, 129]. They should help in delineating the relationship between α-chain disease and Mediterranean type lymphoma.

Radioimmunoelectrophoretic analysis of proteins synthesized *in vitro* by intestinal and mesenteric lymph node cells in the presence of ^{14}C-labelled aminoacids showed α-chain disease protein to be produced by the abnormal plasma cells. No light chains could be detected either in these cells or in their extracts[16, 32, 117].

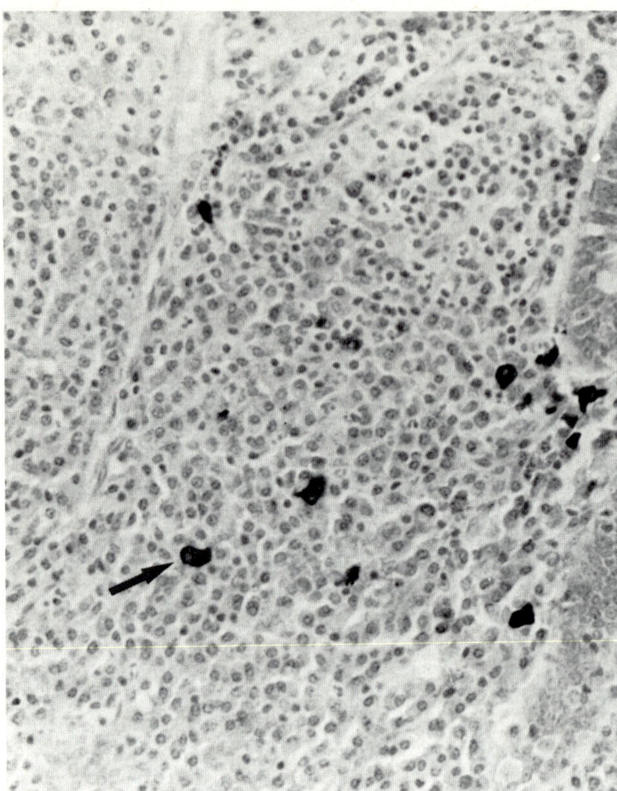

Figure 10.7 Immunoperoxidase staining for IgA: the diffuse benign-appearing plasma cell proliferation in the lamina propria shows strong cytoplasmic positivity; atypical cells infiltrating crypts and assembled in nodules (arrows) exhibit no Ig secretion. Counterstained with haematoxylin (× 98)

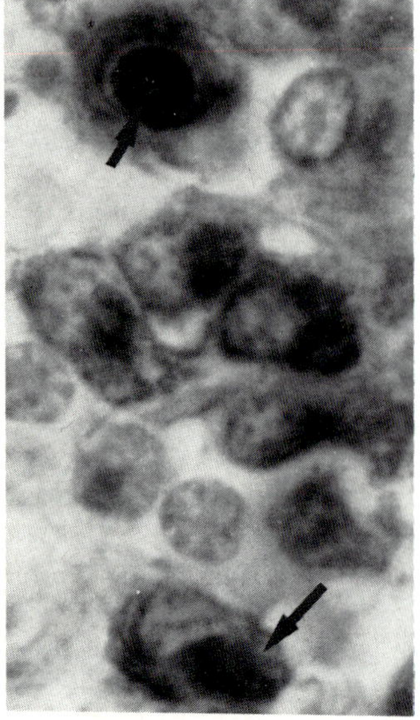

Figure 10.8 Higher power of *Figure 10.7*. Intracytoplasmic (long arrow) and intranuclear (small arrow) IgA positive vacuoles are seen in the plasma cells infiltrating diffusely the small intestinal mucosa in α-chain disease (× 1495)

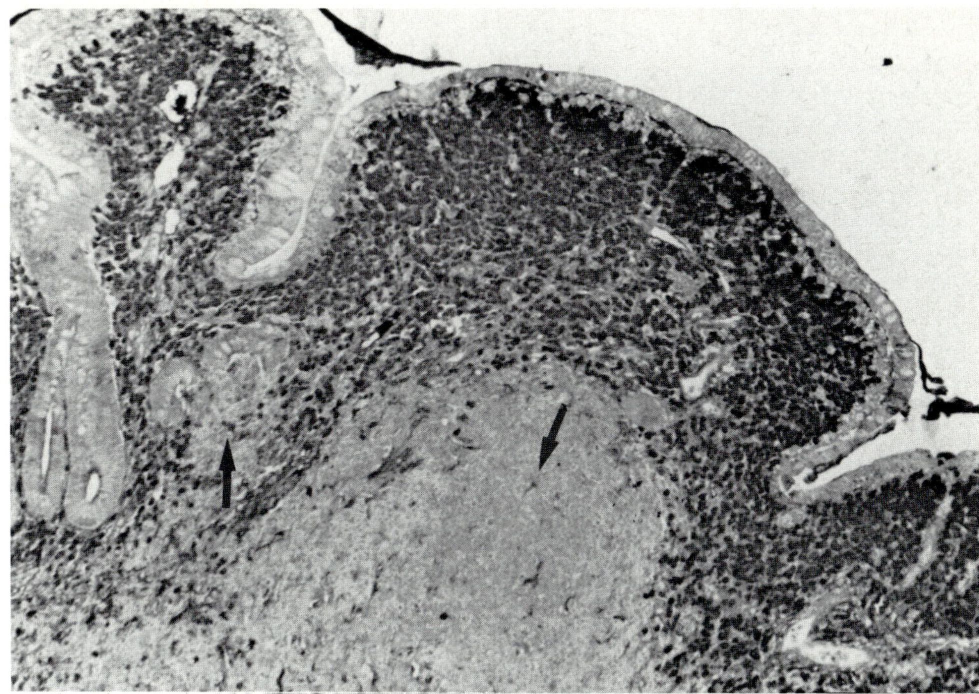

Figure 10.9 Immunoperoxidase staining for κ light chains. No light chains are found in the abnormal plasma cells in the lamina propria except for occasional cells (arrows); the same proportion of cells stained for λ light chains IgG or IgM. Counterstained with haematoxylin (× 140)

CLINICAL ASPECTS

Age and sex distribution

Review of 166 α-chain disease cases shows that the age of patients ranges from 10 to 60 years with an average of 19.7 years. The peak incidence over all patients is situated in the second and third decades and is identical in both sexes. Only 9 per cent of all cases are older than 30 years. The proportion of patients presenting in childhood varies from 9 per cent in published reports to 33 per cent in our own survey, where the mean age at diagnosis was 13 years. The male to female ratio is approximately two to one in this subgroup.

Geographical distribution

Alpha chain disease was originally described in patients from Syria[92], and subsequently in patients from Algeria[4, 6, 12, 61, 66, 74, 75, 86, 95, 97, 117, 125, 127, 131], Tunisia[20, 105, 128], Pakistan[31, 32], Colombia[60], Iraq[1, 2, 139], Greece[32, 35, 71, 124], Italy[14, 19, 28], Spain[13, 22, 38, 54, 55], Iran[11, 32, 56, 73, 79, 138], Lebanon[107, 108], Israel[49, 101, 121], Libya[32], Cambodia[93], South Africa[70, 80], Morocco[125], Argentina[87], Yugoslavia[88], Bangladesh[106], Nigeria[134], Mali[68], Portugal[67]. Recently, the disease has been described in the USA[23] and Finland[109].

Clinical features

Review of the above documented cases shows that the clinical picture is uniform and identical to that described earlier by Ramot *et al.*[100] and Eidelman *et al.*[36] in patients with Mediterranean type lymphoma. The major symptoms were diarrhoea, 97 per cent, weight loss, 99 per cent, and abdominal pain, 94 per cent. The onset of the disorder is usually marked by diarrhoea which may be initially mild and gradual, intermittent or continuous, or occasionally acute. In rare cases, since diarrhoea may not be prominent and since the pain may be relatively acute and localized in the right lower quadrant or in the epigastrium, the physician makes a clinical diagnosis of appendicitis[14, 93], peritonitis[127] or pancreatitis[12]. Subsequently, diarrhoea becomes prominent and consists of three or four stools daily, stools are usually voluminous, bulky and greasy. However, exacerbations often occur, daily bowel movements being greater than ten per day; the discharge may reach fourteen litres a day[139]. Occasionally, stools may contain blood and mucus[1, 6, 131]. Severe weight loss is usual. Emaciation and dehydration are usually prominent at presentation. Anorexia, weakness, lassitude and fatigue are common. Abdominal pain of varying intensity, site, relationship to meal, may be reported as colicky, cramping or more often distension or vague discomfort. Nausea and vomiting occurred in 26 per cent of all the cases. Tetany is reported as a symptom on presentation in up to 8.2 per cent of the cases. Amenorrhoea is not uncommon, seen in 10 per cent of all female patients. Growth retardation may be present. Low grade fever is noticed during the course of the disease in 12 per cent of the cases. Digital clubbing is found at presentation in about 40 per cent of the cases. The abdomen is usually distended. Generalized tenderness is not uncommon. Abdominal masses are found at presentation in about 26 per cent of the cases. Surgical presentation with intestinal obstruction, intussusception, perforation and peritonitis occur in 8 per cent of cases, and usually after a long history of diarrhoea. Oedema and ascites are detectable in 4 and 6 per cent of the cases. An enlarged spleen is exceptional, found in only 2 cases[128, 134]. Hepatomegaly and peripheral lymphadenopathy are not significant features and are found respectively in 8 and 7 per cent of the cases.

Radiological aspects

The radiological aspects of the small intestine have been reported as showing a non-specific malabsorptive pattern in many cases. However, the mucosal pattern may appear abnormal throughout the length of the small intestine with diffuse thickening of mucosal folds. Fold edges may be irregular and their contours may be occasionally nodular. In some cases, strictures and filling defects are associated with coarse mucosal folds and thickened small bowel wall. Occasionally impressions due to circumscribed tumours may be superimposed on the other findings. Oesophagus, stomach and colon are usually normal.

Endoscopic aspects

Oesophagus and stomach are usually normal. However, in two cases seen at an advanced stage (personal observations) gastric involvement with multiple ulcerations was evident. Endoscopic appearance of the duodenum may be normal. In some cases, the mucosa may appear thickened and slightly granular. Cerebriform and mosaic-like mucosa may be seen. In one case (personal observation) the mucosa was cobblestone-like with multiple pseudopolyps of varying size. Sigmoidoscopy is usually normal.

LABORATORY INVESTIGATIONS

Haematological and biochemical tests

Erythrocyte sedimentation rate has been normal in 18 per cent of the cases and elevated above 30 mm/1st hour in 78 per cent of the cases. Haemoglobin is often decreased, due commonly to iron deficiency. In 68 per cent of 117 cases, anaemia is mild; it is moderate in 28 per cent and severe in 4 per cent due to blood loss. The white cell count is normal in 70 per cent of the cases. In 9 per cent, it is elevated above 15 000/mm^3 with a polymorphonuclear leucocytosis. In an 18-year-old male patient (Asselah, unpublished observation), white blood count reached 160 000/mm^3 during the course of the disease, blood picture and bone marrow suggesting a chronic lymphocytic leukaemia. In a few patients, neoplastic cells may be seen in blood and bone marrow[11, 32, 35, 92]. Otherwise, bone marrow is usually normal. Platelet count has been normal. Cholesterol is depressed below 1.5 g/l in 75 per cent of the cases. Serum alkaline phosphatase is increased about two to three times above normal in about 45 per cent of the cases and has been reported to be due to the intestinal isoenzyme increase[29, 32]. No other enzyme abnormalities are noted. Low serum calcium under 9 mg/dl is reported in 57 per cent of the cases. No features of osteomalacia have been described. Serum potassium is decreased in most cases. In 58 per cent, it is below 3.5 mEq/l. In many cases[4, 6, 11, 73, 125, 131], hypokalaemia is severe, as low as 1.3 mEq/l. Hypokalaemic nephropathy with polyuria has been a feature at presentation, in some cases[6, 35, 61].

Protein studies

Serum total protein is depressed in all cases where its value is reported, with an average of about 5.6 g/dl. The depression is due to a decreased level of serum albumin although γ-globulin may also be lowered. Among 81 cases, serum albumin was below 2.5 g/dl in 71 per cent of the cases (range: 0.8 g/dl[87] – 3.6 g/dl[139]; average: 2.5 g/dl). In α-chain disease, the serum concentrations of IgA, IgG and IgM, when tested, are decreased in most cases[2, 4, 6, 11, 12, 14, 32, 32, 35, 38, 49, 56, 70, 73, 74, 80, 87, 93, 109, 134]. In one case, selective IgA deficiency has been reported during a remission of α-chain disease.

The diagnosis of α-chain disease relies upon serum protein immunochemical analysis (*Figure 10.10 and Figure 10.11*). Serum electrophoresis may detect the pathological protein in showing, usually, in the α_2 to β region, an abnormal broad band but in only 50 per cent of the cases[1, 2, 6, 56, 73, 120]. With immunoelectrophoretic analysis using polyvalent antisera to human normal serum, the protein abnormality may escape detection. The analysis using a monospecific antiserum is more reliable[34, 116, 117]. The abnormal protein reacts with antisera to α-heavy chain

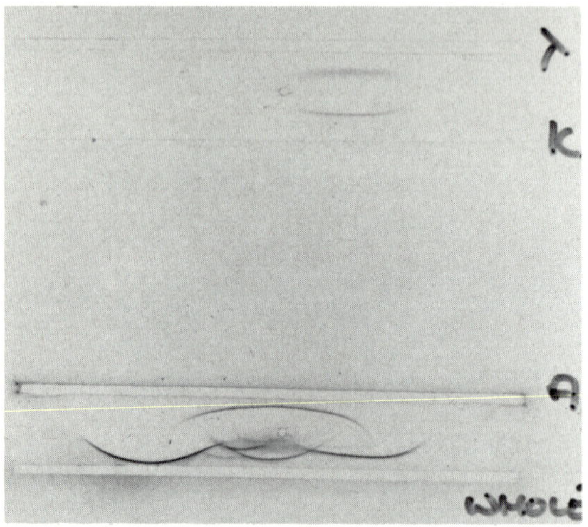

Figure 10.10 Immunoelectrophoretic pattern given by the serum of a patient with α-chain disease, using monospecific anti-IgA serum (note the precipitin line given by the α-chain disease protein) respectively anti-κ anti-λ antisera: the α-chain disease protein does not react with anti-light chains sera

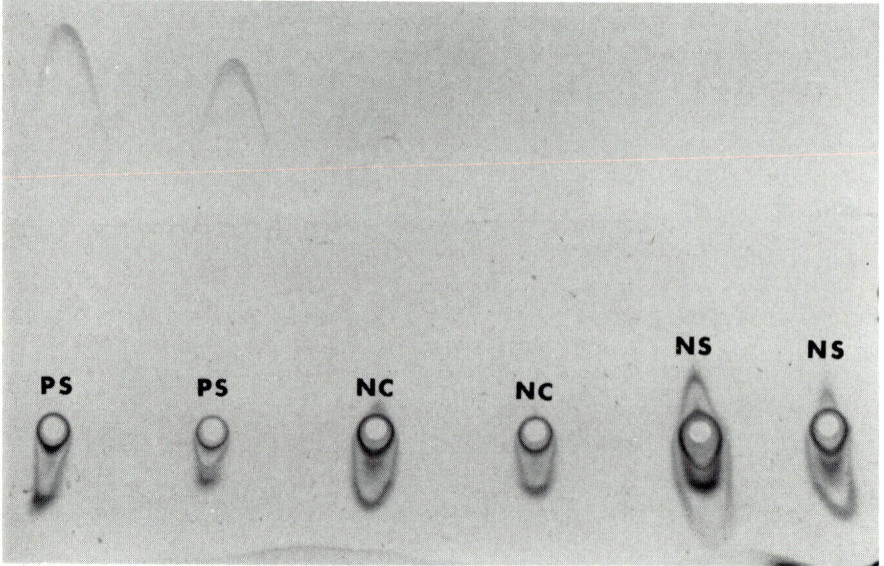

Figure 10.11 Results of investigation for serum α-chain disease protein with rocket immunoselection method; PS: sera from one patient with α-chain disease (sera dilution 1:50 and 1:100) showed the peaks in the upper zones; NC: negative controls (sera dilution 1:5 and 1:20; NS: normal serum

resulting in an abnormal precipitin line in α-globulin to β_2 region and does not react to antisera to κ and λ light chains (*Figure 10.10*). Various patterns have been described[117]. The electrophoretic heterogeneity of α-chain disease protein has been related to its high carbohydrate content, high propensity to polymerize and its aminoterminal heterogeneity[41, 45, 46, 117, 118]. However, since many IgA myelomas may not react with antisera to light chain[34, 45, 117], the failure of light chain antisera to precipitate the abnormal protein is not sufficient evidence for diagnosis. Therefore, a number of methods have been used: urea–acid–starch gel electrophoresis or gel filtration of the purified, reduced and alkylated protein in dissociating solutions[117, 118]; immunoelectrophoresis using selected antisera containing precipitating antibodies to the determinants specific for the Fab region[117, 118]; immunoselection techniques – using anti-light chain antisera[91]; immunoselection combined with immunoelectrophoresis[32]; two dimensional immunoelectrophoresis[25]; rocket immunoelectrophoresis[50] (*Figure 10.11*). Immunoselection combined with immunoelectrophoresis using an antiserum with Fab specificity seems to be the simplest to perform and the most reliable[34]. In all reported cases, the abnormal protein belongs to the α_1 subtype. The abnormal protein may be demonstrated in concentrated urine, and jejunal fluid in all cases. No Bence Jones proteinuria is found.

Structural and immunochemical studies

The present status of knowledge on this subject has been recently reviewed[46, 48, 120, 135]. Studies of heavy chain proteins have shed light on the genetic control of immunoglobulin structure, synthesis and assembly[17, 40, 41, 43, 47]. As in other heavy chain diseases the defect of α-chain disease protein seems to be due to a primary defect in synthesis by abnormal plasma cells rather than to secondary proteolytic degradation of normal immunoglobulin[18, 47, 118, 136, 137]. The incomplete IgA contains the Fc fragment, the hinge region of the α_1 heavy chain and the J chain and is lacking the Fd portion of the heavy chain and the light chains[116, 117]. It consists of dimers and polymers. The molecular weight of the basic monomeric unit has been found to vary between 29 000 and 35 000[117, 118]. The deletion of the Fd portion may result from an abnormality affecting the gene(s) which control its synthesis. However, the synthesis of heavy and light chains is under the control of separate non-linked genes. Therefore, the abnormality may be due to a mutational event[43, 45] or alternatively a defect of a possible regulator which controls the expression of two non-linked genes[47].

Intestinal function

Malabsorption is almost invariable and results from the diffuse and massive cell infiltration of the gut mucosa and the frequently associated bacterial and parasitic infection of the intestinal lumen. However, the mechanisms are not elucidated.

Microscopic and electron miscroscopic studies (*see above*) do not provide convincing evidence of altered epithelial cells, damaged microvilli suggesting microvillous malfunction or of dilated lymphatics suggesting lymphatic obstruction. Small intestinal stasis, caused by plasmacytic infiltration of the underlying lamina propria interfering with intestinal motility or by extrinsic mesenteric lymph node compression, gives rise to massive bacterial overgrowth in the duodeno-jejunum. Overgrowth of aerobes and anaerobes has been demonstrated in many patients[12, 32, 66, 87, 92, 93, 95, 125, 131, 139], accounting for the temporary response of the diarrhoea to antibiotic therapy. On the other hand, bacterial overgrowth and colonization of the intestine by *Giardia lamblia* may result from the immunodeficiency state itself, i.e. the secretion of IgA fragments which lack either the capacity to detect antigen and/or the effective antigen antibody combining sites. Finally, an underlying deficiency of the immune system and/or the IgA secretory system, not yet clearly understood, might be involved in the pathogenesis of the malabsorption in addition to other factors.

Faecal fat excretion

The faecal fat excretion has been abnormal in 91 per cent of the cases (average: 25.3 g/day). Elevation of faecal fat excretion has been found in some cases as high as 50 g/day[75] and 80 g/day[131].

Xylose absorption, vitamin B uptake and protein losing enteropathy

Seventy-six per cent of patients have abnormal xylose absorption. The vitamin B12 uptake is in most cases depressed to levels below 6 per cent, and in some cases to 0.99 per cent[32] and 1.2 per cent[92]. But in most cases, values were not reported after antibiotic therapy. Studies of protein losing enteropathy are recorded only in a few cases[12, 23, 125, 131]. In those cases using i.v. ^{51}Cr albumin test, the test is abnormal.

Microbiology and parasitology

Intestinal parasites and fungi are found in 41 per cent of the cases. They are various, the most common being *Giardia lamblia*[6, 12, 31, 32, 56, 68, 70, 73, 93].

Other parasites include *Entamoeba histolytica*[4, 6], *Trichomonas*[80], *Ascaris lumbricoides*[70, 80], *Trichuris trichiura*[70, 106], *Taenia saginata*[1, 6], *Taenia stronguloides*[134], *Taenia solium*[70], *Anguillula*[68], *Bilharzia*[68], and Coccidia[58]. However, these findings require cautious interpretation since incidences in normal controls among similar populations are lacking. Bacterial overgrowth was found in most cases studied[12, 32, 66, 87, 92, 93, 95, 125, 131, 139] using various methods. When collection of intestinal juice through small bowel intubation was used, different species were found. Virological studies, when performed, showed inconclusive results.

NATURAL HISTORY OF α-CHAIN DISEASE

A history of several years, before diagnosis in some patients (9 years[73], 11 years[128], 14 years[1]) shows the potential chronicity of the disease. The longest follow up of any patient so far reported was 14 years[73]. This patient was treated with abdominal radiation. However, in most cases, the average duration of the disease is less than 4 years. Most patients show periods of remission and relapse. These remissions can last a few months or more than 2 years. It is interesting to note that some patients treated with antibiotics or chemotherapy and/or abdominal radiation have shown a clinical, biological and histological remission of variable duration. However, as the spontaneous course of the disease may be long[1, 6, 128], the beneficial effect of any type of treatment is difficult to assess.

The course of the disease is usually fatal. The prognosis in α-chain disease is usually better than that of Mediterranean type lymphoma, because of the earlier diagnosis of α-chain disease, due to the presence of the marker α-chain disease protein in serum. When α-chain disease patients reach the stage of overt malignant lymphoma, the prognosis is, as in Mediterranean type lymphoma, usually poor. Follow-up information in order to determine the survival rate is, however, not available for most patients. Death occurs in a cachectic condition and is related usually to sepsis, fungal infection, metabolic disturbance or progressive malignancy.

In conclusion, it appears that the course of the disease can be, for some patients initially slow, apparently benign, and suddenly turns to a much more aggressive malignant lymphoma. For others, it is rapidly progressive, leading to death after a few months.

DISEASES ASSOCIATED WITH α-CHAIN DISEASE

Various intercurrent diseases, apart from common intestinal infections, have been documented: bronchopneumonia[1, 6, 14, 35, 87, 125, 132], cytomegalovirus infections[70], tuberculosis of the intestine[6], and/or of the abdominal lymph nodes[6, 66], or of the groin[32], bilharziasis of the urinary bladder[1], hydatid cyst of the liver[6]. Other disorders include ankylosing spondylitis[66], ulcerative colitis[1], thalassaemia[1], nodular non-functioning goitre[14], Meckel's diverticulum[4, 6], cholelithiasis[4], appendicitis[14, 93] gastric ulcer[32] and malacoplakia[51]. These associations, apart from infections which may be related to the immunodeficiency state itself, are probably coincidental.

Malignant neoplasia

Usually, overt malignant lymphomas occur during the course of the disease. Of particular interest are other lymphoid neoplasia apparently without relationship to α-chain disease and which may occur either during a remission or during an active phase of the disease: ileocaecal plasmacytoma with IgA and light chain secretion[124]; a retroperitoneal immunoblastic sarcoma with IgG and κ light chain secretion[55]; a case of Hodgkin's disease in another patient[75]; a blood and bone marrow picture of chronic lymphocytic leukaemia in an 18 year old patient developing 16 months after the onset of the disease (personal observation). The first two cases are most intriguing. The finding of monotypic λ chain in the first case recalls a similar result in two α-chain disease patients[4, 90] and suggests that light chain synthesis may not be restricted to μ-chain disease. The second case is more fascinating and suggests the possibility of a mutation of the neoplastic clone. In the third case, immunological studies have not been performed on the Hodgkin's lymphoma and one must remember that some pleomorphic lymphoplasmacytic lymphoma associated with α-chain disease may simulate a Hodgkin's disease morphologically. However, the possibility of development of other lymphoma neoplasia independent of α-chain disease in immunocompromised patients cannot be ruled out. The fourth case, although extremely fascinating was unfortunately not well documented: immunohistochemical studies in the bone marrow cell infiltrate were not performed.

PATHOGENESIS OF α-CHAIN DISEASE

Serial histological examinations suggest that during its progression, the disease evolves through a highly differentiated slow growing neoplastic process to a less differentiated and highly malignant one. The natural history, which correlates with the histological findings, is remarkably similar to that of other lymphoproliferative disorders, especially some leukaemias and the other heavy chain diseases. Most cases of α-chain disease are associated with a dense and monotonous cell proliferation extensively involving the small intestinal mucosa and the mesenteric lymph nodes. In our experience, this aspect is quite different from the mild and non-specific changes resulting from chronic and massive intestinal microorganism polyinfestations and seems neoplastic rather than merely reactive. However, the monoclonal character of the α-chain disease protein has not yet been demonstrated and the nature of the initial plasma cell proliferation is still controversial.

The cause of the disease is not yet known, but the following have been suggested:

(1) that α-chain disease results from environmental factors;
(2) that α-chain disease is due to genetic factors;
(3) that it is due to an underlying immune deficiency.

Environmental factors were earlier suggested by Ramot *et al.*[100] and Eidelman *et al.*[36] in Mediterranean type lymphoma because of the low socio-economic background of the patients. Alpha chain disease may result from prolonged stimulation of the IgA synthesizing cells by intestinal microorganisms[94, 96, 115, 119]. The benign appearance of the initial cell proliferation and the complete remission achieved in a few patients with antibiotics[66, 74, 95, 101] have added credence to this hypothesis. The concept of persistent immunological stimulation as a factor of oncogenesis was put forward by Dameshek and Schwartz[27] in 1959, Schwartz and Beldotti[112] again in 1959 and O'Connor and Davies[83] in 1960.

This has been supported by various animal studies[72, 76, 84, 89, 110, 111]. However, the relevance of this to the human situation is not clear. On the other hand, by analogy with Burkitt's[84] lymphoma, the possibility of an oncogenic virus has been postulated[94, 96, 115, 119, 120]. However, microbiological studies have failed to demonstrate any specific bacterial, viral, fungal or parasitic agent, although this may have been present in early life[94, 96, 115, 120]. Moreover, the disease has been described in patients with a high standard of living[79] and in developed countries[23, 109]

Genetic predisposition has been assumed to play a role because of the initial confinement of the disease to the Mediterranean area among Arabs and non-Ashkenazi Jews. The data supporting this hypothesis are far from complete. The disease has now been described in widely separated regions. No hereditary basis is yet known. There is no report of α-chain disease in patients' families. Immunochemical studies on IgA of close relatives of patients with α-chain disease are negative. No association with diseases of known genetic transmission has been reported. The chromosome counts performed in a few patients were normal – except for one patient[49]. HLA studies, although as yet to be concluded, from Iran, showed a significant increase of AW19 and B_{12} antigens in α-chain disease and Mediterranean type lymphoma[82].

A primary underlying immunodeficiency state, which paves the way to the development of both α-chain disease and other associated lymphoid neoplasias could be implicated. However, so far, no firm conclusions can be drawn from the immunological data. The progress in hybridoma technology in analysing the steps of development of T-lymphocytes and their subpopulations and a better knowledge of the genetic engineering and the biochemical requirements for normal B-lymphocyte function will contribute much in the future to the understanding of the immunodeficiency states as well as lymphomas.

RELATIONSHIP OF α-CHAIN DISEASE TO MEDITERRANEAN TYPE LYMPHOMA

There has been considerable dispute as to whether α-chain disease and Mediterranean type lymphoma are the same, different or related diseases. The incidence of α-chain disease in Mediterranean type lymphoma has been estimated to be between 25[101] and 60 per cent[96]. Earlier on it was suggested that all cases of Mediterranean type lymphoma may be α-chain disease[93, 96, 115]. In many cases, α-chain disease protein is not detectable in the serum with available techniques because of its very low concentration. Moreover, 'non-secretory forms' of α-chain disease have been described[69, 97]. Studies at a cellular level in order to demonstrate the abnormal protein have not been used largely. On the other hand α-chain disease protein may disappear as the lymphoma develops[4, 79, 132]. Therefore α-chain disease and Mediterranean type lymphoma may represent successive phases of one disease.

However, α-chain disease protein may disappear from serum during remissions induced by antibiotics[71, 74, 95, 101, 131, 195] or chemotherapy[1, 66, 79, 108, 131, 139] or radiotherapy[1, 73, 80] (Asselah unpublished data). The possibility that α-chain disease may represent a subtype of Mediterranean type lymphoma is more conceivable. Mediterranean type lymphoma should be regarded as a well defined group on clinicohistological grounds. It differs in many respects from other primary intestinal lymphomas such as the so-called Western type lymphoma and the malignant histiocytosis associated with adult coeliac disease. Mediterranean type lymphoma may comprise many subtypes which may be associated with immunoglobulin abnormalities. The following associations have been reported.

(1) Mediterranean type lymphoma associated with α-chain disease.
(2) Mediterranean type lymphoma associated with γ-chain disease[10].
(3) Mediterranean type lymphoma associated with IgA monoclonal gammopathy[21, 129].
(4) Mediterranean type lymphoma associated with excessive serum IgA[9].

Other IgA abnormalities may well be reported in the future. The availability of comparable immunohistochemical techniques in medical centres dealing with these patients would allow better delineation of these subtypes and would help to provide a better understanding of the immunoglobulin aberrations associated with this disease.

TREATMENT

General measures and nutrition

In most patients, marked dehydration, electrolyte depletion and hypoalbuminaemia resulting from diarrhoea with malabsorption require prompt and appropriate fluid and electrolyte replacement. This is a crucial factor in management until the patient's nutritional status has been optimally corrected. Steatorrhoea and diarrhoea subside in the majority of patients within 1 or 2 weeks with broad spectrum oral antibiotics. Simultaneously abdominal cramps are relieved. Since in many cases, *Giardia lamblia* and/or intestinal parasites are associated, appropriate agents must be administered. Supplemental iron and folate should be given to anaemic patients and multivitamin therapy is recommended.

Types of treatment

Therapeutic data were available from reports of 110 patients. Unfortunately these are isolated case reports. Careful studies including clear initial staging of lesions, assessment of treatment on histological grounds and complete long term follow up are lacking. Various types of therapy have been used for α-chain disease. They mainly consist of antibiotics alone in 31 per cent of the cases, cytotoxic chemotherapy and/or steroids in about 54 per cent of the cases and radiation in 12 per cent of the cases.

Antibiotics

Patients may gain symptomatic relief from antibiotics and many authors have emphasized dramatic improvement after, for example, tetracycline or ampicillin with weight gain of up to 20 kg over a few months.

It is doubtful whether antibiotics have any effect on the ultimate course of the disease. Even when treated in the early stages many patients respond only temporarily to antibiotics and relapse occurs[11, 32, 55, 71, 73, 79, 80, 131, 139]. According to published reports the duration of improvement is variable ranging from days to years. There are many reports of no long term beneficial effect of antibiotics[1, 5, 35, 55, 71, 79, 87, 139]. Poor responses to antibiotics have been attributed to inadequate initial staging[52]. More impressive, however, are the few reports which showed prolonged remission, in one case up to 7 years, on clinical, immunological and histological grounds[94, 96, 115, 119]. Taking this into account, the non-neoplastic nature of the benign-appearing plasma cell infiltrate has been put forward. However, at this stage of the disease, the spontaneous course may be very slow. The onset of symptoms may precede the date of diagnosis by more than 14 years[1]. Moreover, similar remissions have been achieved with cytotoxic chemotherapy and/or abdominal radiation[5, 66, 73, 80].

Cytotoxic chemotherapy

Chemotherapy, with chlorambucil, cyclophosphamide, melphalan or various combinations, has been used alone or often in association with corticosteroids. Chemotherapy has been given either initially or only after antibiotics proved ineffective. The results are variable, depending on the histological stage of the disease. Only a few patients were treated at the early stage of the disease. One of those patients[66] treated with chlorambucil recovered completely more than 6 years after his treatment had been ceased. However, most patients when treated at the stage of immunosarcoma had only a temporary improvement of variable duration, 1, 2 or 3 years.

Radiation

There are reports of complete 3 year[80], 6 year (Asselah, unpublished data) and 14 year [73] remissions of patients treated with total abdominal radiation at the early stage of the disease. At a more advanced stage, remissions of shorter duration occurred.

Surgery

Palliative resection is indicated in cases presenting with intestinal obstruction or perforation, due to circumscribed tumours either single or multiple.

Miscellaneous

Gluten free diet was administered in 2 cases without any beneficial effect. Finally, the few patients treated with steroids alone showed no response.

In conclusion, antibiotic therapy is in almost all cases followed by temporary improvement. However, the beneficial effect of antibiotics on the disease itself seems doubtful. Unfortunately there is no report to date of controlled studies comparing the effects of oral antibiotics alone versus chemotherapy and/or abdominal radiation, in the early stage of α-chain disease. At present, radiation and chemotherapy seem to be more beneficial. The value of initial staging laparotomy as included in the WHO protocol has been much emphasized. This may lead to a better knowledge of the disease but it has yet to be proved totally safe for the patient.

References

1 AL BAHRANI, Z., AL-SALEEM, T., AL-MONDHIRY H., BAKIR, F., YAHIA, H., TAHA, I. and KING, J. Alpha chain disease: report of 18 cases from Iraq. *Gut*, **19,** 627–631 (1978)

2 AL-SABTI, E. A. K. Paraproteinemia in normal family members of eight cases with primary intestinal lymphoma in Iraq. *Oncology*, **35,** 68–72 (1978)

3 AL-SALEEM and AL-BAHRANI, Z. Malignant lymphoma of the small intestine in Iraq: a pathological study of 145 cases. *Histopathology*, **31,** 921–924 (1973)

4 ASSELAH, F., SLAVIN, G., SOWTER, G. and ASSELAH, H. Mediterranean type lymphoma and alpha chain disease in Algerians: light microscopic and immunochemical studies. *Cancer* (in press)

5 ASSELAH, F., CROW, J., SLAVIN, G., SOWTER, G., SHELDON, C. and ASSELAH, H. Solitary plasmacytoma of the intestine. *Histopathology* (in press)

6 ASSELAH, H. La maladie des chaines alpha en Algérie. Etude de 24 cas observés de 1968 à 1977. *Thèse* (Docent) Université d'Alger (1978)

7 AYED, K., HADDAD, N., TABBANE, S., CHADLI, A. and HAFSIA, M. Lymphome méditerranéen avec maladie des chaines alpha. A propos d'une observation. *Semaine des Hôpitaux de Paris*, **52,** 177–186 (1976)

8 AZAR, H. A. Cancer in Lebanon and the Near East. *Cancer*, **15,** 66–77 (1962)

9 BAKLIEN, K., FAUSA, O., BRANDTZAEG, P., FROLAND, S. S. and GJONE, E. Malabsorption villous atrophy and excessive serum IgA in a patient with an unusual intestinal immunocyte infiltration. *Scandinavian Journal of Gastroenterology*, **12,** 421–432 (1977)

10 BENDER, S. W., DANON, F., PREUD'HOMME, J. L., POSSELET, H. G., ROETTGER, P. and SELIGMANN, M. Gamma heavy chain simulating alpha chain disease. *Gut*, **19,** 1148–1152 (1979)

11 BERNARDOU, A., SEGOUD, P., BILSKY-PASQUIER, G., MIHAESCHO, E., PREUD'HOMME, J. L. and BROUSSET, J. La maladie des chaines alpha. A propos d'une observation. *Nouvelle Revue Française d'Hématologie*, **12,** 333–350 (1972)

12 BOGNEL, J. L., RAMBAUD, J. C., MODIGLIANI, R., MATUCHANSKY, C., BOGNEL, C. and BERNIER, J. J. Etude clinique, anatomopathologique et immunochimique d'un

nouveau cas de maladie des chaines alpha suivi pendant cinq ans. *Revue Européenne d'Etudes Cliniques et Biologiques*, **17,** 362–374 (1972)

13 BONETTI, A., GILEXTREMERA, B., LINARES, J., PENA ANGULO, J. F., CABABBERO PLASENCIA, A., BERMUDES GARCIA, J. M. and PENA YANEZ, A. Enfermedad immunoproliferative del intestino delgado y enfermedad de las cadenas pesadas alfa. A portacion de un neuvo caso de aparicion tardia con respuesta favorable a la tetraciclina. *Revista Española Enfermedades del aparato digestivo y de la nutrición*, **1,** 42–49 (1980)

14 BONOMO, L., DAMMACO, F., MARANO, R. and BONOMO, G. M. Abdominal lymphoma and alpha chain disease. *American Journal of Medicine*, **52,** 73–86 (1972)

15 BOROCHOVITZ, D., DUTZ, W., KOHOUT, E. and VESSAL, K. Gastrointestinal mucosa and primary gastrointestinal lymphoma. *Israel Journal of Medical Sciences*, **15,** 397–404 (1979)

16 BROUET, J. C., MASON, D. Y., DANON, F., PREUD'HOMME, J. L., SELIGMANN, M., REYES, F., NAVAS, F., GALIAN, A., REVE, E. and RAMBAUD, J. C. Alpha chain disease: evidence for common clonal origin of intestinal immunoblastic lymphoma and plasmacytic proliferation. *Lancet*, **1,** 861–863 (1977)

17 BUXBAUM, J. N. The biosynthesis, assembly and secretion of immunoglobulins. *Seminars in Haematology*, **10,** 33–52 (1973)

18 BUXBAUM, J. N. and PREUD'HOMME, J. L. Alpha and gamma heavy chain disease in man: intracellular origin of the aberrant polypeptide. *Journal of Immunology*, **109,** 1131–1137 (1972)

19 CARBONNE, A., VOLPE, R., SALVATORE, T. and GRIGOLETTA, E. Mediterranean limphoma in un adulto Italiano. *Haematologica*, **65,** 251 (1980)

20 CHADLI, A., HAFSIA, M., MAAMOURI, M. T., HADDA, N. and AYED, K. Lymphome Méditerranéen avec maladie des chaines alpha. Etude anatomopathologique du premier cas Tunisien. *Archives d'Anatomie Pathologique*, **21,** 199–210 (1973)

21 CHANTAR, C., EXCARTIN, P., PLAZA, A. G., CORUGEDO, A. F., ARENAS, J. I., SANZ, E., ANAYA, A., BOOTELLO, A. and SEGOVIA, J. M. Diffuse plasma cell infiltrate of the small intestine with malabsorption associated with IgA monoclonal gammopathy. *Cancer*, **34,** 1620–1630 (1974)

22 CHANTAR, C., BOOTELLO, A., ANAYA, A., ARENAS, J. I. and MARCOS, J. Linfoma mediterraneo: estudio de diez casos, tres de ellos asociados a paraproteinemia. *Revista Clinica Espanola*, **148,** 47–52 (1978)

23 COHEN, H. J., GONZALVO, A., KROOK, J., THOMPSON, T. T. and KREMER, W. B. New presentation of alpha chain disease North America polypoid gastrointestinal lymphoma. Clinical and cellular studies. *Cancer*, **41,** 1161–1169 (1978)

24 CRABBE, P. A., HEREMANS, J. F. and CARBONARA, A. B. The normal human intestinal mucosa as a major source of plasma cells containing gamma A immunoglobulin. *Laboratory Investigation*, **14,** 235 (1965)

25 DAMACCO, F., ANTONACI, S. and MIGLIETTA, A. Two dimensional immunoelectrophoresis as a diagnostic tool for heavy chain disease. *Bollettino dell' Istituto sieroterapico Milanese*, **54,** 460–463 (1975)

26 DAMESHEK, W. Immunologic proliferation and its relationship to certain forms of leukemia and related disorders. *Israel Journal of Medical Sciences*, **1,** 1304–1315 (1965)

27 DAMESHEK, W. and SCHWARTZ, R. S. Leukemia and autoimmunization: some possible relationships. *Blood*, **14,** 115–120 (1959)

28 DE LA PIERRE, G. and NAVONE, A. Studio clinico patologico di un caso di alpha chain disease. *Minerva Medica*, **67,** 2588–2597 (1967)

29 DENT, C. E., NOVIS, T. S., SMITH, R., SUTTON, R. A. L. and TEMPERLEY, J. M. Steatorrhea with striking increase of plasma alkaline phosphatase of intestinal origin. *Lancet*, **1,** 1333–1336 (1968)

30 DOE, W. F. Alpha chain disease: clinicopathological features and relationship to the so-called mediterranean lymphoma. *British Journal of Cancer*, **31,** (Suppl. 2) 350–355 (1975)

31 DOE, W. F., HENRY, K. and DOWLING, R. H. Alpha chain disease. *Quarterly Journal of Medicine*, **39,** 619 (1970)

32 DOE, W. F., HENRY, K., HOBBS, J. R., AVERY JONES, E., DENT, C. E. and BOOTH, C. C. Five cases of alpha chain disease. *Gut*, **13,** 945–957 (1972)

33 DOE, W. F., HENRY, K. and DOYLE, F. H. Radiological and histological findings in six patients with alpha chain disease. *British Journal of Radiology*, **49**, 577–580 (1976)

34 DOE, W. F., DANON, F. and SELIGMANN, M. Immunodiagnosis of alpha chain disease. *Clinical Experimental Immunology*, **36,** 189–197 (1979)

35 ECONOMIDOU, J. C., MANOUSOS, O. N. and KATSAROS, D. Alpha chain disease causing kaliopenic nephropathy and fatal intestinal perforation. *American Journal of Digestive Disease*, **43,** 577–585 (1976)

36 EIDELMAN, S., PARKINS, R. A. and RUBIN, C. E. Abdominal lymphoma presenting as malabsorption: a clinicopathological study of nine cases in Israel and review of literature. *Medicine*, **45,** 111–137 (1966)

37 FAUX, J. A., CRAIN, J. D., ROSEN, F. S. and MERLERE An alpha heavy chain abnormality in a child with hypogammaglobulinemia. *Clinical Immunology and Immunopathology*, **1,** 282–285 (1973)

38 FERNANDES RUBIO, E., PASCUAL, E., REVERTE, CEJUDO, J., BERNALDO DE QUIROS GONZALES, J., GALLILEA BAZACO, I., IZQUIERDO DE PABLOS, J., CALVO DELOMO, T., GRAU LINARES, V., MARTIN HERRAEZ, A. and TOVAR DE LA CRUZ, J. M. Linfoma abdominal mediterraneo con cadena pesada alfa, elevada y afection extra-abdominal. *Revista Clinica Espanola*, **149,** 299–302 (1978)

39 FLORIN-CHRISTENSEN, A., DONIACH, D. and NEWCOMB, P. B. Alpha chain disease with pulmonary manifestations. *British Medical Journal*, **2,** 413–415 (1975)

40 FORTE, F. A., PRELLI, F., YOUNT, W. J., JERRY, L., KOCHWAS, S., FRANKLIN, E. C. and KUNKEL, H. G. Heavy chain disease of the mu type: report of the first case. *Blood*, **36,** 137–144 (1970)

41 FRANGIONE, B. and FRANKLIN, E. C. Heavy chain diseases: clinical features and molecular significance of the disordered immunoglobulin structure. *Seminars in Haematology*, **10,** 53–64 (1973)

42 FRANGIONE, B., FRANKLIN, E. C. and SMITHIES, O. Unusual genes at the aminoterminus of human immunoglobulin variants. *Nature*, **273,** 400–415 (1978)

43 FRANGIONE, B. and FRANKLIN, E. C. Split immunoglobulin genes and human heavy chain deletion mutants. *Journal of Immunology*, **122,** 1177–1181 (1979)

44 FRANKLIN, E. C., LOWENSTEIN, J., BIGELOW, B. and MELTZER, M. Heavy chain disease: a new disorder of serum globulins. Report of the first case. *American Journal of Medicine*, **37,** 332–350 (1964)

45 FRANKLIN, E. C. and FRANGIONE, B. Structural variants of immunoglobulins. In *Contemporary Topics in Molecular Immunology*, edited by F. P. Inman, **4,** 89–98 (1975)

46 FRANKLIN, E. C. and BUXBAUM, J. Immunoglobulin structure synthesis, secretion and relation to neoplasma of B cells. *Clinics in Haematology*, **6,** 503–532 (1977)

47 FRANKLIN, E. C., PRELLI, F. and FRANGIONE, B. Human heavy chain disease protein WIS: implications for the organization of immunoglobulin genes. *Proceedings of the National Academy of Sciences*, **76,** 452–468 (1979)

48 FRANKLIN, E. C. Monoclonal immunoglobulins. *Annals of Clinical and Laboratory Science*, **10,** 181–186 (1980)

49 GAFTER, V., KESSLER, E., SHABTAY, F., SHAKED, P. and DJADETTI, M. Abnormal chromosomal marker (D_{14} Q_{+}) in a patient with alpha chain disease. *Journal of Clinical Pathology*, **33,** 136–144 (1980)

50 GALE, D. S., VERSEY, J. M. B. and HOBBS, J. R. Rocket immunoselection for detection of heavy chain disease. *Clinical Chemistry*, **20,** 1292–1295 (1974)

51 GALIAN, A., GALIAN, P., BOGNEL, C. and RAMBAUD, J. C. Association d'une malakoplakie rectale à une maladie des chaines alpha. *Nouvelle Presse Médicale*, **2,** 707–708 (1973)

52 GALIAN, A., LECESTRE, M. G., SCOTTO, J., BOGNEL, C., MATUCHANSKY, C. and RAMBAUD, J. C. Pathological study of alpha chain disease with special emphasis on evolution. *Cancer*, **39,** 2081–2101 (1977)

53 GHADIALLY, F. N. In *Diagnostic Electron Microscopy of Tumours*, 190–197. London, Butterworths (1980)

54 GUARDIA, J., MORAGAS, A., PEDREIRA, J. D., FERRAGUT, A., GOMEZ-PEREZ, J., MARTINEZ-VASQUES, J. M. and LLORENS, V. Enfermedade de las cadenas pesadas alpha. *Revista Clinica Espanola*, **127,** 923–926 (1972)

55 GUARDIA, J., RUBIES-PRAT, J., GALLART, M. T., MORAGAS, A., MARTINEZ-VASQUES, J. M., BACARDI, R. and VILASECA, J. The evolution of alpha chain disease. *American Journal of Medicine*, **60,** 596–601 (1976)

56 HAGHIGHI, P., KHARAZMI, A., GERAMI, C., HAGHSHENASS, M., ABADI, P., OMIDI, H. and MOSTAFAVI, N. Primary upper small intestinal lymphoma and alpha chain disease: report of 10 cases emphasizing pathological aspects. *American Journal of Surgical Pathology*, **2,** 147–156 (1978)

57 HAGHIGHI, P., KHARAZMI, A., GERAMI, C., ABADI, P. and HAGHSHENASS, M. Immunoperoxidase study in alpha chain disease. *Archives of Pathology and Laboratory Medicine*, **102,** 555–557 (1978)

58 HENRY, K., BIRD, R. G. and DOE, W. F. Intestinal coccidiosis in a patient with alpha chain disease. *British Medical Journal*, **1,** 542–543 (1974)

59 HENRY, K. and KARRER BROWN, T. Primary lymphomas of the gastrointestinal tract. I. Plasma cell tumours. *Histopathology*, **1,** 53–76 (1977)

60 IBARA, R., BONDI, J. L., ROSSE, J. C. and DELARECCHIA, I. Alteraciones de la mucosa del intestino delgado en el linfoma intestinal. *Medicina* (Buenos Aeres), **30,** 234–245 (1970)

61 IRUNBERRY, J., BENALLEGUE, A., ILLOUL, G., TIMSIT, G., ABBADI, M., BENABDALLAH, S., BOUCEKKINE, T., OULAOUDIA, J. P. and COLONNA, P. Trois cas de maladie des chaines alpha observés en Algérie. *Nouvelle Revue Française d'Haematologie*, **10,** 609–616 (1970)

62 ISAACSON, P. Malignant histiocytosis of the intestine, its relationship to malabsorbtion and ulcerative jejunitis. *Human Pathology*, **9,** 661–667 (1978)

63 ISAACSON, P. Middle East lymphoma and alpha chain disease: immunohistochemical study. *American Journal of Surgical Pathology*, **3,** 431–441 (1979)

64 JINICH, H. E., ROJAS, J. A., WEBB, J. A. and KELSEY, J. R. Lymphoma presenting as malabsorbtion. *Gastroenterology*, **54,** 421–428 (1968)

65 KHARAZMI, A., REZAIM, H., ABADI, P., NASR, K., HAGHIGHI, P. and HAGHSHENASS, M. T and B lymphocytes in alpha chain disease. *British Journal of Cancer*, **37,** 48–54 (1978)

66 LAROCHE, C., SELIGMANN, M., MERILLON, H., TURPIN, G., MARCHE, C., CERF, M., LEMAIGRE, G., FOREST, M. and HUREZ, D. Nouvelle observation d'une maladie des chaines lourdes alpha au cours d'un lymphome abdominal de type méditerranéen avec tuberculose isolée des ganglions mésentériques et pelvispondilyte. *La Presse Medicale*, **78,** 55–59 (1970)

67 LASCAR, J., CLEMENT, M., ZENNY, J. C. and VALETTE, M. Lesions osseuses dans une maladie des chaines alpha: à propos d'une observation. *Journal de Radiologie et d'Electroradiologie*, **59,** 227–230 (1978)

68 LEMERCIER, Y., VERNAN, D., MECHALI, D., COULAUD, J. P. and MARCHE, C. Alpha chain disease in a young African black. *Nouvelle Presse Médicale*, **7,** 1028–1029 (1978)

69 LENNERT, K., MOHRI, S., STEIN, H., KAISERLINGE, E. and MULLER-HERMELINK, H. K. *Malignant Lymphomas other than Hodgkin's Disease*. Berlin, Springer Verlag (1978)

70 LEWIN, K. J., KAHN, L. B. and NOVIS, B. H. Primary intestinal lymphoma of 'Western' and 'mediterranean' type, alpha chain disease and massive plasma cell infiltration. A comparative study of 37 cases. *Cancer*, **38,** 2511–2528 (1976)

71 MANOUSOUS, D. B. Alpha chain disease. In *Modern Trends in Gastroenterology,* edited by Alan Read. 259–271. London, Butterworths (1975)

72 METCALF, D. Reticular tumours in mice subjected to prolonged antigenic stimulation. *British Journal of Cancer*, **15,** 769–774 (1961)

73 MIR-MADJLESSI, S. H. and MIR AHMADIAN, M. Alpha chain disease: a report of eleven patients from Iran. *Journal of Tropical Medicine and Hygiene*, **11,** 229–236 (1979)

74 MONGES, H., AUBERT, L., CHAMLIAN, A., REMACLE, J. P., MATHIEU, B., COUGARD, A. and ARROYO, H. Maladie de chaines alpha à forme intestinale. Présentation d'un cas traité par antibiothérapie avec remission clinique, histologique et immunologique. *Archives Françaises des Maladies de l'Appareil Digestif*, **64,** 223–231 (1975)

75 MONGES, H., AUBERT, L., REMACLE, J. P., CHAMLIAN, A., MATHIEU, B., GOUGARD, A., QUILICHINI, R. and CHAFFANJOU, P. Survenue d'une maladie Hodgkin 4 ans après remission complète d'une maladie des chaines alpha. *Gastronetérologie Clinique et Biologique*, **4,** 181–187 (1980)

76 MORRISON, J. L. Murine heavy chain diseases. *European Journal of Immunology*, **8,** 194–199 (1978)

77 NASSAR, V. H., SALEM, P. A., SHAID, M. J., ALAMI, S. K., BALIKIAN, J. B., SALEM, A. A. and NASRALLAH, S. M. 'Mediterranean abdominal lymphoma' or immunoproliferative small intestinal disease. Part 2. Pathological aspects. *Cancer*, **41,** 1340–1354 (1978)

78 NASR, K., HAGHIGHI, P., BAKHSHANDEH, K. and HAGUENAS, M. Primary lymphoma of the upper small intestine. *Gut*, **11,** 673–678 (1978)

79 NAVAB, F., MORARHAN, S., BANI SADRE, M. M., RAMBAUD, J. C. and MOJTABAI, A. The evolution of alpha chain disease. *Gastroentérologie Clinique et Biologique*, **2,** 983–988 (1978)

80 NOVIS, B. H., KHAN, L. B. and BANK, S. Alpha chain disease in sub-saharan Africa. *American Journal of Digestive Diseases*, **18,** 679–688 (1973)

81 NOVIS, B. H. Primary intestinal lymphoma in South Africa. *Israel Journal of Medical Sciences*, **15,** 386–389 (1979)

82 NIKBIN, B., BANISADRE, M. ALA, F. and MOJTABAI, A. HLA AW19, B12 in immunoproliferative small intestinal disease. *Gut*, **20,** 226–228 (1979)

83 O'CONNOR, G. T. and DAVIES, J. N. P. Malignant tumours in African children with special references to malignant lymphoma. *Journal of Pediatrics*, **56,** 526–532 (1960)

84 O'CONNOR, G. T. Persistent immunologic stimulation as a factor in oncogenesis with special reference to Burkitt's tumour. *American Journal of Medicine*, **48,** 279–285 (1970)

85 PANGALIS, G. A. and RAPPAPORT, H. Common clonal origin of lymphoplasmacytic proliferation and immunoblastic lymphoma in intestinal alpha chain disease. *Lancet*, **2,** 880–883 (1977)

86 PHILIPPE, N. and MONNET, P. Maladie des chaines alpha: a propos d'un cas. *Semaine des Hôpitaux de Paris*, **54,** 1276–1277 (1978)

87 PITTMAN, F. E., TRIPATHY, K., ISOBE, T., BOLANOS, O., OSSERMAN, E. F., PITTMAN, J. C., LOTERO, H. R. and DUQUE, E. E. IgA heavy chain disease: a case detected in the Western Hemisphere. *American Journal of Medicine*, **58,** 425–430 (1975)

88 PLENISCAR, S., SUMI-KRIZNIK, T. and GOLOUH, R. Abdominal lymphoma with alpha chain disease. *Israel Journal of Medical Sciences*, **11,** 832–835 (1975)

89 POTTER, M. Peritoneal plasmocytomas in mice. *Physiological Reviews*, **52,** 631 –640 (1972)

90 PREUD'HOMME, J. L., BROUET, J. C. and SELIGMANN, M. Cellular immunoglobulins in human gamma and alpha chain disease. *Clinical Experimental Immunology*, **37,** 283–288 (1979)

91 RADL, J. Light chain typing of immunologlobulins in small sample of biology materials. *Immunology*, **19,** 137–141 (1970)

92 RAMBAUD, J. C., BOGNEL, C., PROST, A., BERNIER, J. J., LEQUINTREC, Y., LAMBLING, A., DANON, F., HUREZ, D. and SELIGMANN, M. Clinicopathological study of a patient with 'mediterranean' type of abdominal lymphoma and a new type of IgA abnormality (alpha chain disease). *Digestion*, **1,** 321–326 (1968)

93 RAMBAUD, J. C., MATUCHANSKY, C., BOGNEL, J. C., BOGNEL, C., BERNIER, J. J., SCOTTO, J., PEROL, C., FERRIER, J. P., MIHAESCO, E., HUREZ, D. and SELIGMANN, M. Nouveau cas de maladie des chaines alpha chez un Eurasien. *Annales de Medicine Interne*, **121,** 135–148 (1970)

94 RAMBAUD, J. C. and SELIGMANN, M. Alpha chain disease. *Clinics in Gastroenterology*, **5,** 341–358 (1976)

95 RAMBAUD, J. C., PIEL, J. L., GALIAN, A., LECLERC, J. P., DANON, F., GIRARPIPEAU, F., MODIGLIANI, R. and ILLOUL, G. Remission complète clinique, histologique et immunologique d'un cas de maladie des chaines lourdes alpha traité par antibiothérapie orale. *Gastroenterologie Clinique et Biologique*, **2,** 49–61 (1978)

96 RAMBAUD, J. C., GALIAN, A., MATUCHANSKY, C., DANON, F., PREUD'HOMME, J. L., BROUET, J. C. and SELIGMAN, M. Natural history of alpha chain disease and the so-called 'mediterranean' type lymphoma. In *Lymphoid Neoplasia*, 271–276, Berlin, Springer Verlag (1978)

97 RAMBAUD, J. C., MODIGLIANI, R. and NGUYEN PHUD, G. B. K. Non-secretory alpha chain disease in intestinal lymphoma. *New England Journal of Medicine*, **303,** 53 (1980)

98 RAMBAUD, J. C. Secondes néoplasies et maladie des chaines alpha. *Gastroenterologie Clinique et Biologique*, **4,** 177–180 (1980)

99 RAMOS, L., MANONS, J., ILLANAS, M., HERNANDEZ-MORA, M., PEREZ-PENA, F., PICONTO, J. L., SANTANA, P. and CHANTAR, C. Radiological characteristics of primary intestinal lymphoma of the 'mediterranean' type: observations of twelve cases. *Radiology*, **126,** 379–385 (1978)

100 RAMOT, B., SHAHIN, N. and BUBIS, J. J. Malabsorption syndrome in lymphoma of small intestine. A study of 13 cases. *Israel Journal of Medical Sciences*, **1,** 221–226 (1965)

101 RAMOT, B. and HULU, N. Primary intestinal lymphoma and its relationship to alpha chain disease. *British Journal of Cancer*, **31,** (Suppl. 2) 343–349 (1975)

102 RAMOT, B., LEVANON, M., HALN, Y., LAHAT, N. and MOROZ, C. The mutual clonal origin of the lymphoplasmacytic and lymphoma cells in alpha chain disease. *Clinical Experimental Immunology*, **27,** 440 (1977)

103 RAPPAPORT, H., RAMOT, B., HULU, N. and PARK, J. K. The pathology of the so-called 'mediterranean' abdominal lymphoma with malabsorption. *Cancer*, **29,** 1502 –1511 (1972)

104 RAPPAPORT, H., PANGALIS, G. A., NATHWANI, B. N. The evolution of immunoblastic lymphomas in morphologically non-neoplastic immunoproliferative disease. In *Differentiation of Normal and Neoplastic Hematopoietic Cells*, edited by B. Clarkson *et al.*, 887–895, Cold Spring Harbor, N.Y. (1978)

105 ROGE, J., DRUET, P. and MARCHE, C. Lymphome mediterranéen avec maladie des chaines alpha triple remission clinique, anatomique et immunologique. *Pathologie et Biologie*, **18,** 851–858 (1970)

106 ROS, I. N., JEFFERIES, R., JOHNS, P., THOMPSON, R. A. and ASQUITH, P. Alpha chain disease complicated by a post nasal lymphoma, responding to antibiotics. *Gut*, **17,** 820 (1976)

107 SALEM, S. N., KAHAN, M. W., LARAZOV, B., OMAR, Y. T. and AL-WADY, H. IgA abnormalities in 'Mediterranean' lymphoma (alpha chain disease). *Post Graduate Medical Journal*, **48,** 314–317 (1972)

108 SALEM, P. A., NASSAR, V. H., SHAHID, M. J., HAJJ, A. A., ALAMI, S. Y., BALIKIAN, J. B. and SALEM, A. A. 'Mediterranean' abdominal lymphoma or immunoproliferative small intestinal disease. Part I. Clinical aspects. *Cancer*, **40,** 2941–2947 (1977)

109 SAVILAHTI, E., BRANDTZAEG, P., KUITUNEN, P. Atypical intestinal alpha chain disease evolving into selective immunoglobulin A deficiency in a Finnish boy. *Gastroenterology*, **79,** 1303–1310 (1980)

110 SCHWARTZ, R. S. Immunoregulation, oncogenic viruses and malignant lymphomas. *Lancet*, **1,** 1266–1268 (1972)

111 SCHWARTZ, R. S. Malignant lymphoproliferative diseases: interaction between immunological abnormalities and oncogenic viruses. *Annual Medical Reviews*, **19,** 269–277 (1980)

112 SCHWARTZ, R. S. and BELDOTTI, L. Malignant lymphoma following allogenic disease: transition from an immunological to a neoplastic disorder. *Sciences*, **149,** 1511–1513 (1965)

113 SCOTTO, J., STRALI, N. and CAROLI, J. Ultrastructural study of two cases of alpha chain disease. *Gut*, **11,** 782–788 (1970)

114 SEIJFFERS, M. J., LEVY, M. and HERMANN, G. Intractable watery diarrhea, hypokalemia and malabsorption in a patient with 'mediterranean' type of abdominal lymphoma. *Gastroenterology*, **55,** 118–124 (1968)

115 SELIGMANN, M. Immunobiology and pathogenesis of alpha chain disease. In *Immunology of the Gut*, Ciba Foundation Symposium 46, 261–272, Amsterdam, Elsevier (1976)

116 SELIGMANN, M., DANON, F., HUREZ, D., MIHAESCO, E. and PREUD'HOMME, J. L. Alpha chain disease: a new immunoglobulin abnormality. *Science*, **162,** 1396–1397 (1968)

117 SELIGMANN, M., MIHAESCO, E., HUREZ, D., MIHAESCO, C., PREUD'HOMME, J. L. and RAMBAUD, J. C. Immunochemical studies in four cases of alpha chain disease. *Journal of Clinical Investigation*, **48,** 2374–2389 (1969)

118 SELIGMANN, M., MIHAESCO, E., FRANGIONE, B. Studies on alpha chain disease. *Annals of the New York Academy of Sciences*, **190,** 487–500 (1971)

119 SELIGMANN, M. and RAMBAU, J. C. Alpha chain disease: a possible model for the pathogenesis of human lymphoma. In *Immunopathology of Lymphoreticular Neoplasms*, edited by J. J. Twomen and R. A. Good, 425, New York, Plenum Publishing Corporation (1978)

120 SELIGMANN, M., MIHAESCO, E., PREUD'HOMME, J. L., DANON, F. and BROUET, J. C. Heavy chain diseases: current findings and concepts. *Immunology Reviews*, **48,** 145 –147 (1979)

121 SELZER, G., SHERMAN, G., GALLIHAN, T. R. and SCHWARTZ, Y. Primary small intestinal lymphomas and alpha chain disease. A study of 43 cases from a pathology department in Israel. *Israel Journal of Medical Sciences*, **15,** 111–123 (1979)

122 SELZER, G., SACKS, M., SHERMAN, G. and NAGGAN, L. Primary malignant lymphoma of the small intestine. Changing incidence with time. *Israel Journal of Medical Sciences*, **15,** 382–385 (1979)

123 SHINER, M. Malignant potential of intestinal plasma cells in alpha chain disease. *Lancet*, **1,** 156–157 (1979)

124 SKINNER, J. M., MANOUSOS, O. N., ECONOMIDOU, J., NICOLAOU, A. and MERIKAS, G. Alpha chain disease with localized plasmacytoma of the intestine. Immunoperoxidase study. *Clinical Experimental Immunology*, **25,** 112–113 (1976)

125 SOULE, J. C. La maladie des chaines lourdes alpha. A propos de 4 cas. *These*. Paris (1975)

126 STOOP, J. W., BALLIEUX, R. E., HIGMANS, W. and ZEGERS, B. J. M. Alpha chain disease with involvement of the respiratory tract in a Dutch child. *Clinical Experimental Immunology*, **9,** 625 (1971)

127 TABBAKH, E. Contribution à l'étude clinique et biologique de la maladie des chaines alpha en Algérie. A propos de quatre observations. *Thèse*. Alger (1972)

128 TABBANE, S., TABBANE, F., CAMMOUN, M., MOURALI, N. 'Mediterranean' lymphoma with alpha heavy chain monoclonal gammopathy. *Cancer*, **38,** 1989–1986 (1976)

129 TANGUN, Y., SARACBASI, Z., INCEMAN, S., DANON, F. and SELIGMANN, M. IgA myeloma globulin and Bence Jones proteinuria in a diffuse plasmacytoma of small intestine simulating alpha chain disease. *Annals of Internal Medicine*, **83,** 673–678 (1975)

130 TAYLOR, C. R. and BURNS, J. The demonstration of plasma cells and other immunoglobulin containing cells in formalin fixed paraffin-embedded tissues using peroxidase labelled antibody. *Journal of Clinical Pathology*, **27,** 14–20 (1974)

131 TEULIERES, J. P. La maladie des chaines alpha. *Thèse*. Lyon (1975)

132 TEULIERES, J. P., LAMBERT, R. and VACHON, A. La maladie des chaines alpha. *Semaine des Hôpitaux de Paris*, **54,** 546–553 (1978)

133 VILPO, J. A., IRJALA, K., KLENI, P., KOUVONEN, J., VIANDER, M. and VILJANEN, M. K. A case of malignant plasma cell dyscrasia with delta chain M component. In *Proceedings of the XVII Congress of International Society of Haematology*, (Paris 1978)

134 WICHER, J. T., ADJUKIEWICZ, A. and DAVIS, J. D. Two cases of alpha chain disease from Nigeria. *Journal of Clinical Pathology*, **30,** 678–681 (1977)

135 World Health Organization. Alpha chain disease and related small intestinal lymphoma. *Archives Françaises des maladies de l'Appareil Digestif*, **65,** 591–607 (1976)

136 WOLFENSTEIN-TODEL, C., MIHAESCO, E. and FRANGIONE, B. 'Alpha chain disease' protein DEF: internal deletion of a human immunoglobulin A heavy chain. *Proceedings of the National Academy of Sciences* (Washington), **71,** 974 (1974)

137 WOLFENSTEIN-TODEL, C., MIHAESCO, E. and FRANGIONE, B. Variant of a human immunoglobulin: alpha chain disease protein AIT. *Biochemical Biophysical Research Communications*, **64,** 47 (1975)

138 ZARRABI, M. and ROSNER, R. Middle Eastern lymphoma: report of a case and review of the literature. *American Journal of Medical Sciences*, **272,** 101–119 (1976)

139 ZLOTNICK, A. and EVY, M. Alpha chain disease: a variant of mediterranean lymphoma. *Archives of Internal Medicine*, **128,** 432–436 (1971)

11
Graft-versus-host disease: effects on the intestine

George B. McDonald

Graft-versus-host disease (GVHD) is an immunological illness which results in damage to the skin, liver, and intestinal mucosa. Until recent years, the study of GVHD was a laboratory exercise in animals, but with the advent of bone marrow transplantation in man, it has become a clinical entity as well. Intestinal GVHD is an intriguing illness because it represents an acute but non-infectious insult organs, which is mediated by lymphoid cells from the donor. Thus, the study of an iatrogenic process such as GVHD provides a better understanding of the intestinal lymphoid system and host defense mechanisms; GVHD also provides new insights into the general process of mucosal destruction, as exemplified by inflammatory bowel disease. This chapter will review the acute and chronic effects of GVHD on the intestine in man, including the pathogenesis of mucosal damage. A brief overview of marrow transplantation is provided, to place the intestinal changes in the proper context.

INTRODUCTION: BONE MARROW TRANSPLANTATION IN HUMANS

Transplantation of marrow stem cells is now an accepted treatment for aplastic anemia, refractory leukemias, and certain severe immunodeficiency syndromes[5, 60, 79, 82–84]. Marrow transplantation after ablative therapy for solid tumors and lymphomas is under investigation. Some of the consequences of transplantation, notably GVHD, have been seen in immunosuppressed patients who received donor lymphocytes unintentionally, usually from transfusions of nonirradiated blood products[22, 38, 47]. A GVHD-like illness has also been described as a result of transfer of maternal lymphocytes to the fetus[36].

Conditioning therapy

Patients with aplastic anemia must be given immunosuppressive therapy so that a marrow graft will not be rejected by the host[79, 84]. The usual regimen consists of cyclophosphamide 50 mg/kg on each of four days, followed by donor marrow infusion 36–48 hours later. Conditioning therapy for patients with leukemia[84] also requires total body irradiation (TBI) (10–14 Gy) as well as immunosuppressive drugs. These regimens damage the liver and the intestinal mucosa, higher doses causing more tissue damage[17,75]. The doses of radiation delivered to the mucosa of patients with cancer are significantly higher than those given before marrow transplantation, but because the threshold for mucosal damage by radiation is lowered by concomitant therapy with cytoxic drugs, the acute morphological effects are almost identical[17]. We studied the rectal mucosa in 13 patients undergoing marrow transplantation. Biopsies taken 7–10 days after conditioning were diffusely abnormal, with atypical crypt nuclei, flattened crypt and abnormal surface epithelia, and crypt cell degeneration. These changes persisted in some biopsies taken 16–20 days after conditioning, but all biopsies taken after day 20 were normal unless GVHD was present[7]. In patients who died before day 20, histological features of the small intestine were decreased crypt mitosis, nuclear atypia, and moderate villous blunting; these changes were probably due to conditioning therapy[4]. Clinical symptoms resulting from conditioning therapy include crampy abdominal pain and watery diarrhea, usually present for 10–14 days.

The technique of marrow transplantation

The donor and recipient must have some genetic similarity[84], as determined by tissue typing for the major histocompatibility complex, HLA[2]. Identical twins are matched at all histocompatibility loci; marrow transplantation in such twins is called *syngeneic*. Reinfusion of one's own stored marrow is *autologous* transplantation. Transplantation between nonidentical persons is called *allogeneic*; this usually involves siblings who share haplotypes and who are thus partially matched. However, successful transplantation from phenotypically identical but unrelated donors has been reported[37,56].

The anesthetized donor undergoes multiple marrow aspirations from the iliac crests. The marrow is collected into tissue culture medium, passed through screens to break up particles, and given to the conditioned recipient by intravenous infusion. Marrow stem cells pass through the lungs and then reside almost exclusively in the marrow cavities[84].

Graft-versus-host reactions

The literature in this field uses the term 'GVH reaction' to denote a phenomenon which results from the injection of immunologically competent cells into a genetically different host which is incapable of rejecting these cells[15,73]. In early experiments, the results of lymphoid-mediated cell destruction, immunodeficiency, and infectious processes were not clearly separable, and distinctions were made between 'GVH reaction' and 'GVH disease'. Classic experimental models of GVH reactions include runt disease, secondary disease, parabiosis intoxication, and F_1

hybrid disease; these models are discussed in a recent monograph[73]. For the purposes of this chapter, I will refer to the clinical syndrome GVHD and not the immunological term 'GVH reaction'.

Acute graft-versus-host disease in man

The syndrome of acute GVHD starts 3–7 weeks after transplantation with a red, macular skin rash involving the trunk, palms, soles, and ears. This may be followed by crampy abdominal pain, profuse watery diarrhea, and jaundice[30, 84, 96]. The diagnosis is difficult before day 20, because the histological effects of chemoradiotherapy on the skin and intestinal mucosa can be confused with GVHD[17, 67]. Intestinal infections, especially cytomegalovirus enteritis, can present in an identical fashion to intestinal GVHD. The more severe the organ dysfunction due to GVHD, the worse the prognosis[84, 96]. Grading systems for GVHD have been widely used to guide therapy, and depend on clinical, laboratory, and biopsy data[41, 84]. GVHD occurs in roughly half of HLA-matched allogeneic transplant recipients, and is severe in half of them[96]. Multiple minor histocompatibility loci control GVHD, but methods for identifying these loci are not yet available.

Chronic graft-versus-host disease in man

Chronic GVHD develops insidiously 3 to 12 months after transplanatation in 25 to 40 per cent of long-term survivors of allogeneic marrow transplants[76]. Clinical manifestations include a scleroderma-like skin disease, a generalized 'sicca syndrome', dysphagia due to esophageal mucosal desquamation and webs, pulmonary insufficiency, chronic liver disease, recurrent bacterial infections, and wasting[34, 49, 76, 80]. Striking intestinal changes have occurred in a small number of patients. Treatment with immunosuppressive drugs alters the natural history of this debilitating disease, which differs from acute GVHD in many respects[80].

ACUTE INTESTINAL GRAFT-VERSUS-HOST DISEASE

Clinical presentation

The red, macular skin rash of acute GVHD usually preceeds signs of intestinal involvement, but occasionally the skin changes are apparent only on biopsy[84, 96]. Anorexia, nausea, diarrhea, and crampy abdominal pain appear rapidly. The abdominal pain is widespread over the mid-abdomen, is mild to moderate in severity and worsens after meals. Some patients are very tender in the right lower quadrant, and others have severe, generalized abdominal pain with peritoneal signs on examination. When such signs are present, it is difficult to be sure that bowel perforation and bacterial or fungal peritonitis have not complicated intestinal GVHD. However, signs of peritoneal inflammation are usually due to transmural small bowel involvement with GVHD (*see* X-ray changes in *Figure 11.1*). Intestinal

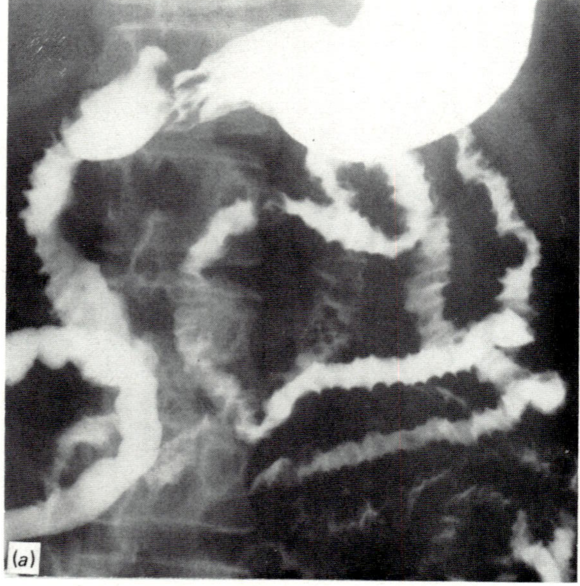

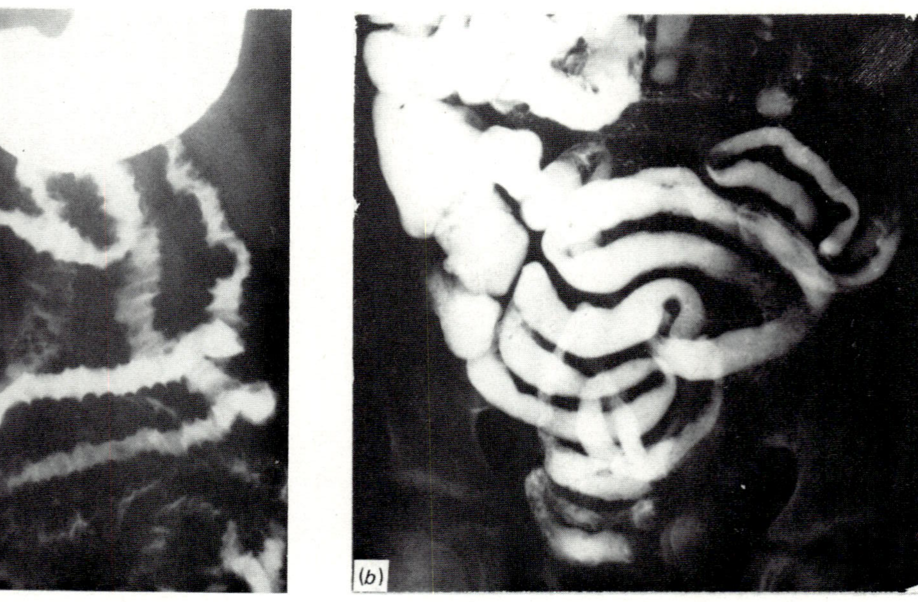

Figure 11.1 Barium X-rays of the intestine during acute graft-versus-host disease in four patients. (*a*) Duodenal and jejunal involvement 33 days after transplantation. There is edema of the intestinal wall, 'thumb-printing,' and effacement of normal folds. (*b*) Ileal involvement 22 days after transplantation. The ileal walls are widened and normal folds effaced to produce this pipe-like appearance

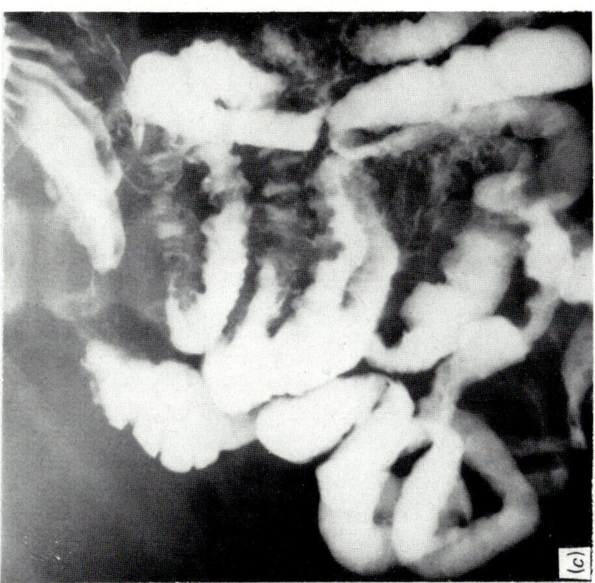

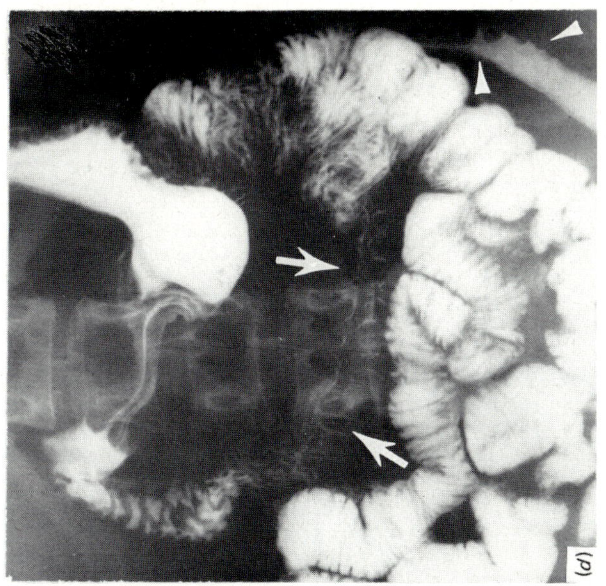

Figure 11.1(*c*) Mid-small intestinal changes 56 days after transplantation. The folds and wall are edematous, with separation of adjacent loops of intestine. (*d*) Colon involvement, seen after rapid transit of barium through the small intestine, 83 days after transplantation. There is mucosal edema and thumb-printing in the transverse colon (large arrows) with edema of the descending colon (small arrows). The stomach and small bowel were normal

ileus may appear with severe GVHD, but this is usually seen only in patients with severe abdominal pain and diarrhea who receive opiates and anticholinergics to control symptoms. (Altered drug metabolism due to venocclusive disease and/or GVHD of the liver may play a role here.) The diarrhea is profuse and watery, persists even when no oral intake is allowed, and can reach 10–15 l/day. Diarrhea volume is a reliable, objective measure of the severity of intestinal GVHD[68, 84]. There is usually occult blood present in the watery stools, but occasionally massive rectal bleeding occurs in amounts of 1–3 liters of blood daily. Such massive bleeding usually occurs in a patient with severe GVHD and thrombocytopenia, and is the result of generalized mucosal oozing. However, isolated ulcers in the stomach, duodenum, small bowel, and right colon can occur in this setting, due either to stress or infectious causes.

Laboratory examinations show the stools to be mucoid and green-colored; ropy 'casts' of mucus and exfoliated debris can be passed. Fecal leukocytes are present in large numbers, but fungal, viral, and bacterial pathogens are absent unless an infection has supervened. Parasites and toxins of *Clostridium difficile* are also absent. Serum albumin levels drop precipitously with severe intestinal GVHD, due to massive protein-losing enteropathy[11, 30, 98]. This can be demonstrated by chromium-51 or α-1-antitrypsin determinations in stool water, but this is not necessary clinically.

Radiology

Barium X-ray studies of the small intestine are useful in establishing a diagnosis of GVHD, particularly in patients with granulocytopenia and thrombocytopenia in whom mucosal biopsy would be dangerous (*Figure 11.1*). Although there are problems with both sensitivity and specificity of X-ray examinations, the finding of a diffusely abnormal small bowel in the absence of pathogens on stool examination in a patient with biopsy-proven GVHD of the skin allows a confident diagnosis of intestinal GVHD. There is mucosal and submucosal edema throughout the intestine in the acute phase: gastric folds are enlarged, the small intestinal wall is thickened, small intestinal circular folds are effaced, and a 'thumb-printing pattern' of bowel-wall edema is common[21, 65, 74]. There is excessive luminal fluid and rapid transit of barium to the colon. Barium enema examinations may show mucosal ulcerations, lack of haustral markings, and transmural thickening[21, 65]. However, very early in the course of GVHD, intestinal X-rays may be normal, presumably because the changes are microscopic. The gross small intestinal changes on X-ray, however, are not specific. Similar findings have been described with acute radiation enteritis, Henoch-Schönlein purpura, and cytomegalovirus enteritis, for example[27, 63, 85].

X-rays taken later, up to 12 weeks after the onset of intestinal symptoms, may show total effacement of folds in the mid- and distal small intestine. These ribbon-like segments of bowel alternate with radiologically normal areas, giving a pattern which is diagnostic of GVHD in the marrow transplant setting[21]. Patients with such severe, untreatable GVHD are unlikely to survive.

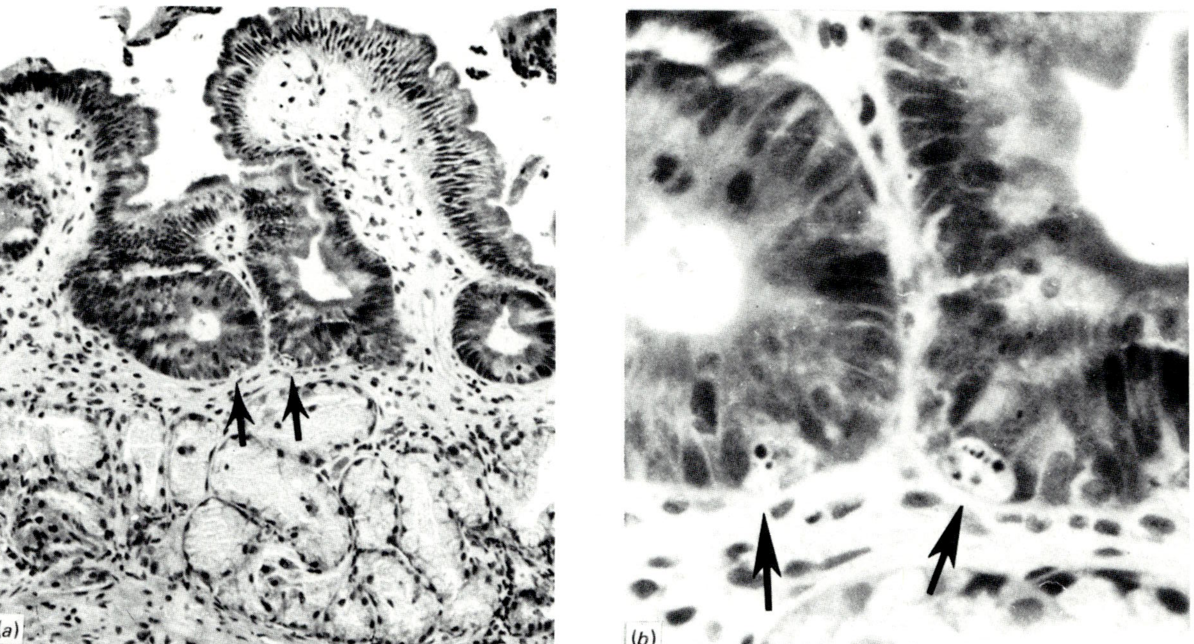

Figure 11.2 Duodenal biopsy taken 42 days after transplantation, showing Grade I graft-versus-host disease. (*a*) Low power view of normal villous architecture overlying Brunner's glands. The arrows point to areas of crypt cell necrosis. (*b*) High power view of the same crypts, illustrating 'apoptotic bodies' (membrane-bound karyolytic fragments resulting from crypt cell necrosis)

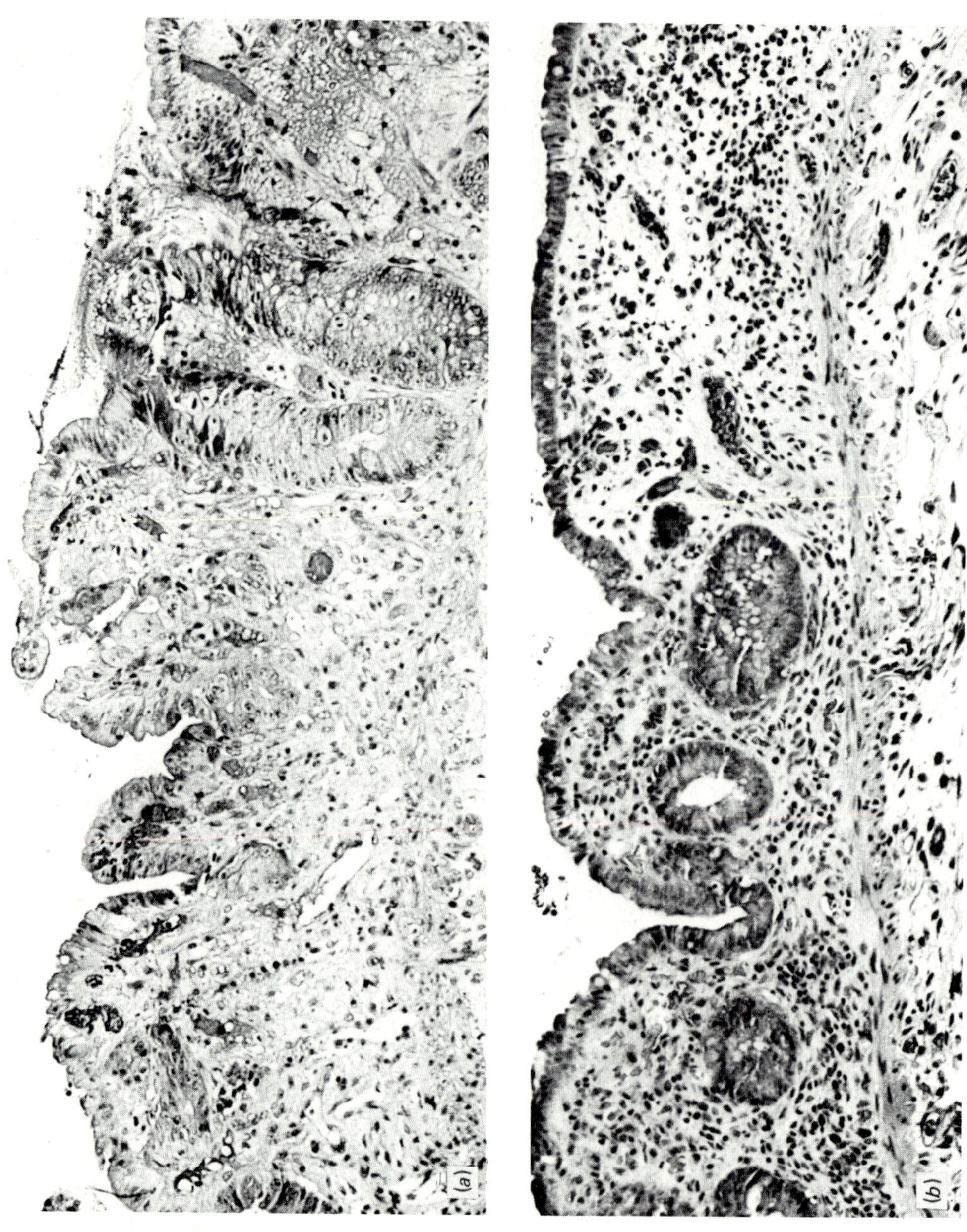

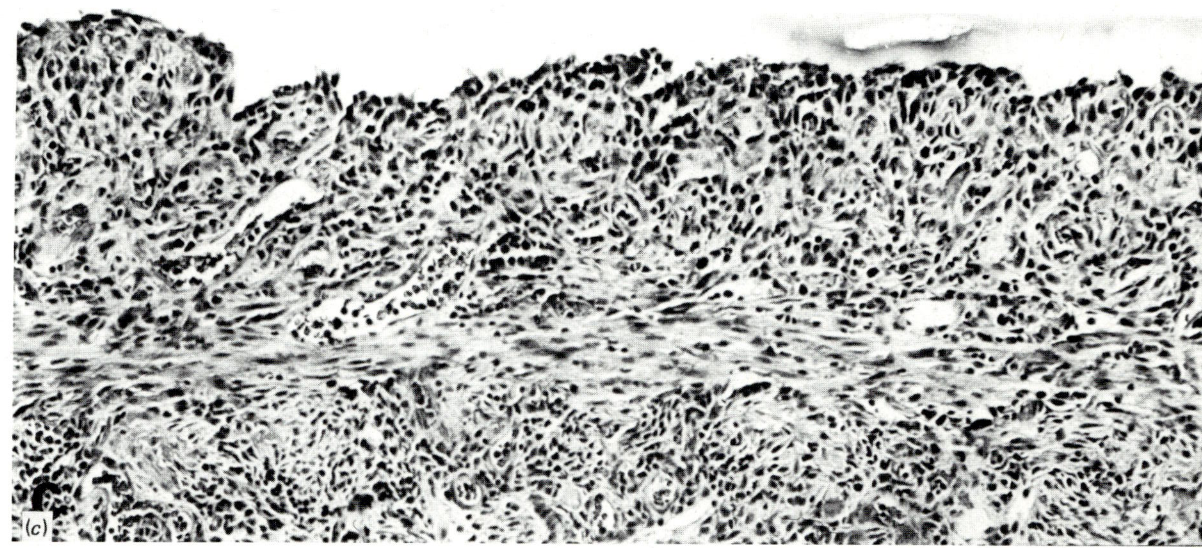

Figure 11.3 Small intestinal biopsies demonstrating more severe graft-versus-host disease in two patients. (*a*) Jejunal biopsy taken 39 days after transplantation, showing Grade III graft-versus-host disease. There is blunting of villi, loss of mucus, and dropout of several crypts. (*b*) Mucosa from resected segment of mid-small intestine, removed at surgery because of intestinal bleeding 75 days after transplantation. There is loss of villous architecture, dropout of crypts, submucosal edema, and a cuboidal surface epithelium. (Grade III GVHD) (*c*) Mucosa from another area of the same resected intestine, showing Grade IV GVHD. There is loss of villi, crypts, and surface cells. Bacteria, viruses and fungi were not identified in this specimen

Endoscopy

Fiberoptic upper endoscopy can be useful in patients with suspected acute intestinal GVHD, but more commonly is used to determine whether infections (CMV, herpes simplex, *Candida*) are the cause of epigastric pain, vomiting, or intestinal bleeding. Autopsy studies, intestinal X-rays, and rectal biopsies show that intestinal GVHD affects all of the intestine, at least at a microscopic level[17, 68]. The duodenal folds may be friable, with punctate areas of intramural hemorrhage. With severe disease, serpiginous areas of mucosal sloughing are apparent in the duodenum, but the stomach is usually spared from gross involvement. Biopsies of normal-appearing duodenal mucosa may show histologic GVHD, reflecting more severe distal intestinal damage. This is analogous to the rectum, where gross changes are uncommon, but biopsies accurately reflect ileal and right colon GVHD[68].

Histology

This is illustrated in *Figures 11.2* and *11.3*. Information about the small intestinal histology of GVHD in man is derived from autopsy material, from a limited number of peroral and endoscopic biopsies, from an occasional surgical specimen, and by inference from rectal histology. A prospective study of intestinal histology is difficult because the ileum is inaccessible and because jejunal biopsies are dangerous in acutely ill patients with few platelets. The lesions of acute GVHD range from necrosis of individual crypt cells to total loss of mucosa, with the most severe involvement in the ileum and right colon[45, 68, 77, 78, 88]. With severe GVHD, there are often sheets of bacteria, fungi, and debris lining the few epithelial cells which remain[4]. One can speculate about the sequence of changes which leads to this end-stage histology, but firm data is lacking.

The earliest event of intestinal GVHD is that of individual crypt cell necrosis. By light microscopy, there are accumulations of membrane-bound-karyolytic fragments at the base or side of crypts. These have been termed 'apoptotic bodies,' 'exploding crypts' and 'karyolytic bodies'[17, 25, 46, 78]. This form of crypt cell necrosis is not specific for GVHD; it has been described with chemoradiation therapy, inflammatory bowel disease, and infectious colitis[1, 13, 17, 25, 32, 57]. However, unlike these diseases, the crypt cell necrosis in early GVHD is usually a very focal finding, unaccompanied by widespread inflammation or cell destruction[17, 25]. A blinded, prospective study of these changes in rectal biopsies showed them to be specific for GVHD if biopsies were done after day 20, by which time the histological effects of chemoradiation therapy had resolved[17]. However, there was neither lymphoid proliferation nor lymphoid cytorrhexis in the vicinity of the 'exploding crypt' lesions on light microscopy[17]. By electron microscopy, lymphocytes indented the cytoplasmic membranes of crypt cells by point contact, and extended broad pseudopods to their nuclear membranes[25]. Both coagulative necrosis and the development of the characteristic membrane-bound karyolytic fragments were evidence of damage to individual crypt cells[25]. These changes are similar to those described with GVHD of the skin and liver[3,24]. Lamina propria lymphocytes appeared viable, in contrast to earlier studies in monkeys, which demonstrated migration of lymphocytes into intestinal crypts, with necrosis of both lymphocytes and crypt cells[78,102]. These monkeys were studied during a time when the effects of conditioning therapy on the mucosa were probably still present. Ultrastructural findings in an F_1 hybrid murine model of GVHD are similar: large lymphocytes contact crypt cells, which become damaged in a manner similar to that described above[73].

The lesions of more extensive GVHD include cystic dilatation of crypts containing cellular debris, hyperplastic crypts with abnormal villous architecture, dropout of whole crypts with a flat overlying villous architecture, and finally total denudation of the epithelium, which may be replaced by a single, cuboidal cell layer[4, 45, 68, 78, 88]. The 'exploding crypt' lesions are disproportionately infrequent in patients with extensive mucosal destruction, leading some to suggest that while the initial insult may be on crypt cells, the more severe destruction is related to either a lamina propria lymphoid reaction or to local immunodeficiency with bacterial invasion of the mucosa[4]. Autopsy material is too crude to allow many definite conclusions about pathogenetic mechanisms.

A grading system for intestinal GVHD based on histology was published in 1979, but did not include the finding of individual crypt cell necrosis[68]. The following is a revised system.

Grade I Individual crypt cell necrosis (apoptosis).
Grade II Crypt abscess, crypt cell flattening, with or without crypt cell necrosis.
Grade III Dropout of one or more whole crypts in a biopsy specimen.
Grade IV Total denudation of epithelium.

The focal crypt changes are probably more specific for GVHD than is extensive mucosal damage, which can result from many destructive processes. Clinically, rectal biopsy will continue to be more useful than proximal small intestinal biopsy.

Intestinal immunodeficiency in graft-versus-host disease

The intestinal lymphoid system in GVHD has been examined in autopsy material from primates and man. Two processes have been described, 'aggressor lymphocyte' destruction which is detailed above, and the 'lymphoid response'[103]. The lymphoid response has been described in lymph nodes, spleen, and Peyer's patches of the intestine, and consists of early lymphoid proliferation, then lymphoid atrophy, then lymphoid reconstitution[9, 12, 103]. However, it is unclear how much of the lymphoid atrophy is due to conditioning therapy and how much to GVHD. Studies in dogs and man do not confirm lymphoid atrophy as an integral part of GVHD[14, 45, 55]. A retrospective autopsy study of lymphoid cellularity in man showed that all graft recipients (including syngeneic and autologous grafts) had depletion of lymphocytes in Peyer's patches and mesenteric lymph nodes in the first 130 days after transplant[4]. Furthermore, severity of GVHD was not related to lymphoid cellularity in these areas. However, patients autopsied after day 130 showed more normal cellularity in Peyer's patches, with good follicles and germinal centers and good cellularity in the B- and T-cell regions of mesenteric lymph nodes[4]. Lymphoid morphology appears more normal about 7 months after marrow grafting[14, 45].

More striking differences between GVHD and non-GVHD patients were apparent on examination of lamina propria plasma cell populations. Patients with acute GVHD had a marked depletion of IgA- and IgM-bearing plasma cells[4]. The same finding has been reported in mice with acute GVHD[31]. Patients with more severe GVHD had a greater depletion, but control patients (those with syngeneic and autologous grafts) had numerous IgA- and IgM-bearing plasma cells in the lamina propria[4]. These studies suggest that local immunodeficiency plays an important role in the severe mucosal destruction of acute GVHD. However, the relative importance of crypt cell destruction by lymphocytes and local immunodeficiency is unclear. A prospective study of marrow grafting in a protected environment (which included non-absorbable antibiotics by mouth) showed no differences in the incidence of GVHD between treatment and control groups, but the onset of clinical GVHD was delayed in treated patients[6]. The severity of GVHD was the same in both groups. Animal studies, however, show that germ-free marrow graft recipients and those 'decontaminated' by antibiotics have less severe GVHD[10, 40, 42, 89–91, 94].

Malabsorption in intestinal graft-versus-host disease

There is gross malabsorption of water, electrolytes, and nutrients when GVHD has caused extensive small intestinal destruction. Malabsorption also occurs with less extensive lesions, but the mechanisms remain unexplored in man. When patients with acute GVHD try to eat, crampy abdominal pain and diarrhea usually result[26]. Sucrose and lactose intolerance are common, particularly during the recovery phase of GVHD when appetite returns[26]. Brush border oligo- and disaccharidases may be diminished, as suggested in a mouse model of GVHD[39]. Malabsorption of fat also occurs clinically and in the grafted mouse[66]. The profuse watery diarrhea may result from isolated crypt damage (increased secretion), villous cell damage (decreased absorption), or loss of ileal absorptive capacity for water and electrolytes. Extensive ileal damage probably leads to bile salt malabsorption and 'cholerrheic enteropathy'; bile salt depletion has been described in the runted mouse[58]. As noted above, protein-losing enteropathy is a common feature of intestinal GVHD in mice as well as in man[11, 98].

Differential diagnosis

In the first 3 weeks after transplantation, the intestinal effects of chemoradiation conditioning therapy may be confused with acute GVHD[17]. This is a problem when a graft has been established or when florid GVHD occurs earlier than usual. Skin and rectal biopsies are less accurate before day 20; but clinically, the occurrence of worsening diarrhea, jaundice, and skin rash at a time when the effects of conditioning therapy should be resolving strongly suggest acute GVHD. Characteristic intestinal X-rays and the absence of pathogens in the stool are additional useful clues.

Intestinal infections remain the most troublesome differential diagnosis. Although many infections can mimic the intestinal symptoms of acute GVHD, the more difficult problem is telling when an infectious process has complicated GVHD. Most of the known intestinal defenses to microbial infection are deranged in patients with GVHD[48]. Clusters and sheets of bacteria (most acquired from the hospital environment) can be found throughout the intestine of such patients at autopsy[4, 68, 70, 100]. The resistant aerobic Gram-negative rods predominate (*Pseudomonas, Serratia, Citrobacter*, etc.), but known bacterial pathogens (*Salmonella, Campylobacter, Yersinia*, etc.) are unusual in the highly protected transplant environment[4, 6, 100]. The concept of diminished 'colonization resistance' has been developed to explain why these aerobic bacteria colonize the bowel[92]. In animals, the anaerobic flora prevent colonization by aerobic organisms. Use of antibiotics suppresses the anaerobic flora, removing the resistance factor and allowing colonization by aerobes and fungi[70, 71]. Clinical studies suggest that selective (rather than total) suppression of the microflora will maintain colonization resistance[93, 99]. Pseudomembranous colitis due to *Clostridium difficile* toxin is occasionally seen, but not as often as one would expect with poly-antibiotic usage[104].

Fungal mucosal infections are commonly due to *Candida* or *Torula* species[18]. Presenting symptoms include fever, diarrhea, and abdominal pain[44]. The diagnosis rests on demonstrating infiltration of mucosa by hyphae, usually by endoscopic biopsy of visible lesions[43, 59]. A presumptive diagnosis can be made by demonstrating hyphae (rather than yeast forms) in the stool or by having large colony counts on stool culture[44, 71].

Cytomegalovirus is the most common viral pathogen after marrow transplantation. There are many sources of CMV in transplant patients: activation of virus in the host, acquisition from donor cells, and infection from blood products[51–53, 101]. CMV infections in the intestine have been described as secondary invaders when mucosal disease was present already[33, 64]. In an immunosuppressed host, however, CMV can clearly be a primary pathogen, producing abdominal pain, ulcerations, watery diarrhea, protein-losing enteropathy, typhlitis, and diffuse colitis[7, 23, 81, 85, 87, 97]. The diagnosis depends on finding typical cytopathic effects in biopsy material and culturing the virus from various secretions. Adenovirus, rotavirus, and coxsackievirus infections have be shown to be a major cause of gastroenteritis in immunodeficient patients[69, 104, 105]. Special enzyme-immunoassay techniques were used to identify these pathogens in a recent prospective survey of marrow graft recipients[104].

Commonly acquired parasites in immunodeficient patients are *Giardia lamblia* and coccidia species[8]. Three species of coccidia can infest the small intestinal and colonic mucosa: these are *Isopora belli*, *Isopora natalensis* and *Cryptosporidium*[8, 50, 54, 97]. Despite the tiny size of these organisms they can be demonstrated in fecal specimens and mucosal biopsies[8, 54, 86, 97]. Dissemination of endogenous parasites such as intestinal protozoa and nematodes is a problem when a patient becomes immunosuppressed[8, 72].

Natural history of intestinal graft-versus-host disease

As might be expected, patients with moderate and severe GVHD do worse than those with mild disease. Clinical grading systems have been used to categorize patients[41, 84, 96]. Treatment of established GVHD is unsatisfactory, especially for severely affected cases. High-dose prednisone and antithymocyte globulin have been widely used[95, 96]. Cyclosporin A and monoclonal antibodies directed against T cells are being studied. However, acute GVHD has a finite life span, suggesting that the relationship between donor lymphocytes and host intestinal cells changes with time. Several theories have been advanced to explain the 'cessation of immunologic hostilities,' such as the loss of aggressor T cells, a loss of antigenic stimulation, and the development of a population of graft lymphocytes tolerant to host histocompatibility antigens[73].

Pathogenesis of intestinal graft-versus-host disease

Three theories have been brought forth to explain mucosal disintegration in acute GVHD. These are the 'innocent bystander' theory; the 'cytotoxic lymphocyte' theory; and the 'immunodeficiency/super-infection' theory.

The first two immunological theories arise from observations that numerous lymphocytes are seen in the mucosa of animals with acute GVHD, as well as in intestinal allografts. The 'innocent bystander' theory states that cell-mediated immune reactions in the lamina propria release lymphokines, which are non-specifically toxic to cells in the vicinity[35]. Support for this theory comes from experiments in which grafts of small intestine which were syngeneic to donor cells were placed either under the kidney capsule of the host, or subcutaneously[16, 89]. When donor cells were infused, a GVHD reaction ensued, damaging the intestinal graft. Since the damaged intestinal cells were histocompatible with donor lymphocytes, they were an unlikely target for an 'aggressor lymphocyte' assault. In human GVHD involving skin and intestine, the most prominent injury occurs in less differentiated cells, but differentiated cells in the vicinity (melanocytes in the skin, enteroendocrine cells in the intestine) are injured as well. This may be an example of the innocent bystander phenomenon[24, 25]. Variations on this theme suggest that viruses and chemicals can alter cell surface antigens, leading to GVH reactions in the vicinity of intestinal epithelial cells[28, 29].

The 'cytotoxic lymphocyte' theory states that donor lymphocytes react against antigens on the surface of host crypt cells, causing their destruction[73, 78, 88]. Our electron microscopic studies of human intestinal GVHD support this theory, which requires demonstration of direct cell-to-cell contact and viable lymphocytes which survive their contact with crypt cells. In acute GVHD, viable lymphocytes are seen near degenerating crypt cells, but they are not present in large numbers[25]. There is point contact by lymphocytes on crypt cells, as mentioned above. This may represent the recognition phase of alloimmune lymphocyte attack on crypt cells. The lysis of target cells by cytotoxic T-lymphocytes probably involves several steps. After recognition of alloantigens, there is conjugation to the membrane, activation of lymphotoxins, and lysis of the target cell. The lymphocyte then detaches, and is presumably capable of another encounter.

The 'immunodeficiency/super-infection' theory suggests that a donor-host lymphoid cell interaction results in immunodeficiency, allowing microbial invasion of the mucosa. Studies in animals show enhanced survival and less crypt cell damage during GVHD when the host is germ-free or 'decontaminated'[10, 40, 42, 89–91, 94]. One hypothesis states that antigens on certain intestinal bacteria cross-react with antigens on intestinal epithelial cells[89]. When bacteria penetrate the mucosa, lymphocytes react against the bacteria and cell antigens. There is little support for this theory in man, and cross-reacting antigens have not been identified. Many patients with florid intestinal GVHD are without evidence of infection, either morphologically or clinically[68]. However, there is evidence that the bacterial flora and intestinal immune defenses play a crucial role in super-infections of established acute GVHD[4].

Each of the 3 theories has some validity in explaining the mucosal denudation in patients dying of acute GVHD, but the primary event seems to be a direct, lymphocyte-mediated crypt cell lysis. Neighboring cells may be damaged in the process. The immunodeficiency which results from depletion of lamina propria IgA- and IgM-bearing plasma cells may lead to bacterial colonization, further mucosal destruction, and sepsis.

To make this field even more complex, some have suggested that GVHD lesions can occur in patients receiving syngeneic marrow grafts[15, 61]. The hypothesis offered to explain this phenomenon states that a deficiency of suppressor T cells after transplantation allows syngeneic 'aggressor lymphocytes' to damage host target cells[61, 62]. However, clinically significant GVHD is unusual in recipients of syngeneic marrow for either malignancy or aplasia[19, 20].

CHRONIC INTESTINAL GVHD IN MAN

Clinical presentation

Small intestinal involvement is uncommon in patients with chronic GVHD, but we have seen five such patients with malabsorption. Most patients who develop chronic GVHD have had acute GVHD earlier in their post-transplant course. In some, the acute process melds into the chronic disease. In others, the acute process resolves completely before chronic GVHD becomes apparent. In yet others, chronic GVHD develops *de novo*, without antecedent acute GVHD[76].

Patients whose severe acute GVHD does not respond to treatment do not usually survive to develop chronic GVHD. Four patients with chronic GVHD developed intractable diarrhea, pan-malabsorption, crampy abdominal pain, and severe malnutrition. In two of them, acute GVHD never really resolved before signs of chronic GVHD were noted; in two, acute GVHD had resolved before chronic GVHD appeared. Each of these patients was seen early in our experience with chronic GVHD, before effective therapy was recognized[76]. Treatment of chronic GVHD with immunosuppressive drugs alters the natural history of this disease, such that we have not seen extensive intestinal disease in recent years[80]. The fifth patient was a recent case with moderately severe chronic GVHD who had chronic diarrhea and moderate malabsorption.

Intestinal structure and function

The patients with severe malabsorption had coefficients of fat absorption of 30–50 percent, but small intestinal X-rays and jejunal biopsies were normal. In one well-studied patient, intraluminal digestion of a Lundh test meal was normal, adequate bile salt concentrations were achieved in luminal water, and a Schilling test with intrinsic factor was normal. At autopsy, there was normal villous architecture, focal fibrosis in the lamina propria, and segmental fibrosis of the submucosal and serosal layers, extending from stomach to colon[76]. There was also hyalinization of serosal and submucosal blood vessels, with subendothelial basal lamina replication. The smooth muscle layers were normal. We suspect that lymphatic blockade due to fibrosis in the submucosa led to severe malabsorption. In two patients whose acute GVHD became chronic GVHD, widespread colonic submucosal fibrosis and mucosal calcification was present at autopsy[76].

The fifth patient with malabsorption demonstrated less severe disease, with a coefficient of fat absorption of 62 percent. Intestinal X-rays and biopsies were normal, but cultures of jejunal fluid showed $>10^4$ *Pseudomonas* and *Candida* species. He had cholestasis due to chronic GVHD of the liver, giving two likely explanations for his steatorrhea (bacterial overgrowth and deficient bile salts). However, his steatorrhea responded dramatically to ingestion of non-absorbable antibiotics and nystatin.

CONCLUSIONS

Intestinal graft-versus-host disease remains an enigma despite recent descriptions of the clinical and pathologic process. Although lamina propria lymphocytes are involved in crypt cell destruction and mucosal disintegration, the way in which they effect cytolysis is unknown. Extensive mucosal denudation probably results from lymphocyte-mediated cell destruction from one side and from the action of luminal constituents (microorganisms, pancreatic enzymes) from the other. The immunological assault on target organs is finite, a phenomenon which is also unexplained. The return of local immune defenses is long delayed after allogeneic marrow transplantation, which leads to problems in the diagnosis of GVHD. Microorganisms can cause an enteritis which mimics GVHD, or can superinfect already damaged mucosa. Some patients develop extensive submucosal fibrosis as part of their chronic GVHD, a process whose pathophysiology is poorly understood.

There are more questions than answers at this point. However an arcane disease such as GVHD is a model which might bring understanding to other intestinal diseases in which mucosal disintegration is prominent. The relationship between epithelial cells and their lamina propria lymphocytes not only provides a barrier to luminal organisms, but may also be important in maintaining cell integrity. Developments in our understanding of intestinal immunology will come rapidly in the next decade, answering many of these questions.

References

1 ALUWIHARE, A. P. Electron microscopy in Crohn's disease. *Gut*, **12,** 509–518 (1971)

2 BACH, F. H. and VAN ROOD, J. J. The major histocompatibility complex – genetics and biology. *New England Journal of Medicine*, **295,** 806–813, 871–878 and 927–936 (1976)

3 BERNUAU, D., GISSELBRECHT, C., DEVERGIE, A., FELDMANN, G., GLUCKMAN, E., MARTY, M. and BOIRON, M. Histological and ultrastructural appearance of the liver during graft-versus-host disease complicating bone marrow transplantation. *Transplantation*, **29,** 236–244 (1980)

4 BESCHORNER, W. E., YARDLEY, J. H., TUTSCHKA, P. J. and SANTOS, G. W. Deficiency of intestinal immunity with graft-versus-host disease in humans. *Journal of Infectious Diseases*, **144,** 38–46 (1981)

5 BLUME, K. G., BEUTLER, E., BROSS, K. J., CHILLAR, R. K., ELLINGTON, O. B., FAHEY, J. L., FARBSTEIN, M. J., FORMAN, S. J., SCHMIDT, G. M., SCOTT, E. P. *et al.* Bone marrow ablation and allogeneic marrow transplantation in acute leukemia. *New England Journal of Medicine*, **302,** 1041–1046 (1980)

6 BUCKNER, C. D., CLIFT, R. A., SANDERS, J. E, MEYERS, J. D., COUNTS, G. W., FAREWELL, V. T., THOMAS, E. D. and THE SEATTLE MARROW TRANSPLANT TEAM. Protective environment for marrow transplant recipients. A prospective study. *Annals of Internal Medicine*, **89,** 893–901 (1978)

7 CAMPBELL, D. A., PIERCEY, J. R., SCHNITKA, T. K., GOLDSAND, G., DEVINE, R. D. O. and WEINSTEIN, W. M. Cytomegalovirus-associated gastric ulcer. *Gastroenterology*, **72,** 533–535 (1977)

8 CATTY, D. and ROSS, I. N. Immunological aspects of infection with gastrointestinal parasites (protozoa and nematodes). In *Immunology of the Gastrointestinal Tract*, edited by P. Asquith, 246–267. Edinburgh, Churchill Livingstone (1979)

9 CHOMETTE, G., MATHE, G., AURIOL, M., BROCHERIOUS, C. and PINAUDEAU, Y. Le syndrome secondaire chez l'homme. Etudes anatomique de six case de leucemie traites par greffe allogenique de moelle osseuse apres irradiation totale. *Virchows Archiv* (*Pathologische Anatomie*), **349,** 98–114 (1970)

10 CONNELL, M. S. and WILSON, R. The treatment of x-irradiated germfree CFW and C3H mice with isologous and homologous bone marrow. *Life Science*, **4,** 721–729 (1965)

11 CORNELIUS, E. A. Protein-losing enteropathy in the graft-versus-host reaction. *Transplantation*, **9,** 247–252 (1970)

12 De VRIES, M. J. Pathology of secondary disease in primates. In *Proceedings of the International Symposium on Bone Marrow Therapy and Chemical Protection in Irradiated Primates*, 101–111 The Netherlands, Krips, (1962)

13 DOBBINS, W. O. Diagnostic pathology of the intestine and colon. In *Diagnostic Electron Microscopy*, Volume 1, edited by B. F. Trump and R. T. Jones, 253–339. New York, John Wiley & Sons (1978)

14 DRENGUIS, W. R. and SALE, G. E. Lymph node repopulation after bone marrow transplantation (abstract). *Clinical Research*, **26,** 161A (1978)

15 ELKINS, W. L. An immunogenetic approach to the graft-versus-host reaction and secondary disease. In *Biology of Bone Marrow Transplantation*, edited by R. P. Gale and C. F. Fox, 195–207. New York, Academic Press (1980)

16 ELSON, C. O., REILLY, R. W. and ROSENBERG, I. H. Small intestinal injury in the graft-versus-host reaction: an innocent bystander phenomenon. *Gastroenterology*, **72,** 886–889 (1977)

17 EPSTEIN, R. J., McDONALD, G. B., SALE, G. E., SHULMAN, H. M. and THOMAS, E. D. The diagnostic accuracy of the rectal biopsy in acute graft-versus-host disease: a prospective study of thirteen patients. *Gastroenterology*, **78,** 764–771 (1980)

18 ERAS, P., GOLDSTEIN, M. J. and SHERLOCK, P. *Candida* infection of the gastrointestinal tract. *Medicine*, **51,** 367–379 (1972)

19 FEFER, A., BUCKNER, C. D., THOMAS, E. D., CHEEVER, M. A., CLIFT, R. A., GLUCKSBERG, H., NEIMAN, P. E. and STORB, R. Cure of hematologic neoplasia with transplantation of marrow from identical twins. *New England Journal of Medicine*, **297,** 146–148 (1977)

20 FEFER, A., EINSTEIN, A. B., THOMAS, E. D., BUCKNER, C. D., CLIFT, R. A., GLUCKSBERG, H., NEIMAN, P. E. and STORB, R. Bone-marrow transplantation for hematologic neoplasia in 16 patients with identical twins. *New England Journal of Medicine*, **290,** 1390–1393 (1974)

21 FISK, J. D., SHULMAN, H. M., GREENING, R. R., McDONALD, G. B, SALE, G. E. and THOMAS, E. D. Gastrointestinal radiographic features of human graft-versus-host disease. *American Journal of Roentgenology*, **136,** 329–336 (1981)

22 FORD, J. M., LUCEY, J. J., CULLEN, M. H., TOBIAS, J. S. and LISTER, T. A. Fatal graft-versus-host disease following transfusion of granulocytes from normal donors. *Lancet*, **2,** 1167–1169 (1976)

23 FREEMAN, H. J., SCHNITKA, T. K., PIERCEY, J. R. and WEINSTEIN, W. M. Cytomegalovirus infection of the gastrointestinal tract in a patient with late onset immunodeficiency syndrome. *Gastroenterology*, **73,** 1397–1403 (1977)

24 GALLUCCI, B. B., SHULMAN, H. M., SALE, G. E., LERNER, K. G., CALDWELL, L. E. and THOMAS, E. D. The ultrastructure of the human epidermis in chronic graft-versus-host disease. *American Journal of Pathology*, **95,** 643–662 (1979)

25 GALLUCCI, B., SALE, G. E., McDONALD, G. B., EPSTEIN, R., SHULMAN, H. M. and THOMAS, E. D. The fine structure of human rectal epithelium in acute graft-versus-host disease. *American Journal of Surgical Pathology* (in press)

26 GAUVREAU, J. M., LENSSEN, P., DHENEY, C. L., AKER, S. N., HUTCHINSON, M. L. and BARALE, K. V. Nutritional management of patients with intestinal graft-versus-host disease. *Journal of the American Dietetic Association*, **79,** 673–677 (1981)

27 GLASIER, C. M., SIEGEL, M. J., McALISTER, W. H. and SHACKELFORD, G. D. Henoch-Schonlein syndrome in children: gastrointestinal manifestations. *American Journal of Roentgenology*, **136,** 1018–1085 (1981)

28 GLEICHMANN, H. Studies on the mechanism of drug sensitisation: T-cell-dependent popliteal lymph node reaction to diphenylhydantoin. *Clinical Immunology and Immunopathology*, **18,** 203–211 (1981)

29 GLEICHMANN, E. and GLEICHMANN, H. Spectrum of disease caused by autoreactive T cells, mode of sensitization to the drug diphenylhydantoin, and possible role of SLE-typical self antigens in B-cells triggering. In *Immunoregulation and Autoimmunity*, edited by R. S. Krakauer and M. K. Cathcard, 73–83. North Holland, Elsevier (1980)

30 GLUCKSBERG, H., STORB, R., FEFER, A. BUCKNER, C. D., NEIMAN, P. E., CLIFT, R. A., LERNER, K. A. and THOMAS, E. D. Clinical manifestations of graft-versus-host disease in human recipients of marrow in HLA-matched sibling donors. *Transplantation*, **18,** 295–304 (1974)

31 GOLD, J. A., KOSEK, J., WANEK, N. and BAUR, S. Duodenal immunoglobulin deficiency in graft-versus-host disease (*GVHD*) mice. *Journal of Immunology*, **117,** 471–476 (1976)

32 GONZALEZ-LICEA, A. and YARDLEY, J. H. A comparative ultrastructural study of the mucosa in idiopathic ulcerative colitis, shigellosis and other human colonic disease. *Bulletin of the Johns Hopkins Hospital*, **118,** 444–461 (1966)

33 GOODMAN, Z. D.,BOITNOTT, J. K. and YARDLEY, J. H. Perforation of the colon associated with cytomegalovirus infection. *Digestive Diseases and Sciences*, **24,** 376–380 (1979)

34 GRAZE, P. R. and GALE, R. P. Chronic graft-versus-host disease: a syndrome of disordered immunity. *American Journal of Medicine*, **66,** 611–620 (1979)

35 GREBE, S. C. and STREILEN, J. W. Graft-versus-host reaction: a review. *Advances in Immunology*, **22,** 119–221 (1976)

36 GROGAN, T. M., BROUGHTON, D. D. and DOYLE, W. F. Graft-versus-host reaction (GvHR): a case report suggesting GvHR occurred as a result of a maternofetal cell transfer. *Archives of Pathology*, **99,** 330–334 (1975)

37 HANSEN, J. A., CLIFT, R. A., THOMAS, E. D., BUCKNER, C. D., STORB, R. and GIBLETT, E. R. Transplantation of marrow from an unrelated donor to a patient with acute leukemia. *New England Journal of Medicine*, **303,** 565–567 (1980)

38 HATHAWAY, W. E., BRANGLE, R. W., NELSON, T. L. and ROECKEL, I. E. Aplastic anaemia and alymphocytosis in an infant with hypogammaglobulinemia: graft-versus-host reaction? *Journal of Pediatrics*, **68,** 713–716 (1966)

39 HEDBERG, C. A., REISER, S. and REILLY, R. W. Intestinal phase of the runting syndrome in mice. *Transplantation*, **6,** 104–110 (1968)

40 HEIT, H., WILSON, R., FLIEDNER, T. M. and KOHNE, E. Mortality of secondary disease in antibiotic-treated mouse radiation chimeras. In *Germfree Research: Biological Effects and Gnotobiotic Environment*, edited by J. B. Henneghan, 477–485. New York, Academic Press (1973)

41 HERSHKO, C. and GALE, R. P. GVHD scoring system for predicting survival and specific mortality in bone marrow transplant recipients. In *Biology of Bone Marrow Transplantation*, edited by R. P. Gale and C. F. Fox, 59–67 New York, Academic Press (1980)

42 JONES, J. M., WILSON, R. and BEALMEAR, P. M. Mortality and gross pathology of secondary disease in germfree mouse radiation chimeras. *Radiation Research*, **45,** 577–588 (1971)

43 JOSHI, S. N., GARVIN, P. J. and SUNWOOD, Y. C. Candidiasis of the duodenum and jejunum. *Gastroenterology*, **80,** 829–833 (1981)

44 KANE, J. G., CHRETIEN, J. H. and GARAGUSI, V. F. Diarrhoea caused by *Candida. Lancet*, **1,** 335–336 (1976)

45 KOLB, H., SALE, G. E., LERNER, K. G., STORB, R. and THOMAS, E. D. Pathology of acute graft-versus-host disease in the dog. *American Journal of Pathology*, **96,** 581–592 (1979)

46 LERNER, K. G., KAO, G. F., STORB, R., BUCKNER, C. D., CLIFT, R. A. and THOMAS, E. D. Histopathology of graft-versus-host reaction (GvHR) in human recipients of marrow from HLA-matched sibling donors. *Transplant Proceedings*, **6,** 367–371 (1974)

47 LOWENTHAL, R. M., MENON, C. and CHALLIS, D. R. Graft-versus-host disease in consecutive patients with acute myeloid leukemia treated with blood cells from normal donors. *Australia New Zealand Journal of Medicine*, **11,** 179–183 (1981)

48 McCLELLAND, D. B. L. Bacterial and viral infections of the gastrointestinal tract. In *Immunology of the Gastrointestinal Tract*, edited by Asquith, P., 214–245 Edinburgh, Churchill Livingstone (1979)

49 McDONALD, G. B., SULLIVAN, K. M., SCHUFFLER, M. D., SHULMAN, H. M. and THOMAS, E. D. Esophogeal abnormalities in chronic graft-versus-host disease in humans. *Gastroenterology*, **80,** 914–921 (1981)

50 MEISEL, J. L., PERERA, D. R., MELIGRO, C. and RUBIN, C. E. Overwhelming watery diarrhoea associated with a cryptosporidium in an immunosuppressed patient. *Gastroenterology*, **70,** 1156–1160 (1976)

51 MEYERS, J. D., FLOURNOY, N. and THOMAS, E. D. Cytomegalovirus infection and specific cell-mediated immunity after marrow transplant. *Journal of Infectious Diseases*, **142,** 816–824 (1980)

52 MEYERS, J. D. and THOMAS, E. D. Infection complicating bone marrow transplantation. In *Clinical Approach to Infection in the Immunocompromised Host*, edited by R. H. Rubin and L. S. Young, 507–551. Plenum Press, New York (1982)

53 NEIMAN, P. E., THOMAS, E. D., REEVES, W. C., RAY, C. G., SALE, G., LERNER, K. G., BUCKNER, C. D., CLIFT, R. A., STORB, R., WEIDEN, P. L. *et al.* Opportunistic infection and interstitial pneumonia following marrow transplantation for aplastic anemia and hematologic malignancy. *Transplantation Proceedings*, **8,** 663–667 (1976)

54 NIME, F. A., BUREK, J. D., PAGE, D. L., HOLSCHER, M. A., and YARDLEY, J. H. Acute enterocolitis in a human being infected with the protozoan cryptosporidium. *Gastroenterology*, **70,** 592–598 (1976)

55 OCHS, H. D., STORB, R., THOMAS, E. D., KOLB, H. J., GRAHAM, T. C., MICKELSON, E., PARR, M. and RUDOLPH, R. H. Immunologic reactivity in canine marrow graft recipients. *Journal of Immunology*, **113,** 1039–1057 (1974)

56 O'REILLY, R. J., DUPONT, B., PAHWA, S., GRIMES, E., SMITHWICK, E. M., PAHWA, R., SCHWARTZ, S., HANSEN, J. A., SIEGAL, F. P., SORELL, M. *et al.* Reconstitution in severe combined immunodeficiency by transplantation of marrow from an unrelated donor. *New England Journal of Medicine*, **297,** 1311–1318 (1977)

57 OTTO, H. F. The interepithelial lymphocytes of the intestine: morphological observations and immunological aspects of intestinal enteropathy. In *Current Topics in Pathology,* Volume 57, edited by E. Grundmann and W. H. Kirsten, 81–121. New York, Springer-Verlag (1973)

58 PALMER, R. H. and REILLY, R. W. Bile salt depletion in the runting syndrome. *Transplantation*, **12,** 479–483 (1971)

59 PETERS, M., WEINER, J. and WHELAN, G. Fungal infection associated with gastroduodenal ulceration: endoscopic and pathologic appearances. *Gastroenterology*, **78,** 350–354 (1980)

60 POWLES, R. L., MORGENSTERN, G., CLINK, H. M., HEDLEY, D., BANDINI, G., LUMLEY, H., WATSON, J. G., LAWSON, D., SPENCE, D., BARRETT, A. *et al.* The place of bone-marrow transplantation in acute myelogenous leukemia. *Lancet*, **1,** 1047–1050 (1980)

61 RAPPEPORT, J., REINHERZ, E., MIHM, M., LOPANSRI, S. and PARKMAN, R. Acute graft-versus-host disease in recipients of bone-marrow transplants from identical twin donors. *Lancet*, **1,** 717–720 (1979)

62 REINHERZ, E. L. and SCHLOSSMAN, S. F. Regulation of the immune response-inducer and suppressor T-lymphocyte subsets in human beings. *New England Journal of Medicine*, **303,** 370–373 (1980)

63 ROGERS, L. F. and GOLDSTEIN, H. M. Roentgen manifestations of radiation injury to the gastrointestinal tract. *Gastrointestinal Radiology*, **2,** 281–291 (1977)

64 ROSEN, P., ARMSTRONG, D. and RICE, N. Gastrointestinal cytomegalovirus infection. *Archives of Internal Medicine*, **132,** 274–276 (1973)

65 ROSENBERG, H. K., SEROTA, F. T., KOCH, P., BORDEN, S. IV and AUGUST, C. S. Radiographic features of gastrointestinal graft-versus-host disease. *Radiology*, **138,** 371–374 (1981)

66 ROSENBERG, J. L., WALL, A. J., SCANU, A. M. and REILLY, R. W. Fat malabsorption in the immunologically runted mouse (Abstract). *Gastroenterology*, **64,** A-109 (1973)

67 SALE, G. E., LERNER, K. G., BARKER, E. A., SHULMAN, H. M. and THOMAS, E. D. The skin biopsy in the diagnosis of acute graft-versus-host disease in man. *American Journal of Pathology*, **89,** 621–635 (1977)

68 SALE, G. E., SHULMAN, H. M., McDONALD, G. B. and THOMAS, E. D. Gastrointestinal graft-versus-host disease in man: a clinicopathologic study of the rectal biopsy. *American Journal of Surgical Pathology*, **3,** 291–299 (1979)

69 SAULSBURY, F. T., WINKELSTEIN, J. A. and YOLKEN, R. H. Chronic rotavirus infection in immunodeficiency. *Journal of Pediatrics*, **97,** 61–65 (1980)

70 SCHIMPFF, S. C. Infection prevention during profound granulocytopenia: new approaches to alimentary canal microbial suppression. *Annals of Internal Medicine*, **93,** 358–361 (1980)

71 SCHIMPFF, S. C. Surveillance cultures. *Journal of Infectious Diseases*, **144,** 81–84 (1981)

72 SCOWDEN, E. B., SCHAFFNER, W. and STONE, W. J. Overwhelming strongyloidiasis: an unappreciated opportunistic infection. *Medicine*, **57,** 527–544 (1978)

73 SEEMAYER, T. A. The graft-versus-host reaction: a pathogenetic mechanism of experimental and human disease. In *Perspectives in Pediatric Pathology*, edited by M. S. Rosenberg and R. P. Bolande, 93–136. New York, Masson Publishing Company (1979)

74 SHIMKIN, P. M., DeLELLIS, R. A., CAROLLA, R. L. and WEINSTEIN, M. A. Graft-versus-host disease. Radiographic findings in a patient with severe intestinal involvement. *Radiology,* 102, 623–624 (1972)

75 SHULMAN, H. M., McDONALD, G. B., MATTHEWS, D., DONEY, K. C., KOPECKY, K. J., GAUVREAU, J. M. and THOMAS, E. D. An analysis of hepatic venocclusive disease and centrilobular hepatocyte degeneration following bone marrow transplantation. *Gastroenterology*, **79,** 1178–1191 (1980)

76 SHULMAN, H. M., SULLIVAN, K. M., WEIDEN, P. L., McDONALD, G. B., STRIKER, G. E., SALE, G. E., HACKMAN, R., TSOI, M. S., STORB, R. and THOMAS, E. D. Chronic graft-versus-host syndrome in man: a clinical pathological study of 20 long-term Seattle patients. *American Journal of Medicine*, **69,** 204–217 (1980)

77 SLAVIN, R. E. and SANTOS, G. W. The graft-versus-host reaction in man after bone marrow transplantation: pathology, pathogenesis, clinical features, and implications. *Clinical Immunology and Immunopathology*, **1,** 472–498 (1973)

78 SLAVIN, R. E. and WOODRUFF, J. M. The pathology of bone marrow transplantation. In *Hematologic and Lymphoid Pathology Decennial 1966–1975*, edited by S. C. Sommers, 69–124, Appleton-Century-Crofts, New York. (1975)

79 STORB, R., THOMAS, E. D., BUCKNER, C. D., CLIFT, R. A., DEEG, H. J., FEFER, A., GOODELL, B. W., SALE, G. E., SANDERS, J. E., SINGER, J. *et al.* Marrow transplantation in thirty 'untransfused' patients with severe aplastic anemia. *Annals of Internal Medicine*, **92,** 30–36 (1980)

80 SULLIVAN, K. M., SHULMAN, H. M., STORB, R., WEIDEN, P. L., WITHERSPOON, R. P., McDONALD, G. B., SCHUBERT, M. M., ATKINSON, K. and THOMAS, E. D. Chronic graft-versus-host disease in fifty-two patients: adverse natural course and successful treatment with combination immunosuppression. *Blood*, **57,** 267–276 (1981)

81 SUTHERLAND, D. E. R., CHAN, F. Y., FOUCAR, E. SIMMONS, R. L., HOWARD, R. J. and NAJARIAN, J. S. The bleeding cecal ulcer in transplant patients. *Surgery*, **86,** 386–398 (1979)

82 THOMAS, E. D., BUCKNER, C. D., CLIFT, R. A., FEFER, A., JOHNSON, F. L., NEIMAN, P. E., SALE, G. E., SANDERS, J. E., SINGER, J. W., SHULMAN, H. *et al.* Marrow transplantation for acute nonlymphoblastic leukemia in first remission. *New England Journal of Medicine*, **301,** 597–599 (1979)

83 THOMAS, E. D., SANDERS, J. E., FLOURNOY, N., JOHNSON, F. L., BUCKNER, C. D., CLIFT, R. A., FEFER, A., GOODELL, B. W., STORB, R. and WEIDEN, P. L. Marrow transplantation for patients with acute lymphoblastic leukemia in remission. *Blood*, **54,** 468–476 (1979)

84 THOMAS, E. D., STORB, R., CLIFT, R. A., FEFER, A., JOHNSON, F. L., NEIMAN, P. E., LERNER, K. G., GLUCKSBERG, H. and BUCKNER, C. D. Bone marrow transplantation. *New England Journal of Medicine*, **292,** 832–843, 895–902 (1975)

85 TYTGAT, G. N., HUIBREGTSE, K., SCHELLEKENS, P. T. and FELTKAMP-VROOM, T. H. Clinical and immunologic observations in a patient with late onset immunodeficiency. *Gastroenterology*, **76,** 1458–1465 (1979)

86 TZIPORI, S., ANGUS, K. W., GRAY, E. W. and CAMPBELL, I. Vomiting and diarrhea associated with cryptosporidial infection (letter). *New England Journal of Medicine*, **303,** 818 (1980)

87 UNDERWOOD, J. C. E. and CORBETT, C. L. Persistent diarrhoea and hypoalbuminemia associated with cytomegalovirus enteritis. *British Medical Journal*, **1,** 1029–1030 (1978)

88 VAN BEKKUM, D. W. and DE VRIES, M. J. *Radiation Chimeras*. 146–150. New York, Academic Press (1967)

89 VAN BEKKUM, D. W. and KNAAN, S. Role of bacterial microflora in development of intestinal lesions from graft-versus-host reaction. *Journal of the National Cancer Institute*, **58,** 787–790 (1977)

90 VAN BEKKUM, D. W., ROODENBURG, J., HEIDT, P. J. and VAN DER WAAIJ, D. Mitigation of secondary disease of allogeneic mouse radiation chimeras by modification of the intestinal microflora. *Journal of the National Cancer Institute*, **52,** 401–404 (1974)

91 VAN BEKKUM, D. W. and VOS, O. Treatment of secondary disease in radiation chimaeras. *International Journal of Radiation Biology*, **3,** 173–181 (1961)

92 VAN DE WAAIJ, D., BERGHUIS, J. M. and LEKKERKERK, J. E. C. Colonization resistance of the digestive tract of mice during systemic antibiotic treatment. *Journal of Hygiene (Cambridge)*, **70,** 605–610 (1972)

93 WADE, J. C., SCHIMPFF, S. C., HARGADON, M. T., FORTNER, C. L., YOUNG, V. M. and WIERNIK, P. H. A comparison of trimethoprim-sulfamethoxazole plus nystatin with gentamicin plus nystatin in the prevention of infections in acute leukemia. *New England Journal of Medicine*, **304,** 1057–1062 (1981)

94 WAGEMAKER, G., VRIESENDORP, H. M. and VAN BEKKUM, D. W. Successful bone marrow transplantation across major histocompatibility barriers in Rhesus monkeys. *Transplantation Proceedings*, **13,** 875–880 (1981)

95 WEIDEN, P. L., DONEY, K., STORB, R. and THOMAS, E. D. Anti-human thymocyte globulin (ATG) for prophylaxis and treatment of graft-versus-host disease in recipients of allogeneic marrow grafts. *Transplantation Proceedings*, **10,** 213–216 (1978)

96 WEIDEN, P. L. and THE SEATTLE MARROW TRANSPLANT TEAM. Graft-versus-host disease in allogeneic marrow transplantation. In *Biology of Bone Marrow Transplantation*, edited by R. P. Gale and C. F. Fox, 37–48. New York, Academic Press (1980)

97 WEINSTEIN, L., EDELSTEIN, S. M., MADARA, J. L., FALCHUK, K. R., McMANUS, B. M. and TRIER, J. S. Intestinal cryptosporidiosis complicated by disseminated cytomegalovirus infection. *Gastroenterology*, **81,** 584–591 (1981)

98 WEISDORF, S. A., LONGSDORF, J. A., SALATI, L. M., RAMSAY, N. K. and SHARP, H. L. Intestinal graft-versus-host disease: a new protein losing enteropathy (abstract). *Gastroenterology*, **80,** 1313 (1981)

99 WEISER, B., LANGE, M., FIALK, M. A., SINGER, C., SZATROWSKI, T. H. and ARMSTRONG, D. Prophylactic trimethoprim-sulfamethoxazole during consolidation chemotherapy for acute leukemia: a controlled trial. *Annals of Internal Medicine*, **95,** 436–438 (1981)

100 WINSTON, D. J., GALE, R. P., MEYER, D. V., YOUNG, L. S. and THE UCLA BONE MARROW TRANSPLANTATION GROUP. Infectious complications of human bone marrow transplantation. *Medicine*, **58,** 1–31 (1979)

101 WINSTON, D. J., HO, W. G., HOWELL, C. L., MILLER, M. L., MICKEY, R., MARTIN, W. J., LIN, C. H. and GALE, R. P. Cytomegalovirus infections associated with leukocyte transfusions. *Annals of Internal Medicine*, **93,** 671–675 (1980)

102 WOODRUFF, J. M., BUTCHER, W. I. and HELLERSTEIN, L. J. Early secondary disease in the Rhesus monkey. II. Electron microscopy of changes in mucous membranes and external epithelia as demonstrated in the tongue and lip. *Laboratory Investigation*, **27,** 85–98 (1972)

103 WOODRUFF, J. M., HANSEN, J. A., GOOD, R. A., SANTOS, G. W. and SLAVIN, R. E. The pathology of the graft-versus-host reaction (GVHR) in adults receiving bone marrow transplants. *Transplantation Proceedings*, **8,** 675–684 (1976)

104 YOLKEN, R. H., BISHOP, C. A., TOWNSEND, T. R., BOLYARD, E. A., BARTLETT, J., SANTOS, G. W., SARAL, R. Infectious gastroenteritis in bone-marrow-transplant recipients. *New England Journal of Medicine*, **306,** 1009–1012 (1982)

105 ZAHRADNIK, J. M., SPENCER, M. J. and PORTER, D. D. Adenovirus infection in the immunocompromised patient. *American Journal of Medicine*, **68,** 725–732 (1980)

12
Vasculitis and the intestine

M. Camilleri, C. D. Pusey, V. S. Chadwick and A. J. Rees

INTRODUCTION

Involvement of the gastrointestinal tract is a recognised but poorly characterised complication of the systemic vasculitides and there are relatively few centres with sufficient numbers of patients with such conditions to allow detailed study of the clinical, pathological and radiological features.

Hammersmith Hospital, London, is a tertiary referral centre for the treatment of systemic vasculitis and this has facilitated the prospective study of a series of 65 patients over the last 7 years; 18 (27 per cent) have had major gastrointestinal manifestations. These occurred in 13/25 patients with polyarteritis (4 of these 13 patients having macroscopic aneurysms and being grouped as polyarteritis nodosa), 4 of 36 patients with Wegener's granulomatosis and 1 of 4 with Churg–Strauss syndrome. There was evidence of gastrointestinal involvement at presentation in 50 per cent of these and it developed subsequently in the remaining patients; it was directly responsible for death in 27 per cent. *Table 12.1* shows some of the clinical and investigational features in the group of patients reviewed during the past 7 years.

Gastrointestinal manifestations also occur in giant cell arteritis and thromboangiitis obliterans, and in vasculitis complicating other diseases such as rheumatoid arthritis, systemic lupus erythematosus and Behçet's syndrome.

In patients with primary systemic vasculitis, a pathological diagnosis of necrotising vasculitis was most commonly made on the basis of compatible renal (94 per cent) or skin (40 per cent) biopsies. Diagnosis of gut involvement in such patients depends on a high index of suspicion when gastrointestinal symptoms occur in the setting of an active vasculitis. Radiological investigations may be helpful, showing paralytic ileus on plain abdominal radiographs; segmental abnormalities showing mucosal ulceration or bowel stricture on contrast radiology of the gut; or the presence of angiographic abnormalities such as aneurysms of medium-sized arteries (polyarteritis nodosa group) or organ infarcts. The role of endoscopy and intestinal biopsy is considered below.

Table 12.1 Clinical features of 18 patients seen at Hammersmith Hospital, London, with gastrointestinal manifestations of systemic vasculitis (denominator indicates number of patients who underwent the investigation)

Disease group	*Total No.*	*No. with GI manifestations*	*Abdominal pain*	*Diarrhoea*	*Blood*	*Abnormal LFTs*	*Positive radiology*		*Positive gut biopsy*
							Plain or contrast	*Angiography*	
Polyarteritis nodosa	8	4	3	2	3	2	1/3	4/4	4/4
Microscopic polyarteritis	17	9	8	4	3	4	4/7	0/7	2/2
Wegener's granulomatosis	36	4	3	2	1	3	2/4	0/1	1/1
Churg-Strauss syndrome	4	1	0	1	1	0	1/1	1/1	1/1

In the 73 per cent of our own patients who survived, gastrointestinal manifestations remitted with improvements in the systemic illness following treatment with steroids, cyclophosphamide or plasma exchange.

Aetiology

Vasculitis is a relatively common pathological finding characterised by inflammation and necrosis of blood vessels, that may follow infection or allergy[26]. Usually symptoms are mild, transient, confined to the skin and demand no specific treatment. Much less commonly extensive vasculitis affecting blood vessels in many organs may cause life-threatening disease. This may occur in isolation or may complicate other diseases such as infective endocarditis, rheumatoid arthritis and systemic lupus erythematosus (*Table 12.2*). Although there is presumptive evidence that an unusual response to hepatitis B virus may be responsible in some patients, the aetiology can rarely be ascertained.

Table 12.2 Classification of systemic vasculitides affecting the gut

Vessels affected	*Granulomas*	
	Absent	*Present*
Large	Takayasu's	Giant cell arteritis
Medium	Polyarteritis nodosa	Churg-Strauss syndrome
Small	Microscopic polyarteritis	Wegener's granulomatosis
	Henoch-Schönlein purpura	

Associated diseases (usually small vessels): systemic lupus erythematosus (SLE), rheumatoid arthritis, essential mixed cryoglobulinaemia, carcinoma, lymphoma, leukaemia, Behçet's syndrome.

Pathogenesis

In most cases, by analogy to experimental acute serum sickness, the pathogenesis is thought to be due to deposition of immune complexes in the walls of blood vessels – a type III hypersensitivity reaction. However deposits of immunoglobulins are only rarely detected in the walls of affected blood vessels and using current assays circulating immune complexes are found in less than half the patients[54]. These negative findings can be explained: immunoglobulin deposits may be very rapidly degraded; it is known that in experimental cutaneous vasculitis, immunoglobulins found within two hours of the development of a lesion can no longer be detected four hours later[20]. Secondly in experimental models, trivial amounts of immune complexes deposited in the vessel wall can provoke vasculitis. And finally, the insensitivity of present assays for immune complex-like activity may account for this failure to detect such activity. Thus, although other mechanisms such as antibody-mediated injury (a type II response), or cell-mediated injury by cytotoxic T lymphocytes (a type IV response) have been postulated, deposition of immune complexes remains the most attractive hypothesis to explain development of systemic vasculitis.

Until more is known of the pathogenesis of these conditions it will not be possible to develop a rational approach to classificiation.

Pathology

The pathological hallmark of systemic vasculitis is inflammation and necrosis of the walls of blood vessels. In general the vessels are surrounded by acute inflammatory cells, particularly neutrophils and monocytes, which infiltrate surrounding tissues. There is destruction of the vessel wall and prominent 'fibrinoid necrosis' (*Figure 12.1*). In certain types of systemic vasculitis, the injury to the blood vessels is associated with granulomas and numerous giant cells. Unfortunately it is frequently impossible to obtain unequivocal evidence of vasculitis in biopsies from patients, even when taken from affected organs, and the diagnosis has to be based on clinical presentation, a compatible biopsy, and an apparent response to treatment.

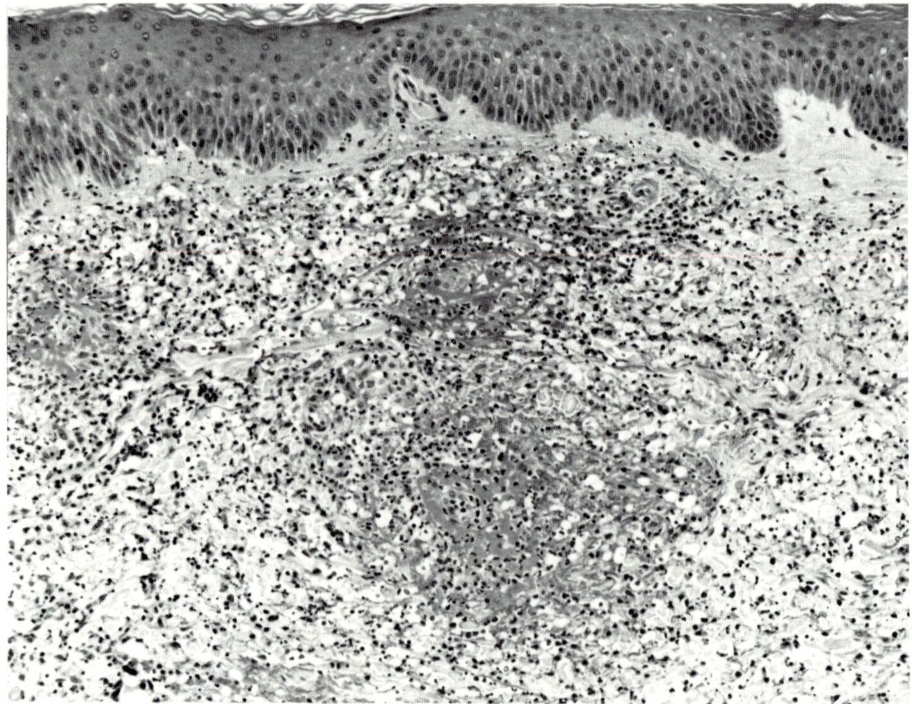

Figure 12.1 Leucocytoclastic angiitis of a dermal small vessel showing leucocyte infiltration of vessel wall and perivascular cuffing and fibrinoid necrosis (H and E × 150)

Classification

Distinct clinical syndromes such as polyarteritis nodosa, microscopic polyarteritis, Churg-Strauss syndrome and Wegener's granulomatosis have been described and reflect the size of the vessel involved and the presence of granulomas (*Table 12.2*). Such divisions are useful as a guide to treatment and prognosis but it is essential to realise that they provide only a working classification and do not imply that each syndrome is a distinct entity. Indeed there is strong evidence to suggest that conditions such as microscopic polyarteritis and Wegener's granulomatosis are merely parts of a spectrum. There are no serological investigations specific for systemic vasculitis. But the following non-specific findings are common: anaemia (which may be severe), leucocytosis (usually neutrophilia, except in Churg-Strauss syndrome, in which eosinophilia is the rule); and thrombocytosis. Tests for circulation immune complexes and for rheumatoid factor may be weakly positive but other autoantibodies are uncommon, and serum complement levels are usually normal.

Clinical features

Inevitably the clinical presentation of systemic vasculitis depends on the organs involved and may vary considerably from patient to patient. Despite this, many clinical features are common to all patients, allowing the condition to be suspected clinically. Most patients become increasingly sick with fever, malaise, weight loss and arthralgia which are often complicated by the development of peripheral neuropathy (either mononeuritis multiplex or symmetrical peripheral neuropathy), a rash and evidence of glomerulonephritis.

Treatment

For many years, corticosteroids have been the main drugs used in management of polyarteritis[32, 56, 70], and most authors have advocated starting with a dose of 40–60 mg prednisolone daily (or its equivalent). Most patients respond to this treatment, and more recently, Fauci *et al.*[27] and Lieb *et al.*[51] have documented additional benefit when steroids are combined with cyclophosphamide. Repeated plasma exchange has also been advocated, particularly for the most severely affected patients[53, 54].

Patients with Churg-Strauss syndrome usually respond to corticosteroids alone, but these agents seem to have little effect on the progression of Wegener's granulomatosis[39, 86] and it is now generally accepted that cytotoxic drugs, in particular cyclophosphamide, have greatly improved the prognosis of this disease[27, 28, 41, 66, 68]. The dose of cyclophosphamide is usually 1–3 mg per kg per day.

POLYARTERITIS NODOSA

Case history

D.D. presented at the age of 42 years with headaches and malaise and was found to be hypertensive. Five years later he developed muscle and joint pains and proximal muscle weakness, and over the next year, anorexia, weight loss (6 kg) and epigastric pain. General physical examination revealed a 'livido reticularis' rash, tender nodules on the knees and tender limb muscles. On abdominal examination, he was tender on the left side of the abdomen.

Investigations revealed a prolonged erythrocyte sedimentation rate (ESR) 43 mm 1st hour; necrotising vasculitis in the dermis on skin biopsy; impaired renal function (creatinine clearance 28 ml/min) and a low plasma albumin (28 g/l). Selective visceral angiography showed multiple aneurysms in medium-sized arteries. Over the next few months, he developed several gastrointestinal complications. These included: an episode of subacute intestinal obstruction which responded to intravenous fluids, nasogastric suction and intravenous corticosteroid therapy; and chronic iron deficiency anaemia (Hb. 6.9 g/dl, MCV 72 f1), the cause of which was not evident on a barium radiological series.

Following a massive gastrointestinal bleed, a laparotomy showed that the small and large intestine were filled with blood, though no mass lesion or palpable ulcer could be found in the bowel. A lymph node biopsy revealed a necrotising vasculitis. Following a further episode of massive gastrointestinal bleeding, requiring transfusion of 25 pints of blood in two days, repeat selective superior mesenteric arteriography confirmed the presence of multiple aneurysms in medium-sized arteries, one of which was bleeding into the mid–small bowel (*Figure 12.2*). There were no other episodes of bleeding after resection of this loop of lower jejunum (which showed histological evidence of vasculitis) until his death a few months later from acute pancreatitis (serum amylase 3000 iu/l), at a time when he was taking 50 mg prednisolone daily.

Macroscopic polyarteritis (polyarteritis nodosa, or classical polyarteritis) presents as a systemic illness of rapidly increasing severity. Non-specific symptoms often include malaise, profound weight loss, muscle and joint aches and pains. These are frequently associated with severe abdominal pain, which may be due to local pressure from an expanding aneurysm or to ischaemia. The pain may derive from liver, gallbladder, pancreas, kidneys or intestine and may be accompanied by intestinal infarction and severe intraabdominal or gastrointestinal haemorrhage. The skin is involved much less commonly than in patients with microscopic polyarteritis and glomerulonephritis is relatively unusual. Severe hypertension occurring in a patient suspected of having systemic vasculitis strongly suggests involvement of medium-sized vessels. Organ biopsies are frequently unhelpful in making the diagnosis and visceral angiography is the investigation of choice.

Most patients respond to treatment with large doses of corticosteroids, starting with about 60 mg prednisolone each day, and there is increasing evidence that cytotoxic drugs, and in particular cyclophosphamide (3 mg per kg per day), confer additional benefit in recalcitrant patients.

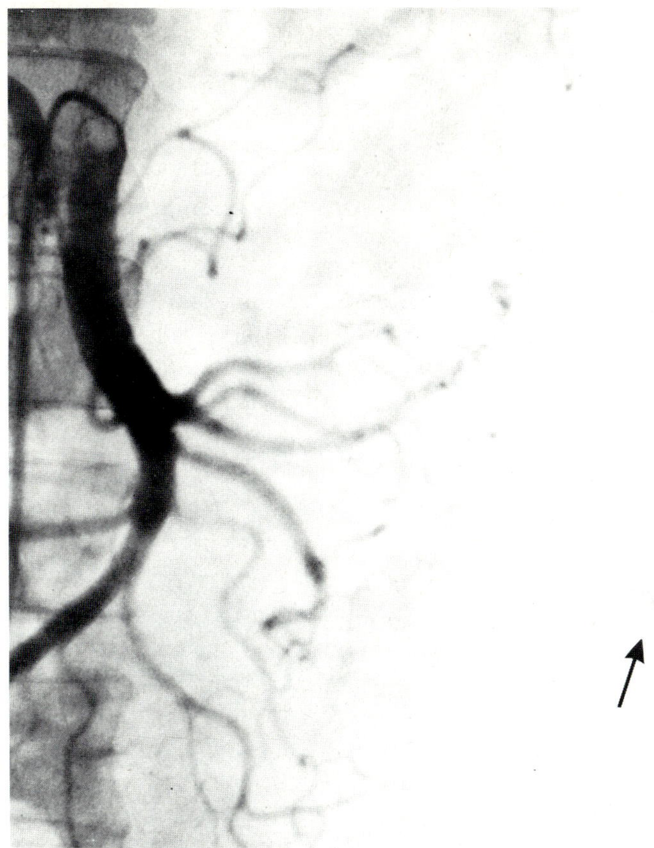

Figure 12.2 Subtraction angiograph of superior mesenteric artery showing aneurysms on medium-sized vessels and appearance of contrast within bowel lumen (arrowed) due to haemorrhage from a ruptured aneurysm

The case report above illustrates many of the important features of the gastrointestinal complications of polyarteritis nodosa. Around 50–70 per cent of patients with this syndrome will develop abdominal manifestations during the course of their disease[59, 84]. These manifestations vary with the severity of the vasculitis and are associated with inflammation, ulceration, or perforation of the affected abdominal organ.

The clinical presentation is usually with abdominal pain, nausea, vomiting and diarrhoea (which may be bloody). Intestinal infarction (which occurs in about 6 per cent of all patients[59] results in haemorrhage, or in perforation with peritonitis, fever, leucocytosis and ileus[30]. Less severe vasculitis may result in changes in the small intestine which may be mistaken for coeliac disease[83] or Crohn's disease[49], and may cause diarrhoea and steatorrhoea[16, 49]. Colonic mucosal infarction may cause bloody diarrhoea that may be mistaken for ulcerative colitis[34, 42]. The occurrence of systemic features suggestive of polyarteritis nodosa together with intestinal disease should alert the clinician to the possibility that polyarteritis is the cause of the intestinal disorder. A careful review of reports in the literature of associations of inflammatory bowel disease (usually Crohn's) with cutaneous, articular or neuro-muscular[23] manifestations suggests that many of these are primary vasculitic disorders affecting the gut rather than systemic complications of classical inflammatory bowel disease.

A histopathological diagnosis may rarely be made by biopsies from any target organ including the gut showing a non-granulomatous necrotising vasculitis. Radiological diagnosis is by visceral angiography, which can be expected to show macroscopic aneurysms in about 60 per cent of cases[84]. This group of patients with macroscopic aneurysms may have a high incidence of gastroenterological complications, and mortality (often due to a combination of intestinal infarction and renal failure[84]).

ALLERGIC GRANULOMATOUS ANGIITIS OR CHURG-STRAUSS SYNDROME

Case history

I.C. developed asthma at 18 years of age. Ten years later she presented with bloody diarrhoea associated with eosinophilia in the peripheral blood. Barium enema and rectal biopsy suggested a non-specific colitis. One year later, she developed nasal polyps, arthralgia, paraesthesiae, a rash, mouth ulcers and diarrhoea. Investigations showed elevated ESR (90 mm 1st hour), eosinophil count (18.3×10^9/l), serum IgG (21.4 g/l) and IgE (151 iu/ml; N<122). Scattered pulmonary infiltrates were seen on the chest X-ray; and a skin biopsy showed perivascular eosinophilic infiltration. There was evidence of circulating immune complexes by the Clq assay. A non-specific colitis was confirmed radiologically and the rectal biopsy showed a predominance of mononuclear cell and eosinophil infiltration. Visceral arteriography revealed infarcts in the kidneys and spleen. Treatment with oral prednisolone (60 mg daily) produced a striking improvement.

This patient suffers from the Churg-Strauss syndrome[19] which typically presents in patients with a history of atopy with asthma, eosinophilia and pulmonary infiltrates in middle life. A disseminated necrotising vasculitis affecting all sizes of vessels in the lungs, skin and nerves and the gastrointestinal tract is the pathological hallmark of the condition, and it can be differentiated from polyarteritis nodosa by the findings of extravascular granulomas in association with the necrotising vasculitis, and eosinophilic infiltration of the tissues[18]. The Churg-Strauss syndrome has also been regarded as being half way along the broad spectrum of disease that includes polyarteritis nodosa and hypereosinophilic syndrome at its two extremes[81]. About 20 per cent of patients with this syndrome have abdominal manifestations, usually pain, the cause of which is often difficult to establish. Other clinical manifestations are: diarrhoea, perforation and cholecystitis. In a large series reported from the Mayo Clinic[18], one such patient had a gastric ulcer; another had pseudopolyps in the colon consistent with chronic ulcerative colitis; a third patient had allergic granulomas in the stomach, liver and omentum; a fourth patient had an allergic granulomatous process massively involving the ascending colon and mimicking a neoplasm; and a fifth patient died of septicaemia following perforation of the small bowel affected by necrotising vasculitis and allergic granulomatosis. The gallbladder may rarely be affected and presents the picture of acute cholecystitis[48].

Thus, as with polyarteritis nodosa, the severity of the vasculitis probably determines the gastrointestinal complications, which range from ulceration and inflammation to frank infarction and perforation. The characteristic eosinophilic infiltration may be detected if multiple deep rectal biopsies are taken, and this may be a valuable and simple diagnostic procedure in the Churg-Strauss syndrome[57]. Sometimes, however, the diagnosis is only made at laparotomy, which may reveal vasculitic nodules on the peritoneal surfaces. This suggests that laparoscopy and biopsy of such nodules may be an alternative diagnostic procedure[57].

The gastrointestinal manifestations of Churg-Strauss usually respond to high dose corticosteroid therapy unless organ infarction and perforation have occurred.

MICROSCOPIC POLYARTERITIS

Case history

A.S. first presented with diarrhoea at the age of 58 years. Examination and sigmoidoscopy were initially normal; however, two years later, after a flare up of diarrhoea associated with passage of fresh blood, the rectal mucosa was found to be inflamed, friable and bled on contact. He presented to this hospital six years after first developing diarrhoea. A maculopapular rash on the trunk and ulcerating nodules on the limbs were biopsied and revealed epidermal necrosis with an acute necrotising vasculitis of medium-sized vessels in the dermis. Although his renal function was normal (serum creatinine 122 μmol/l), he passed an average of 6 grams of protein in his urine daily and a percutaneous renal biopsy showed a focal necrotising glomerulonephritis with capsular adhesions and only one glomerulus showed evidence of crescent formation. The major clinical presentation, however, was with diarrhoea and rectal bleeding. A barium enema examination was normal; however, colonoscopy showed purpura of the rectal and colonic mucosa, particularly from the splenic flexure to the rectum where purpuric lesions were confluent whereas they were scattered in the transverse and ascending colons (*Figure 12.3*). Ulceration was also seen in the rectum and biopsies from the rectum and colon showed acute and chronic inflammatory cellular infiltration and free pus on the surface of the mucosa. The liver function tests were normal and tests for circulating immune complexes were negative. Treatment with high dose corticosteroids resulted in striking improvement in the systemic and intestinal disorders.

Microscopic polyarteritis shows many of the features of the macroscopic disease or polyarteritis nodosa. Fever, weight loss, and cutaneous vasculitis are all common but unlike the macroscopic form glomerulonephritis is the rule; pulmonary vasculitis (without granulomas) is not uncommon whilst severe hypertension and gut involvement are rare. Biopsies of affected tissue may be positive but more

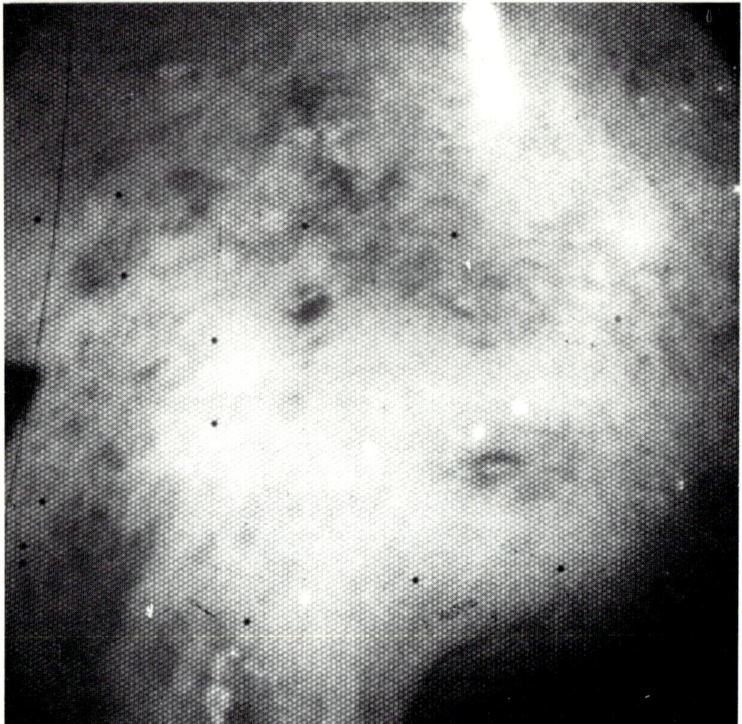

Figure 12.3 Colonic purpura in a patient with microscopic polyarteritis

commonly the diagnosis is inferred from the combination of a compatible clinical presentation and a renal biopsy showing focal necrotising glomerulonephritis. Renal biopsy is the investigation of choice in any patient with clinical evidence of glomerulonephritis. Treatment with steroids and cytotoxic drugs is usually effective.

The gastrointestinal features of this form of systemic vasculitis have been described in the section regarding polyarteritis nodosa since it is difficult to differentiate the macro- and microscopic forms of polyarteritis in the cases reported with gastrointestinal manifestations in the literature. In our group of patients mortality from gut complications of the two groups did not appear to be different: two out of four with macroscopic disease and three out of nine patients with microscopic disease developed a fatal gastrointestinal complication.

WEGENER'S GRANULOMATOSIS

Case history

P.R. was 43 years old when she presented with sinusitis, deafness, mouth ulcers, conjunctivitis and arthralgia. One year later, she developed bloody diarrhoea with oral and anal ulcers, a vasculitic skin rash and oliguria. Her renal function was severely impaired (serum creatinine 394 μmol/l), and she had proteinuria of 1.3 g per day. Renal biopsy showed a focal necrotising glomerulonephritis. The serum alkaline phosphatase was raised at 261 iu/l, and circulating immune complexes were detected by Clq and monoclonal rheumatoid factor binding assays. She subsequently developed radiological evidence of pulmonary cavitating granulomas and lesions in the ileum and caecum were seen on a barium radiological series. Non-specific proctitis was identified on rectal biopsy. No aneurysms were visible on a selective visceral arteriogram.

Wegener's granulomatosis has many similarities to the microscopic form of polyarteritis: the skin, kidneys and peripheral nerves are usually all involved but in addition there is much emphasis on the lungs and upper airways. Granulomas are frequently in evidence on chest X-rays and in addition there is often ulceration of mouth and nose, and deafness. It may be associated with immune complex-tissue injury[87].

Gastrointestinal involvement appears exceedingly uncommon. Only one of 18 patients had evidence of gastrointestinal involvement, and this was a small bowel perforation identified at post mortem, in one large series[28].

In the group of 36 patients seen at Hammersmith, London, with this condition in the past seven years, four patients had evidence of gut involvement in the setting of a severe multisystem disorder.

In the past ten years it has been shown that this disease is sensitive to cyclophosphamide therapy[26, 27]. The patient whose case history is described above responded remarkably well to a combination of immunosuppressive agents (with corticosteroids and cyclophosphamide), and plasma exchange.

HENOCH-SCHÖNLEIN PURPURA

Case history

D.W. presented at the age of 28 years with a two week history of colicky abdominal pain which was insidious in onset. This was associated with a severe symmetrical arthritis involving the ankles, knees, elbows, wrists and hands. Four days prior to admission, he also noticed a rash on the left leg and both buttocks and forearms. Physical examination revealed a low grade fever (temp. 38C), swelling of the metacarpophalangeal joints of both hands and the left ankle, and a macular erythematous rash over both buttocks, arms and forearms. On abdominal examination, he was generally tender with some rebound tenderness.

Investigations showed: ESR 80 mm 1st hour; neutrophil leucocytosis; tests for circulating immune complexes negative (Clq binding assay); alkaline phosphatase (hepatic isoenzyme) raised at 241 iu/l; urine protein was less than 1 g per day, though the serum albumin was 27 g/l; urinary sediment contained red cells and red cell casts and a mesangial IgA nephropathy was found on percutaneous renal biopsy. Abdominal X-rays showed dilated small gut loops and multiple fluid levels. Extensive mucosal abnormalities and pronounced luminal narrowing in the proximal ileum were seen on a barium follow through. He was treated with intravenous fluids, nasogastric suction and systemic corticosteroids, and made a rapid recovery. Repeat barium follow through at four weeks was entirely normal.

Henoch-Schönlein purpura is a small vessel vasculitis typically occurring in children (usually six months to seven years old[29]), involving joints, skin, kidneys and intestine; exceptional patients additionally have pulmonary vasculitis. There is prominent deposition of IgA within glomeruli and less commonly in blood vessels and the diagnosis should not be made when these are absent. Colicky abdominal pain is the commonest gut presentation and it may mimic an acute abdominal emergency[3, 4, 29, 37]. Gastrointestinal bleeding may be found in up to 80 per cent of cases if tests for occult blood are performed serially[44]. Rarely, abdominal surgery is necessary due to complications such as perforation[5, 44] or intussusception[13, 88], the latter occurring in about 2–3 per cent of all cases of the syndrome. Chronic small bowel obstruction has been reported in a single case[89]. The necrotising arteritis that underlies the bowel complications may also cause acute cholecystitis[44] and acute pancreatitis[55, 65], and abnormalities of liver enzymes suggest hepatic involvement by the same process.

The diagnosis of Henoch-Schönlein purpura is usually made on clinical grounds. The gastrointestinal features present with non-specific mucosal abnormalities that may simulate Crohn's disease radiologically. The pathognomonic skin rash and associated renal involvement (with a characteristic IgA mesangial nephropathy on biopsy) form the basis for a positive clinical diagnosis. This disorder usually responds to treatment with high dose corticosteroids alone, and there is a tendency in a few cases to a relapse of the disorder often while tailing down the steroid dose.

VASCULITIS COMPLICATING OTHER DISEASES

A systemic vasculitis, usually involving small vessels, may also occur as a complication of other diseases including bacterial endocarditis, connective tissue diseases (such as SLE, rheumatoid arthritis and Behçet's syndrome) and essential mixed cryoglobulinaemia.

Systemic lupus erythematosus

Case history

T.C. suffered from epilepsy at the age of 16 years. Seven years later she presented with acute abdominal pain, suggestive of peritonitis, that settled with conservative therapy. At 33 years of age, she had a cholecystectomy and two years later developed subacute intestinal obstruction due to adhesions. When she was 38 years old she developed a mild right-sided stroke and two years later presented after having passed a 10 cm 'cast' of bowel mucosa per rectum. This occurred after a few weeks' history of lower abdominal pain, particularly after meals. On physical examination she had evidence of a right-sided stroke, polyarthritis and Raynaud's phenomenon, and had tenosynovitis of the hands. In the abdomen, the liver was enlarged and there was tenderness, guarding and rebound tenderness in the left iliac fossa. Investigations revealed a high ESR (30 mm 1st hour), a positive antinuclear factor and DNA binding titre (80 per cent). Her renal function was normal although urine protein excretion was 1.9 g/day; urinary sediment showed red cells and red cell casts. Renal biopsy showed a proliferative glomerulonephritis with diffuse positive immunofluorescence for IgG in both mesangium and capillary walls, and IgM and C_3 in the mesangium. Her serum albumin was 29 g/l and she excreted 3 g of D-xylose in five hours after a 25 gram oral load. A barium enema revealed a stricture of the sigmoid colon (*Figure 12.4*) and a lateral aortogram showed proximal occlusion of the inferior mesenteric and coeliac arteries.

This case illustrates some of the gastrointestinal manifestations of systemic lupus erythematosus, such as abdominal pain, peritonitis, adhesions, bowel ulceration and mucosal infarcts. Other presenting features in SLE include cholecystitis, pancreatitis and malabsorption or a protein-losing enteropathy[11, 12, 55].

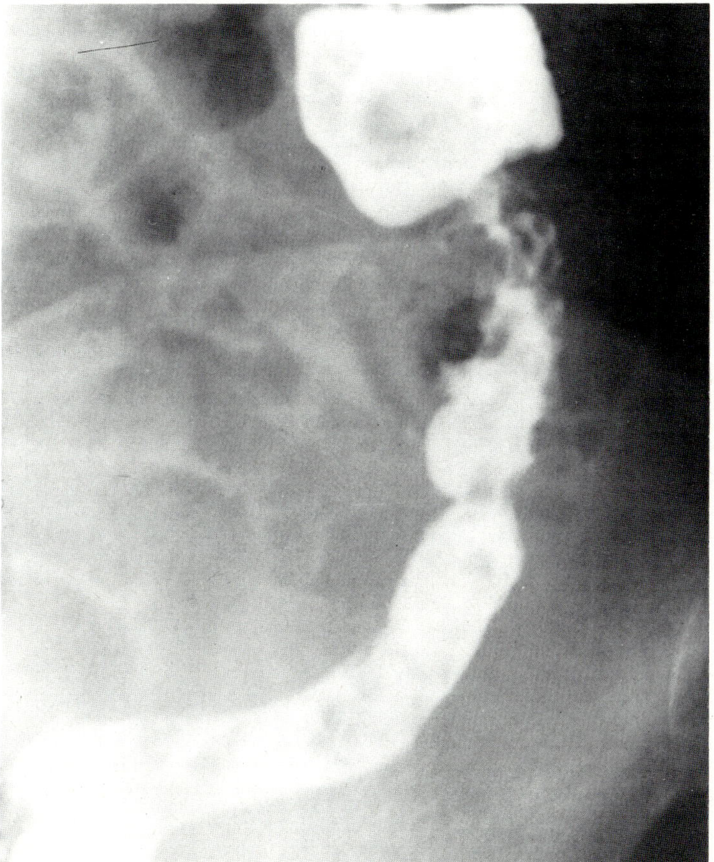

Figure 12.4 Stricture of descending and sigmoid colon in a patient with systemic vasculitis complicating systemic lupus erythematosus

Lupus 'enteritis' presents a range of clinical features in the stomach and intestine: ulceration[30, 64a], inflammation[35, 47, 75], oedema (often with ileus[12]), inflammatory polyposis[58] and perforation[7, 30, 46, 90]. The presentation with acute abdominal symptoms may be due to the above mentioned inflammation and perforation[64] but SLE may also cause a peritonitis[25, 60]. Ascites[9, 43, 73] may be painless or associated with serositis.

Lupus arteritis affecting the bowel tends to involve small arteries, though larger vessels may also be affected[63]. Gut manifestations of SLE are often associated with vasculitis outside the gut, particularly the skin. Arteriography is, in general, unable to demonstrate the arteritis though occasional reports have recorded positive arteriography[63]. Abdominal paracentesis may aid detection of peritonitis due to perforated bowel, spontaneous bacterial infection or serositis[52, 76]. However, exploratory laparotomy may be necessary if bowel perforation cannot be excluded.

There are four well documented cases of malabsorption secondary to SLE[6, 77] and this may be associated with villous flattening. Two cases of protein-losing enteropathy[62, 85] due to SLE have been reported.

Rheumatoid arthritis

Systemic vasculitis (commonly involving skin, nerves and kidneys) is associated with longstanding rheumatoid arthritis (usually of the nodular and erosive variety)[5]. This vasculitis is often accompanied by high titres of IgM rheumatoid as well as IgE rheumatoid factor, 7S IgM, cryoglobulins, and evidence of complement consumption[74]. The gastrointestinal tract is affected in about 10 per cent of patients with systemic rheumatoid vasculitis[74]. The usual presentation is with acute abdominal pain[1, 8, 74], associated with intestinal ulceration and sometimes perforation and peritonitis. The necrotising vasculitis of small arteries may be detected by rectal biopsy[72, 74]. Occasionally, subacute vasculitic changes or a capillaritis are seen in the rectal biopsy. In one series, the presence of a necrotising arteritis on rectal biopsy was associated with a poor prognosis, a motor neuropathy and low levels of anticomplementary activity, suggesting widespread systemic vascular involvement. Rarely, rheumatoid disease may be complicated by a malabsorption syndrome[22, 40]. Treatment with high dose corticosteroids usually results in improvements of both systemic vasculitis and the gut manifestations.

Behcet's syndrome

There are at least 60 cases in the world literature of Behçet's disease involving the gastrointestinal tract. Most have appeared in the Japanese literature[2]. The typical gastrointestinal complications are ulceration, inflammation or perforation of the ileum or right side of the colon and common clinical presentations are with abdominal pain, diarrhoea or bleeding. Recurrent perforation is not uncommon, and some authors recommend extensive resection of gut segments which contain such perforations[2]. Macroscopically there may be colitis, indistinguishable from chronic ulcerative colitis[10] except for the distribution, which in Behçet's disease often spares the rectum, and the greater depth of ulcers (75 per cent reaching muscular or serosal layers) that are often multiple and circumscribed in Behçet's disease. This renders colonoscopy rather dangerous because of the risk of colonic perforation. The absence of granulomas on histological analysis may help differentiate Behçet's from Crohn's disease[2]. Radiological assessment of the colon, showing multiple, discrete, large deep ulcers predominantly on the right side of the colon has been regarded as characteristic of the condition and when associated with the other clinical features (ocular, mucocutaneous and articular) allows a positive diagnosis to be made[24].

Microangiographic studies[2] have revealed impaired submucosal microcirculation in the vicinity of ulcers while histological analysis often reveals chronic inflammatory cell infiltration predominantly around small vessels (capillary and venule).

Treatment with corticosteroids may help to reverse the gut inflammation though most authors advocate surgical resection (*see above*) if gut manifestations become prominent.

Essential mixed cryoglobulinaemia (EMC)

There is a single case, reported by Reza *et al.*[67] of a patient with recurrent abdominal pain, peripheral neuropathy and arthralgias occurring chiefly in the winter months, who was found to have an essential IgG–IgM mixed cryoglobulinaemia. Contrast radiology revealed strictures in the ileum and colon. However, there was no evidence of inflammatory bowel disease at colonoscopy, whereas histological examination of the surgically resected ileum and proximal colon showed severe vasculitis without evidence of inflammatory bowel disease. Gastrointestinal involvement in essential mixed cryoglobulinaemia is exceedingly rare and careful radiological and histological assessment is important to exclude the commoner phenomenon of cryoglobulinaemia occurring as a complication of gut disorders such as coeliac disease[21].

GIANT CELL ARTERITIDES

Takayasu's arteritis

Takayasu's arteritis may be associated with inflammatory bowel disease which may present features suggestive of ulcerative colitis or Crohn's disease[17, 31, 61, 79]. Most associated arterial lesions are of the occlusive type except for the case described by Owyang *et al.*[61] which was characterised by the development of large artery aneurysms of the superior mesenteric and left hepatic arteries. It is unclear whether these are chance associations or whether the arteritis resulted in the inflammatory bowel disease.

Giant cell arteritis

Case history

L.F. was a 62 year old Polish woman who had been taking steroids intermittently for six years for temporal arteritis. She presented with a six month history of constant pain in the left upper quadrant of the abdomen. She had not taken steroids for eighteen months prior to this presentation with abdominal pain. There was associated anorexia and some dysphagia. Physical examination revealed a systemic blood pressure of 160/110 mmHg and in the abdomen there was a prominent abdominal aorta, and a loud epigastric bruit. Investigations revealed a high ESR (85 mm 1st hour) but otherwise normal haematological, biochemical and serological indices apart from a weak positive antinuclear factor (1/40 speckled). Aortography showed an aneurysm of the ascending aorta but no other aneurysms of medium or large sized arteries. The affected aorta was replaced with a graft and histological analysis revealed cystic medial necrosis and atheromatous changes. Treatment with high dose oral steroids resulted in a dramatic response of her abdominal pain, which was then controlled with modest maintenance doses.

There are at least 14 cases (recorded in the world literature) of this disorder affecting the mesenteric vessels. It is usually associated with temporal arteritis and presents with a clinical picture suggestive of small bowel ischaemia or frank infarction necessitating laparotomy and resection of the involved small bowel[50, 80]. In a large review of 248 patients with giant cell arteritis, it was noted that about 15 per cent had evidence of disease affecting the aorta and its major branches[45], including the superior mesenteric artery. Rarely, Crohn's disease may be complicated by a giant cell arteritis affecting the bowel vessels. These lesions are thought to be different from arterial involvement by the granulomatous reaction of Crohn's disease[82].

THROMBOANGIITIS OBLITERANS (BUERGER'S DISEASE)

Thromboangiitis obliterans rarely affects the gastrointestinal tract. However, there are a few well documented cases in the literature (including one report by Buerger[14]) of mesenteric involvement. Rob[69] recorded one patient with small bowel necrosis necessitating resection; other workers reported a patient who required resection of two feet of infarcted jejunum and postoperatively developed melaena with evidence of mucosal ulceration of a large segment of the ileum[38]. Similarly, segmental colonic involvement (with inflammation and ulceration of transverse and sigmoid colon) have been reported[38, 71]. One case of colonic involvement has been complicated by perforation and peritonitis[36]. When the disease affects the coeliac artery, infarction of the organs supplied may result – liver, spleen and pancreas[78].

CLOSING REMARKS

The diverse clinical presentations of systemic vasculitis makes confident diagnosis difficult for the inexperienced clinician; even when suspected, it is often impossible to obtain unequivocal confirmatory evidence. Morphological evidence of vasculitis is frequently missing from biopsy specimens taken from affected tissues, but severe necrotising glomerulonephritis in a patient with systemic disease strongly suggests the diagnosis. Angiography is not always helpful and aneurysms are found only in those patients (the minority) with involvement of medium sized vessels. The investigation of choice in patients with evidence of glomerulonephritis (that is, severe proteinuria and erythrocytes and red cell casts in the urinary sediment) is a percutaneous renal biospy, whereas patients with severe abdominal pain, marked hypertension and lack of evidence of glomerulonephritis are more likely to have involvement of medium-sized arteries, and should have visceral angiography to identify aneurysms and organ infarction. The diagnosis of the gastrointestinal manifestations is largely based on the occurrence of abdominal pain, diarrhoea or gut haemorrhage in patients with a systemic disorder where corroborative evidence of an underlying vasculitis is achieved as outlined above. Treatment of these patients is aimed at controlling the underlying systemic vasculitis and dealing with any surgical complications in the gut such as perforation or uncontrollable haemorrhage.

Acknowledgements

We would like to express our thanks to several colleagues at Hammersmith Hospital: Professor D. K. Peters and Dr G. R. V. Hughes for allowing us to study their patients; Drs D. J. Allison, A. P. Hemmingway and N. B. Bowley, Department of Diagnostic Radiology for help in radiological assessment of these patients; Professor N. A. Wright, Department of Histopathology for allowing us to consult records in his department and Miss Ann Love for excellent secretarial assistance.

References

1 ADLER, R. H., NORCROSS, B. M. and LOCKIE, L. M. Arteritis and infarction of the intestine in rheumatoid arthritis. *Journal of the American Medical Association*, **180,** 922–926 (1962)

2 BABA, S., MARUTO, M., ANDO, K., FERAMOTO, T. and ENDO, I. Intestinal Behçet's disease: report of five cases. *Diseases of the Colon and Rectum*, **19**, 428–440 (1976)

3 BAILEY, H. Purpura as an acute abdominal emergency. *British Journal of Surgery*, **18,** 234–240 (1930)

4 BALF, C. L. The alimentary lesions in anaphylactoid purpura. *Archives of Diseases in Childhood*, **26,** 20–27 (1951)

5 BASU, R. Perforation of the bowel in Henoch-Schönlein purpura. *Archives of Diseases in Childhood*, **34,** 342–343 (1959)

6 BAZINET, P. and MARIN, G. A. Malabsorption in systemic lupus erythematosus. *American Journal of Digestive Diseases*, **16**, 460–466 (1971)

7 BERG, P., POSTEL, A. H. and LEE, S. L. Perforation of the ileum in steroid-treated systemic lupus erythematosus. *American Journal of Digestive Diseases*, **5**, 274–282 (1960)

8 BIENENSTOCK, M., MINICK, R. and ROGOFF, B. Mesenteric arteritis and intestinal infarction in rheumatic disease. *Archives of Internal Medicine*, **119**, 359–364 (1967)

9 BITRAN, J., McSHANE, D. and ELLMAN, M. H. Ascites as the major manifestation of systemic lupus erythematosus. *Arthritis and Rheumatism*, **19**, 782–785 (1976)

10 BOE, J., DALGAARD, J. B. and SCOTT, D. Micro-cutaneous-ocular syndrome with intestinal involvement. A clinical and pathological study of four fatal cases. *American Journal of Medicine*, **25**, 857–867 (1958)

11 BROWN, C. H., SHIRLEY, E. K. and HASERICK, J. R. Gastrointestinal manifestations of systemic lupus erythematosus. *Gastroenterology*, **31**, 649–666 (1956)

12 BRUCE, J. and SIRCUS, W. Disseminated lupus erythematosus of the alimentary tract. *Lancet*, **1**, 795–797 (1959)

13 BRUST, N. M. Ileo-ileal intussusception associated with Henoch-Schönlein purpura. *Archives of Paediatrics*, **69**, 212–218 (1952)

14 BUERGER, L. *The Circulating Disturbances of the Extremities Including Gangrene, Vasomotor and Trophic Disorders*. Philadelphia, W. B. Saunders Co. (1924)

15 BYWATERS, E. G. L. and SCOTT, J. T. The natural history of vascular lesions in rheumatoid arthritis. *Journal of Chronic Disease*, **16**, 905–914 (1963)

16 CARRON, D. B. and DOUGLAS, A. P. Steatorrhoea in vascular insufficiency of small intestine. Five cases of polyarteritis nodosa and allied disorders. *Quarterly Journal of Medicine*, **34**, 331–340 (1965)

17 CHAPMAN, R., DAWE, C. and WHORWELL, P. J. Ulcerative colitis in association with Takayasu's disease. *American Journal of Digestive Diseases*, **23**, 660–662 (1978)

18 CHUMBLEY, L. C., HARRISON, E. G. and De REMEE, R. A. Allergic granulomatosis and angiitis (Churg-Strauss syndrome). *Mayo Clinic Proceedings*, **52**, 477–484 (1977)

19 CHURG, J. and STRAUSS, L. Allergic granulomatosis, allergic angiitis and periarteritis nodosa. *American Journal of Pathology*, **27**, 277–302 (1951)

20 CREAM, J. J., BRYCESON, A. D. M. and RYDER, G. Disappearance of immunoglobulin and complement from the Arthus reaction and its relevance to studies of vasculitis in man. *British Journal of Dermatology*, **84**, 106–109 (1971)

21 DOE, W. F., EVANS, D., HOBBS, J. R. and BOOTH, C. C. Coeliac disease, vasculitis and cryoglobulinaemia. *Gut*, **13**, 112–123 (1972)

22 DYER, N. H., KENDALL, M. J. and HAWKINS, C. F. Malabsorption in rheumatoid disease. *Annals of Rheumatic Disease*, **30**, 626–630 (1971)

23 DYER, N. H., VERBOV, J. L., DAWSON, A. M., BORRIE, P. F. and STANSFELD, A. G. Cutaneous polyarteritis nodosa associated with Crohn's disease. *Lancet*, **1**, 648–650 (1970)

24 ENG, K., RUOFF, M. and BYSTRYN, J.-C. Behçet's syndrome: an unusual cause of colonic ulceration and perforation. *American Journal of Gastroenterology*, **75**, 57–59 (1981)

25 ESTES, D. and CHRISTIAN, C. J. The natural history of systemic lupus erythematosus by prospective analysis. *Medicine (Baltimore)*, **50**, 885–895 (1971)

26 FAUCI, A. S., HAYES, B. F. and KATZ, P. The spectrum of vasculitis: clinical, pathologic, immunologic and therapeutic considerations. *Annals of Internal Medicine*, **89,** 660–676 (1978)

27 FAUCI, A. S., KATZ, P., HAYNES, B. F. and WOLFF, S. M. Cyclophosphamide therapy of severe necrotising vasculitis. *New England Journal of Medicine*, **301,** 235–238 (1979)

28 FAUCI, A. S. and WOLFF, S. M. Wegener's granulomatosis: studies in eighteen patients and a review of the literature. *Medicine* (*Baltimore*), **52,** 535–561 (1973)

29 FELDT, R. H. and STICKLER, G. B. The gastrointestinal manifestations of anaphylactoid purpura in children. *Staff Meetings of the Mayo Clinic*, **37,** 465–473 (1962)

30 FINKBINER, R. B. and DECKER, J. P. Ulceration and perforation of the intestine due to necrotising arteritis. *New England Journal of Medicine*, **268,** 14–18 (1963)

31 FRIEDMAN, C. J. and TEGTMEYER, C. J. Crohn's disease associated with Takayasu's arteritis. *Digestive Diseases and Sciences*, **24,** 954–958 (1979)

32 FROHNERT, P. P. and SHEPS, S. G. Long term follow up study of periarteritis nodosa. *American Journal of Medicine*, **43,** 8–14 (1967)

33 GARNER, J. A. M. Acute pancreatitis as a complication of anaphylactoid (Henoch-Schönlein) purpura. *Archives of Diseases of Childhood*, **52,** 971–972 (1977)

34 GOLDMAN, B. A., DICKENS, K. L., SCHONKEN, J. R. Quoted by O'Neill, P. B. Gastrointestinal abnormalities in collagen disease. *American Journal of Digestive Diseases*, **6,** 1069–1083 (1942)

35 GRAY, N., MACKAY, I. R., TAFT, L. I., WEIDEN, S. and WOOD, I. J. Hepatitis, colitis and lupus manifestations. *American Journal of Digestive Diseases*, **3,** 481–489 (1958)

36 GUAY, A., JANOWER, M. L., BAIN, R. W. and McCREADY, F. J. A case of Buerger's disease causing ischaemic colitis with perforation in a young male. *American Journal of Medical Science*, **271,** 239–240 (1976)

37 HANDLE, J. and SWARTZ, G. Gastrointestinal manifestations of Schönlein-Henoch syndrome. *American Journal of Roentgenology*, **78,** 643–652 (1957)

38 HERRINGTON, J. L. Jr. and GROSSMAN, L. A. Surgical lesions of the small and large intestine resulting from Buerger's disease. *Annals of Surgery*, **168,** 1079–1087 (1968)

39 HOLLANDER, D. and MANNING, R. T. The use of alkylating agents in the treatment of Wegener's granulomatosis. *Annals of Internal Medicine*, **67,** 393–398 (1967)

40 HOULI, J. and REZEK, J. Digestive and articular manifestations of collagen diseases. *Annals of Rheumatic Disease*, **24,** 52–56 (1965)

41 ISRAEL, H. L., PATCHEVSKY, A. S. and SALDANA, M. J. Wegener's granulomatosis, lymphomatoid granulomatosis and benign lymphocyte angiitis and granulomatosis of lung. *Annals of Internal Medicine*, **87,** 691–699 (1977)

42 JERNSTROM, P. and STASNEY, J. Acute ulcerative enteritis due to polyarteritis. *Journal of the American Medical Association*, **148,** 544–546 (1952)

43 JONES, P. E., RAWCLIFFE, P., WHITE, N., SEGAL, A. W. Painless ascites in systemic lupus erythematosus. *British Medical Journal*, **1,** 1513 (1977)

44 KATZ, A. J. and GANG, D. L. A five year old girl with a skin rash and abdominal pain. MGH Case Records. 14/80. *New England Journal of Medicine*, **302,** 853–858 (1980)

45 KLEIN, R. G., HUNDER, G. G., STANSON, A. W. and SHEPS, S. G. Large artery involvement in giant cell arteritis. *Annals of Internal Medicine*, **83,** 806–812 (1975)

46 KLEINMAN, P., MEYERS, M. A., ABBOTT, G. and KAZAM, E. Necrotising enterocolitis with pneumatosis intestinalis in systemic lupus erythematosus and polyarteritis. *Radiology*, **121,** 595–598 (1976)

47 KURLANDER, D. J. and KIRSNER, J. B. The association of chronic 'non-specific' inflammatory bowel disease with lupus erythematosus. *Annals of Internal Medicine*, **60,** 799–813 (1964)

48 LASSER, A. and GHOFRANY, S. Necrotising granulomatous vasculitis and allergic granulomatosis of the gallbladder. *Gastroenterology*, **71,** 660–662 (1976)

49 LAWRIE, T. D. V. Polyarteritis nodosa – a report of two cases presenting with abdominal symptoms and signs. *Glasgow Medical Journal*, **36,** 220–221 (1955)

50 LIE, J. T. Disseminated visceral giant cell arteritis. Histopathologic description and differentiation from other granulomatous vasculitides. *American Journal of Pathology*, **69,** 299–305 (1978)

51 LIEB, E. S., RESTIVO, C. and PAULUS, H. E. Immunosuppressive and corticosteroid therapy of polyarteritis nodosa. *American Journal of Medicine*, **67,** 941–947 (1979)

52 LIPSKY, P. E., HARDIN, J. A., SCHOUR, L. and PLOTZ, P. H. Spontaneous peritonitis and systemic lupus erythematosus. Importance of accurate diagnosis of Gram-positive bacterial infections. *Journal of the American Medical Association*, **233,** 929–931 (1975)

53 LOCKWOOD, C. M., REES, A. J., PINCHING, A. J., PUSSELL, B., SWENY, P., UFF, J. and PETERS, D. K. Plasma exchange and immunosuppression in the treatment of fulminating immune complex nephritis. *Lancet*, **1,** 63–67 (1977)

54 LOCKWOOD, C. M., PUSEY, C. D., REES, A. J. and PETERS, D. K. Plasma exchange in the treatment of immune complex disease. *Clinics in Immunology and Allergy*, **1,** 433–455 (1981)

55 MATOLO, N. M. and ALBO, D. Jr. Gastrointestinal complications of collagen vascular diseases: surgical implications. *American Journal of Surgery*, **122,** 678–682 (1971)

56 MEDICAL RESEARCH COUNCIL. Treatment of polyarteritis nodosa with cortisone: results after three years. *British Medical Journal*, **1,** 1399–1400 (1960)

57 MODIGLIANI, R., MUSCHART, J.-M., GALIAN, A., CLAUVEL, J.-P. and PIEL-DES RUISSEAUX, J.-L. Allergic granulomatous vasculitis (Churg-Strauss syndrome). Report of a case with widespread digestive involvement. *Digestive Disease Science*, **26,** 264–270 (1981)

58 MORTON, R. E., MILLER, A. I. and KAPLAN, R. Systemic lupus erythematosus: unusual presentation with gastric polyps and vasculitis. *Southern Medical Journal*, **69,** 507–509 (1976)

59 MOWREY, F. H. and LUNDBERG, B. A. Clinical manifestations of periarteritis nodosa with emphasis on hepatic and visceral manifestations. *Annals of Internal Medicine*, **40,** 1145–1164 (1954)

60 MUSHER, D. Systemic lupus erythematosus: a cause of medical peritonitis. *American Journal of Surgery*, **124,** 368–372 (1972)

61 OWYANG, C., MILLER, L. J., LIE, J. T. and FLEMING, C. R. Takayasu's arteritis in Crohn's disease. *Gastroenterology*, **76,** 825–828 (1979)

62 PACHAS, W. N., LINSCHEER, W. G. and PINELS, R. S. Protein losing enteropathy in systemic lupus erythematosus. *American Journal of Gastroenterology*, **55,** 166–167 (1971)

63 PHILLIPS, J. C. and HOWLAND, W. J. Mesenteric arteritis in systemic lupus erythematosus. *Journal of the American Medical Association*, **206,** 1569–1570 (1968)

64 POLLACK, V. E., GROVE, W. J., KARK, R. M., MUEHRCKE, R. C., PIRANI, C. L. and STECK, I. E. Systemic lupus erythematosus simulating acute surgical condition of the abdomen. *New England Journal of Medicine*, **259,** 258–266 (1958)

64a PSUCHIGA, M., OKAZAKI, I., ASAKURA, H. and OHKUBO, T. Radiographic and endoscopic features of colonic ulcers in systemic lupus erythematosus. *American Journal of Gastroenterology*, **67,** 277–285 (1975)

65 PUPPALA, A. R., CHENG, J. C. and STEINHEBER, F. U. Pancreatitis – a rare complication of Schönlein-Henoch purpura. *American Journal of Gastroenterology*, **69,** 101–104 (1978)

66 RAITT, J. W. Wegener's granulomatosis: treatment with cytotoxic agents and adrenocorticoids. *Annals of Internal Medicine*, **74,** 344–356 (1971)

67 REZA, M. J., ROTH, B. E., POPS, M. A. and GOLDBERG, L. S. Intestinal vasculitis in essential mixed cryoglobulinaemia. *Annals of Internal Medicine*, **81,** 632–634 (1974)

68 REZA, M. J., DORNFIELD, L., GOLDBERG, L. S., BLUESTONE and PEARSON, C. M. Wegener's granulomatosis: long term follow up of patients treated with cyclophosphamide. *Arthritis and Rheumatism*, **18,** 501–506 (1975)

69 ROB, C. Surgical diseases of the celiac and mesenteric arteries. *Archives of Surgery*, **93,** 21–32 (1966)

70 ROSE, G. A. and SPENCER, M. Polyarteritis nodosa. *Quarterly Journal of Medicine*, **26,** 43–79 (1957)

71 SACHS, I. L., KLIMA, T. and FRANKEL, N. B. Thromboangiitis obliterans of the transverse colon. *Journal of the American Medical Assocation*, **238,** 336–337 (1977)

72 SCHNEIDER, R. E. and DOBBIN, W. O. Suction biopsy of rectal mucosa for the diagnosis of arteritis in rheumatoid arthritis and related disorders. *Annals of Internal Medicine*, **68,** 561–568 (1968)

73 SCHOCKET, A. L., LAIN, D. and KOHLER, P. E. Immune complex vasculitis as a cause of ascites and pleural effusions in systemic lupus erythematosus. *Journal of Rheumatology*, **5,** 33–38 (1978)

74 SCOTT, D. G. I., BACON, P. A. and TRIBE, C. R. Systemic rheumatoid arthritis: a clinical and laboratory study of 50 cases. *Medicine* (*Baltimore*), **60,** 288–297 (1981)

75 SHAFER, R. B. and GREGORY, D. H. Systemic lupus presenting as regional ileitis. *Minnesota Medicine*, **53,** 789–792 (1970)

76 SHESOL, B. F., ROSATO, E. F. and ROSATO, F. E. Concomitant acute lupus erythematosus and primary pneumococcal peritonitis. *American Journal of Gastroenterology*, **63,** 324–326 (1975)

77 SIURALA, M., JULKUNEN, H., TOIVONEN, S., POLKINEN, R., SAXEN, E. and PITKANEN, E. Digestive tract in collagen disease. *Acta Medica Scandinavica*, **178,** 13–25 (1965)

78 SOBEL, R. A. and RUEBNER, B. H. Buerger's disease involving coeliac artery. *Human Pathology*, **10,** 112–115 (1979)

79 SOLOWAY, M., MUIR, T. W. and LINTON, D. W. Takayasu's arteritis: report of a case with unusual findings. *American Journal of Cardiology*, **25,** 258–263 (1970)

80 SRIGLEY, J. R. and GARDINER, G. W. Giant cell arteritis with small bowel infarction. A case report and review of the literature. *American Journal of Gastroenterology*, **73,** 157–161 (1980)

81 SUEN, K. C. and BURTON, J. D. The spectrum of eosinophilic infiltration of the gastrointestinal tract and its relationship to other disorders of angiitis and granulomatosis. *Human Pathology*, **10,** 31–42 (1979)

82 TEJA, K., CRUM, C. P. and FRIEDMAN, C. Giant cell arteritis and Crohn's disease: an unreported association. *Gastroenterology*, **78,** 796–802 (1980)

83 TOIVONEN, S., PITKANEN, E. and SIURALA, M. Collagen disease associated with intestinal malabsorption and sprue-like changes in the intestinal mucosa. *Acta Medica Scandinavica*, **175,** 91–95 (1964)

84 TRAVERS, R. L., ALLISON, D. J., BRETTLE, R. P. and HUGHES, G. R. V. Polyarteritis nodosa: a clinical and angiographic analysis of 17 cases. *Seminars in Arthritis and Rheumatism*, **8,** 184–199 (1979)

85 TRENTHAM, P. E. and MASI, A. J. Systemic lupus erythematosus with a protein-losing enteropathy. *Journal of the American Medical Association*, **236,** 287–288 (1976)

86 WALTON, E. W. Giant cell granuloma of the respiratory tract (Wegener's granulomatosis). *British Medical Journal*, **2,** 265–276 (1958)

87 WOLFF, S. M., FAUCI, A. S., HORN, R. G. and DALE, D. C. Wegener's granulomatosis. *Annals of Internal Medicine*, **81,** 513–525 (1974)

88 WOLFSOHN, H. Purpura and intussusception. *Archives of Diseases in Childhood*, **22,** 242–247 (1947)

89 YOUNG, D. G. Chronic intestinal obstruction following Henoch-Schönlein disease. *Clinical Pediatrics*, **3,** 737–740 (1964)

90 ZIZAC, J. M., SHOLMAN, L. E. and STEVENS, M. B. Colonic perforations in systemic lupus erythematosus. *Medicine (Baltimore)*, **54,** 411–426 (1975)

13
'Atopy' and the gut

J. Pepys

INTRODUCTION

The role of allergy in gastrointestinal disease is controversial, so much so as to justify the dictum that 'gastrointestinal allergy is a diagnosis frequently entertained, occasionally evaluated and rarely established'[40]. Where causal agents are identified, allergic disorders are classified as 'extrinsic', and regarded almost exclusively until recent years as 'atopic', or where causal agents are not identified on an atopic basis as 'cryptogenic', a preferable term to 'intrinsic' or 'non-allergic'. Studies in allergic asthma show that extrinsic agents can mediate clinical reactions on an atopic or non-atopic basis, and that both mechanisms may operate together and even be interdependent[67, 68, 71, 74]. The respiratory tract and the skin are readily accessible models for direct observation and characterization of allergic reactions under controlled conditions.

In this analysis of 'atopy and the gut', emphasis will be laid on the definition of terms; on certain basic aspects of related immunopathology and their possible clinical relevance; on the roles of IgE and IgE antibody, mast cells and basophils and other cell types including eosinophils, lymphocytes and plasma cells; on the relationship of atopy to other types of allergic reaction and on the role in such analysis of the effects of sodium cromoglycate.

DEFINITIONS

Allergy

The problems about the roles of 'allergy' and 'atopy' are complicated by the use and abuse of these terms. 'Allergy' as defined by von Pirquet can be summarised as the 'acquired, specific altered capacity to react', covering both decreased reactivity or immunity, and increased reactivity or hypersensitivity, with their often complex interrelationships. The term 'allergy' is commonly used to describe hypersensitivity, and is often used in a still more restricted sense to mean Type I, immediate allergy or atopy. The types of allergy each have characteristic features determined by their antibody mechanism. They are, Type I, immediate allergy mediated mainly by IgE antibody, but also and less commonly by IgG subclass (short term sensitizing, STS) antibody[65,72]; Type II, allergy relevant to autoallergy; Type III, immune-complex complement-dependent, allergy; and Type IV, delayed tuberculin-type, lymphocyte-dependent allergy. The types of allergy often coexist, and may be interdependent. An important example is the introductory role Type I plays in the development after some hours of the more severe tissue-damaging, Type III reaction[20,67]. There is, also, an indistinguishable dual reaction, compatible with a Type III reaction, in which neither precipitins nor immune-complexes are found and which appears to be attributable to IgE antibody alone[24].

Atopy

A familial tendency to develop, in a natural way, immediate type allergy to common environmental allergens was recognised by Cooke and van der Veer in 1916 who called it 'human protein hypersensitiveness[20]. They estimated a prevalence of about 10 per cent. The term 'atopy' introduced by Coca and Cooke[16] to describe this included: hay fever; asthma; infantile, flexural, eczema; urticaria and gastrointestinal disorders. They claimed that the immediate allergy was not passively transferable, although Prausnitz and Kuestner had reported their observations two years previously[76]. Coca and Grove later coined the term 'reagin' to describe the heat-labile, passively transferable substance[17]. Anaphylaxis, regarded as a phenomenon of experimental animals, was excluded and lessening of sensitivity by injection of the specific agent was included. They distinguished atopy from contact sensitivity and emphasized the differences of atopy due to natural sensitization, that is, via mucosal membranes, from sensitization by injection.

This complex definition of 'atopy' is responsible for the confusion with which it is associated. There are differences in the clinical definition of the disorders and in only a proportion can evidence of allergic sensitivity be found. The use of the term 'atopy' to describe a defining characteristic – the capacity to develop (in a natural way) Type I, immediate, IgE-mediated allergy in response to the ordinary exposures to common allergens[69] – gives it a more precise meaning.

CLASSIFICATION OF ATOPY

The polar-atopic group can be identified by skin prick tests with three or four relevant allergen extracts, such as house dust, the house dust allergy mite (*Dermatophagoides* spp.), grass pollen and cat[36]. Positive wealing reactions to one or more of these is evidence of the production of specific IgE antibody, with some limited reservation for Type I reactions mediated by IgG-STS (short term-sensitizing) antibody[71]. The prick test can be supported or replaced by the radioallergosorbent test (RAST) for specific IgE antibodies. In subjects giving negative reactions to prick tests and positive reactions to intracutaneous tests, there is little correlation with specific IgE antibody[84] and, where sought, IgG-STS antibody has been found. These findings may explain differences dependent on the mode of testing for evidence of IgE antibody and atopy.

Prick tests show that about 40 per cent of the population are atopic in the immunological sense without symptoms. They are more likely to become sensitized, and more rapidly sensitized, under certain conditions, for example in occupational exposure to enzymes of *B. subtilis*[70] in the manufacture of detergents and to the salts of platinum[72] in the refining of the metal. The presence of IgE antibodies in the absence of symptoms is nevertheless associated with decreased β-adrenergic, and increased α-adrenergic and cholinergic activity[45] acting as a 'priming' effect which could result in increased responses to specific and non-specific stimuli.

Atopic status determined by the number of common allergens, from nil to three or more, to which propositi react shows highly significant correlations with the presence in first degree relatives of allergic respiratory disorders and infantile eczema[69]. Routine classification of all patients as described above is recommended. It places them in atopic or non-atopic groups and shows their, and their families', atopic status in addition to whatever causally related information is provided.

Atopic sensitization

IgE reaginic antibody

The identification of immunoglobulin E as the heat-labile, passively transferable, long-term sensitizing antibody greatly advanced the understanding of atopy[42]. It is a normal immunoglobulin present in minute amounts in the serum, about 1/10,000th to 1/40,000th that of IgG. It is to be expected that IgE antibody could also be induced by highly potent allergens in those regarded, by definition, as non-atopic. IgE-producing *plasma cells* lie mainly in mucosal related lymphoid tissues, probably relevant to the mucosae as portals of entry for allergen in atopics and also for local sensitization[85]. Its production is dependent on T-lymphocyte function, being increased when T- suppressor lymphocyte activity is decreased[15].

IgE owes its biological importance to the presence on mast and basophil cells of receptors for the heat-labile footpiece (Fc). The bridging of two molecules of IgE initiates the release and production of potent mediators of tissue reactions. IgE is not transmitted through the placenta, and it is formed during embryonic development[59]. Specific IgE antibodies to food allergens, different from those of the mother, have been found in neonates[47]. These include antibodies to egg allergen as indicated by J. Pepys (personal communication). These findings may have bearing on the acute, often severe, reactions of infants on first eating of egg although they may also have ingested egg allergen through breast-milk. These infants are frequently highly atopic. Control of maternal diet during pregnancy and breast feeding merits study for its potential preventive value.

Serum total IgE levels are higher the larger the number of allergens to which the subject is sensitive[84], though the amounts of specific IgE antibody do not account for the total values. Increases in total IgE levels are seen in response to potent allergenic stimulation, with very high levels, for example, in allergic bronchopulmonary aspergillosis in relation to episodes of pulmonary eosinophilia, an acute allergic pneumonitis, in which the amounts of specific IgE antibody to the causal allergen, *A. Fumigatus*, play only a small part[55]. High values are found in gastrointestinal parasitic infestations in man and animals. Potentiation of pre-existing IgE antibody levels to unrelated allergens by parasitic infestation has also been found[44]. Such changes could be expected to increase the overall severity of reactions to both specific and non-specific stimuli. An increase of total IgE after challenge in a patient with wheat sensitivity was associated with abnormal numbers of IgE-producing plasma cells in the jejunum[11]. Monitoring of serum IgE antibody and total levels might therefore be useful clinically.

Passive sensitization of human ileum and colon for Type I, immediate reactions has long been known. Biopsy specimens of human jejunum passively sensitized with IgE antibody showed degranulation of mast cells on allergen challenge[80].

Mucosa as the portal of entry for allergens in atopy

A role for mucosal permeability in sensitization by the 'natural' route in atopics is postulated. Nasal instillation of allergen induced immediate-type allergy in atopics but not in non-atopics, whereas with injection there were no differences[78]. In patients with cystic fibrosis a high proportion have IgE antibodies to a number of allergens, although they do not give histories of 'atopic' eczema[91], a stigma of highly atopic subjects. These findings suggest that increased mucosal permeability is related to IgE antibody production.

Other factors associated with increased absorption of food allergens and antibody responses are gastroenteritis[33] and low IgA levels. Infants from atopic families and with a tendency to low IgA levels are more readily sensitized to cows' milk and more likely to develop 'atopic' eczema[86].

In patients with 'atopic' eczema increased mucosal permeability and absorption of food allergens has been found, apparently unrelated to causal foods[43]. Penetration of allergens through epithelial tight junctions as in the bronchus is attributed to mucosal damage. This could be induced by reactions of sensitised basophils on the mucosal surface with liberation of histamine and other mediators[38]. This concept is of clinical importance in relation to the preservation of the integrity of mast and basophil cells by topical sodium cromoglycate. This could explain the decrease in absorption of food allergens from the gut by oral sodium cromoglycate (Nalcrom), and the decrease in total serum IgE levels in patients with 'atopic' eczema so treated[54], presumably because of decreased stimulation by allergenic foods of the mucosally related IgE producing plasma cells.

Mast/basophil cells and atopy

Mast cells are pre-eminent in the immunopathology of Type I, IgE-mediated reactions. Their role in homeostasis is probably associated with their close relationship to the microcirculation and to smooth muscle, on which their content of tissue mediators can exert rapid and vigorous action. Amongst these are, preformed mediators, such as histamine with its effects on H_1 and H_2 receptors and 5-hydroxytryptamine (serotonin), and newly generated ones such as platelet activating factor, and the leukotrienes, with their potent inflammatory effects, derived from cyclo- and lipo-oxygenase breakdown of arachidonic acid, and including the prostaglandins and slow-reacting substance of anaphylaxis (SRS-A)[92]. They also liberate preformed eosinophil chemotactic factor (ECF-A) and neutrophil chemotactic factor (NCF), and other chemotactic factors such as histamine and newly generated lipid factors[93].

The IgE mediated mast cell reaction initiates an enzyme cascade in the cell membrane which causes an energy-dependent influx of calcium ions into the cell, by acting on the 'calcium gate', with resultant release of histamine. Calcium ion flux is assuming major importance in the sequence of events of mast cell reactions. It has been suggested that sodium cromoglycate may exert its protective action on the integrity of the mast cell by modifying calcium ion flux. Indirect support for such a possibility is the finding that nifedipine[13] and verapamil[65], both used in cardiology for their action on calcium ion flux, can block exercise-induced asthma, as does sodium cromoglycate[66].

A further effect of increase in calcium ion flux in the cell membrane is the increase in cytosol calcium with the formation of calmodulin. This, in turn, induces calcium dependent production of neurotransmitters such as noradrenaline, acetylcholine and dopamine with their effects on nerve receptors[22]. Mast cells are present at nerve terminals and it may be that they act as a 'buffer' to irritant stimuli which would otherwise act directly upon the nerves themselves. Agents acting on mast cells and on calcium ion flux are of interest for clinical studies of their effects on specific and non-specific stimuli in the gut.

Increased numbers of mast and basophil cells are found in chronic inflammation, for example in duodenal ulcer, granulomatous polyps, ulcerative colitis, proctitis, amoebiasis and giardiasis, but not in Crohn's disease[87]. It is not clear whether they play a primary causal role or whether this is an epiphenomenon. Mast cell infiltration is a feature of the later stages of the classical Type IV, tuberculin reaction. Another example is the basophil-rich lymphocyte-mediated reaction elicited in the early stages of sensitization demonstrable in skin tests and termed 'cutaneous basophil hypersensitivity'.

Increased populations of mast cells could serve as sites for IgE mediated reactions because of their receptor affinity for IgE, thus contributing to the overall immunopathology. Mast cells in the gut may contain IgE and a marked increase in their number is found in untreated as compared with treated coeliac disease[81]. Suggestive indirect evidence for the role of mast cells and possibly IgE is provided by the beneficial effect of oral sodium cromoglycate on the gastrointestinal manifestations in patients with systemic mastocytosis, though this could take several weeks[25, 79, 83].

'Priming' of mast/basophil cells

Increased sensitivity of mast cells to non-specific agents correlates directly with increased levels of serum total IgE, as shown by the sizes of weals elicited by skin prick tests with a histamine liberator, but, as might be expected, not with histamine itself[84]. Priming of basophil cells is shown by the greater spontaneous release of histamine from separated circulating cells in subjects with food sensitivity[6, 58]. This was most marked in those sensitive to peanuts and other nuts. There is no evidence that this spontaneous release occurs *in vivo*. That such priming might play a part *in vivo*, however, is suggested by the finding of increased spontaneous release of histamine from the basophils of patients with exercise-induced asthma[60].

In vitro evidence of priming is provided by the greater release of SRS-A from chopped guinea-pig lung of sensitized as compared with non-sensitized animals[75].

Eosinophil cells

The association of eosinophil responses with atopy is not as exclusive as was once thought. Eosinophilia is suggestive of allergy and of a possible beneficial response to corticosteroids, which have little effect on Type I allergic reactions but are very effective on Type III, immune-complex reactions[68].

Eosinophil cell infiltrations of the gastrointestinal tract, in the absence of clinical features, are not necessarily evidence of disease[63]. Two phases of tissue eosinophilia have been described in allergen challenge; an early one peaking at 4–6 h, and a later one, progressive over several days, starting after 12–18 h[37]. The early response is mediated by a heat-stable, low molecular weight product probably derived from mast cells[48] and the late response by a heat-labile, high molecular weight product, probably a lymphokine.

There are a number of eosinophil chemotactic factors (ECF) ranging from preformed low molecular weight (500 daltons) ECF-A from specifically sensitized mast and basophil cells, to intermediate weight agents (1500–2500 daltons) found in rat mast cells, to activated components of C5a resulting from immune-complex reactions[4, 7, 8, 90]. There are other serum chemotactic factors, mainly for neutrophils, but also for eosinophils such as kallikrein, plasminogen activator of neutrophil proteases, and tissue enzymes.

Eosinophilia, like IgE antibody, is T-cell dependent and there are lymphokines which stimulate eosinopoiesis[19]. Eosinophilis are commonly associated with mast cells and can digest mast cell granules before mediator release occurs[93]. Prostaglandins, PGE_1 and PGE_2 inhibit the release of granules from mast cells and may be derived from allergen stimulated eosinophils[39]. In addition to a basic cationic protein which potentiates inflammatory responses[29], they contain histaminase, arylsulphatase and phospholipase, which can inactivate histamine, SRS-A and PAF (platelet activating factor) respectively[93].

The killing of schistosomulae by eosinophils suggests a defense response against parasites[10]. Eosinophilia and IgE antibody production are both features of parasitic infestation and a role has also been claimed for IgE in the natural cure of parasitic infestation in animals[14, 44].

ALIMENTARY ALLERGY

Foods and atopy

Food intolerance comprises food allergy, with relevant immunological mechanisms; or food idiosyncrasy, as in gut or systemic enzyme defects. Reactions to foods can be classified as reaginic, i.e. atopic, with anaphylaxis, gastrointestinal, skin and respiratory symptoms; or non-reaginic, with malabsorption and protein-losing enteropathy.

The subject of food allergy is highly controversial, except where the reactions, systemic or gastrointestinal, are clearly related to ingestion of a particular food already, as a rule, known to the patient. In these cases the reactions, with few exceptions, are of an acute, immediate reproducible nature, and with supporting evidence of atopy.

Food allergens

The dictum that 'common things apply commonly' is particularly relevant to food allergy and is the basis for attempts at aetiological diagnosis. The usual foods responsible are cows' milk, egg, nuts, cheese, corn, fish, shellfish, chocolate, coffee, tomato, mushroom, chicken, strawberry, soy protein and food additives. The common gastrointestinal manifestations are abdominal pain and distension, diarrhoea and vomiting. They are probably due to oedema, hypersecretion and smooth muscle contraction elicited by the mediators from allergic reactions, not necessarily IgE mediated.

Among the causes of differences of opinion with regard to food allergy are: the wide range between acceptance based on unproven preconceived ideas and highly restricted, critical observation; the use of intracutaneous tests which are more likely to give immediate reactions without evidence of IgE antibody, and the present uncertain quality of allergen extracts.

Characterisation and standardisation of allergens are only at an early stage and validation in clinically proven cases is needed. Better test results have been obtained with freshly prepared food extracts[6] and even with digests of cows' milk[34], for example, than with commercial preparations. Prick tests with freshly prepared extracts gave positive reactions in all the children in whom a blind food challenge was positive, whereas intracutaneous tests gave many more positive reactions than could be proven clinically[6]. Allergenic moieties have been characterised for only few foods and of these codfish protein in crystalline form is probably the purest,[1] and in cows' milk, β-lactoglobulin is more reactive than casein, lactalbumin and serum albumin respectively[5].

The wholly justified statement that 'the proof of the pudding is in the eating' applies to definitive proof in food allergy. Attempts at avoidance, guided by knowledge of allergenic interrelationships and the content of daily foodstuffs, are commonly made, with deliberate challenge for confirmation. In principle, basic trial diets exclude already proven or suspect foods and those commonly listed. One example consists of fresh fruit and vegetables, fresh fruit juice, tea, coffee, sugar, rice, gluten-free bread, olive oil, barley sugar and a margarine free of added milk products. Persistence of symptoms on such a diet after a trial period of 1–2 weeks could mean that possible causes are included in this diet and exclusion of one food at a time is indicated. The use of an elemental diet as the basis for food avoidance would appear to be worthwhile. Control of symptoms permits the testing of additional single foods. Confirmation of allergic sensitivity by at least three exposures has been suggested[30]. Food challenges should be double-blind, if possible, to exclude the all too common subjective assessment by both patient and doctor. Food challenges should not be made or made only with great care where the history suggests that immediate, potentially severe, reactions may occur. Symptomatic reactions with small bowel biopsy abnormalities may be present within 24 h, and in others may take days or weeks to develop[41,89]. Attempts to identify food allergens by exclusion and trial diets are a necessary part of investigation, with the proviso that they are not an additional burden. Confirmation is usually readily available in atopy, but in other cases patient observation over long periods is needed.

Indirect support for atopy in food reactions is provided by the growing number of reports of the blocking by sodium cromoglycate of both gut and systemic reactions in challenge tests, and by responses to its use in clinical management. The beneficial responses occur mainly in subjects with demonstrable atopy. Sodium cromoglycate (in man and experimental animals) decreases the absorption of food allergens from the gut[8,21]. In some patients diarrhoea and vomiting due to foods are associated with increases in the venous levels of prostaglandins[52]. Administration of prostaglandin synthetase inhibitors, such as aspirin and indomethacin, effectively blocked the reactions in most of the subjects with and without evidence of atopy. Prostaglandin synthesis is a feature of IgE mediated mast cell reactions, but is not confined to it.

Direct observation of tissue changes in biopsy specimens can help to confirm the food reaction. Jejunal biopsies after ingestion of cows' milk have shown eosinophil infiltration and villous atrophy together with increases in IgA, IgM and IgE producing plasma cells[50]. Precipitins may also be present and the question is whether the reactions are of Types I and/or III, or even Type IV allergy, the flattening of the intestinal mucosa being attributed by some to a T cell-mediated reaction[26]. All the types of allergy can be present and be involved together, thus complicating the analysis of the 'end' inflammatory changes.

ALLERGIC GASTROENTEROPATHY

It is under this heading that the features suggestive of or compatible with allergy in general or with atopy in particular can be considered. Some of the disorders are characterised by eosinophilia, such as eosinophilic gastroenteritis and others by inflammatory changes in which the participation of allergic mechanisms is sought, such as coeliac disease, Crohn's disease and ulcerative colitis.

Coeliac disease

Increases in IgE producing plasma cells have been reported in untreated patients with decreases on avoidance of gluten[81]. There is, however, no definitive evidence of atopy as a mechanism in coeliac disease, although mast cells and IgE containing cells are present in the mucosa. If a Type III, immune complex mechanism were involved, Type I allergy could provide the introductory mechanism.

Eosinophilic gastroenteritis

The mucosa and/or muscle layer of the stomach, small bowel and oesophagus can be heavily infiltrated with eosinophils. An association of the mucosal form with food allergy and the presence of allergic respiratory and skin disorders is reported[11,46]. Intense eosinophil infiltration of the stomach has been reported together with raised IgE levels, positive skin tests and other features of atopy[12]. Allergic children with chronic diarrhoea may show eosinophil infiltration and necrosis and regeneration of glandular epithelium in gastric biopsies, which are recommended in atopic children with diarrhoea and growth retardation[46].

Eosinophilic oesophagitis in some subjects with allergic respiratory disease responds to corticosteroids[23,51]. This is unlikely to be due to an effect on Type I allergy, though it does not exclude a role for it.

Inflammatory bowel disease

Studies of atopy in Crohn's disease and in ulcerative colitis have given conflicting results, partly based on differences in criteria for atopy[4, 35, 74, 88]. Some report that hay fever, rhinitis and asthma were twice as common in ulcerative colitis than in controls, whereas only eczema was more common in Crohn's disease. Others have found atopic features in both and yet others no significant difference. Comparison based on immunological classification of atopy, namely IgE production to common allergens, as shown by skin prick tests, showed no significant differences from controls[74]. Some patients with inflammatory bowel disease had raised serum total IgE levels without evidence of atopy, and there was no significant difference between the groups.

Acute immediate reactions confirmed by biopsy have been elicited by intramucosal injection of food allergen in ulcerative colitis. Local IgE production or the presence of higher local concentrations could be responsible[31, 32, 77].

SODIUM CROMOGLYCATE AND GASTROINTESTINAL ALLERGY

Sodium cromoglycate has a potent inhibitory effect on Type I, IgE mediated reactions in the respiratory tract, and atopics tend to respond best to it. It can also block the non-immediate reactions compatible with Type III reactions[68]. It also blocks clinical and mast cell reactions to non-specific stimuli such as exercise, cold, SO_2 and histamine liberators[2]. These effects are attributed to preservation of the integrity of the mast cell and possibly to an effect on irritant receptors. Long term use in asthma decreases the non-specific hyper-reactivity of the bronchi[2].

In most studies of sodium cromoglycate in food allergy, an improvement has been shown in gastrointestinal and other reactions[25, 27, 28, 49, 62, 94]. Most patients were selected because of demonstrable or suspected intolerance with or without positive skin tests or RASTs[94]. In one report only few gave positive reactions to prick and most to intracutaneous tests, suggesting that antibodies other than IgE were present.

Sodium cromoglycate decreases absorption of food allergens from the gut and also the IgE complexes found in the serum after ingestion of food allergens[8, 21, 64]. These findings are valuable additions to the paucity of objective immunological support in food allergy.

The effects of oral sodium cromoglycate in inflammatory bowel disease, reported in a symposium on the mast cell, showed a beneficial effect in a limited number of patients with mild to moderately severe ulcerative colitis and proctitis, with morphological support, particularly in those with eosinophilia[9, 53, 56, 57, 60, 82]. It might be more effective given as continuous instillation of a solution in patients with ileostomies. A 6-month trial of oral sodium cromoglycate in Crohn's disease showed no beneficial effect. There is scope for further studies of sodium cromoglycate in inflammatory bowel disease, since immunological mechanisms such as Types I and III allergy may be involved primarily or become involved secondarily through increased mast cell populations, because of its effects in food allergy and because of its possible role in gastrointestinal mucosal reactions.

References

1 AAS, K. and JEBSEN, J. W. Studies of hypersensitivity to fish. Partial purification and crystallization of a major allergenic component of cod. *International Achives of Allergy and Applied Immunology*, **32,** 1–20 (1967)

2 ALTOUNYAN, R. Review of the clinical activity and modes of action of sodium cromoglycate. In *The Mast Cell*, edited by J. Pepys and A. M. Edwards, 199–216. Tunbridge Wells, Pitman Medical Publishing Co. Ltd. (1979)

3 BASTEN, A. and BEESON, P. Mechanism of eosinophilia. II. Role of the lymphocyte. *Journal of Experimental Medicine*, **131,** 1288–1305 (1905)

4 BINDER, V. and HVIDBERG, E. Histamine content of rectal mucosa in ulcerative colitis. *Gut*, **8,** 24–28 (1973)

5 BLEUMINK, E. and YOUNG, E. Identification of the atopic allergen in cow's milk. *International Archives of Allergy and Applied Immunology*, **34,** 521–543 (1968)

6 BOCK, S., MAY, D. and REMIGIO, L. Clinical manifestations and immunological findings in food sensitivity confirmed objectively. In *The Mast Cell*, edited by J. Pepys and A. M. Edwards, 411–415. Tunbridge Wells. Pitman Medical Publishing Co. Ltd. (1979)

7 BOSWELL, R. N., AUSTEN, K. F. and GOETZL, E. J. Intermediate molecular weight eosinophil chemotactic factors in rat peritoneal mast cells: immunologic release, granule association, and demonstration of structural heterogeneity. *Journal of Immunology*, **120,** 15–20 (1978)

8 BROSTOFF, J., CARINI, C., WRAITH, D. G. and JOHNS, P. Production of IgE complexes by allergen challenge in atopic patients and the effect of sodium cromoglycate. *Lancet*, **1,** 1286–1270 (1979)

9 BROWN, P. and BLAYNEY, K. A therapeutic trial of disodium cromoglycate in the treatment of ulcerative colitis. In *The Mast Cell*, edited by J. Pepys and A. M. Edwards, 673–676. Tunbridge Wells. Pitman Medical Publishing Co. Ltd. (1979)

10 BUTTERWORTH, A. E., STURROCK, R. F., HOUBA, V., MAHMOUD, A. A. F.,SHER, A. and REES, P. H. Eosinophils as mediators of antibody-dependent damage to schistosomula. *Nature*, **256,** 727 (1975)

11 CALDWELL, J. H., SHARMA, H. M. and HURTUBISE, P. E. Eosinophilic gastroenteritis and extreme allergy: immunopathological comparison with nonallergic gastrointestinal disease. *Gastroenterology*, **74,** 1016 (1978)

12 CALDWELL, J. H., TENNENBAUM, J. I. and BRONSTEIN, H. A. Serum IgE in eosinophilic gastroenteritis. Response to intestinal challenge in two cases. *New England Journal of Medicine*, **292,** 1388–1390 (1975)

13 CARRINA, J., DENJEAN, A., ALEXANDRE, G., LOCKHART, A. and DUROUX, P. Inhibition of exercise-induced asthma by a calcium-antagonist, nifedipine. *American Review of Respiratory Disease*, **123,** 156–160 (1981)

14 CATTY, D. Immunology of nematode infection-trichinosis in guinea-pigs. In *Monographs in Allergy*, Volume 5 Basel, Karger (1969)

15 CHIORAZZI, N., FOX, D. A. and KATZ, D. H. Hapten-specific IgE antibody responses in mice. Conversion of IgE 'non-responder' strains to IgE 'responders' by elimination of suppressor T-cell activity. *Journal of Immunology*, **118,** 48–54 (1977)

16 COCA, A. F. and COOKE, R. A. On the classification of the phenomena of hypersensitiveness. *Journal of Immunology*, **8,** 163–174 (1923)

17 COCA, A. F. and GROVE, E. F. Studies in hypersensitiveness. XIII. A study of the atopic reagins. *Journal of Immunology*, **10,** 445–464 (1925)

18 COCHRANE, C. G. Mechanisms involved in the deposition of immune complexes in tissues. *Journal of Experimental Medicine*, **134,** (Suppl.) 75–89 (1971)

19 COLLEY, D. G. Eosinophils and immune mechanisms. I. Eosinophil stimulation promoter (ESP). A lymphokine induced by specific antigen or PHA. *Journal of Immunology*, **110,** 1419–1423 (1973)

20 COOKE, R. A. and VAN DER VEER, A. Jr. Human sensitisation. *Journal of Immunology*, **1,** 201–305 (1916)

21 DANNAEUS, A., FOUCARD, T. and JOHANSSON, S. G. O. The effect of orally administered sodium cromoglycate on symptoms of food allergy. *Clinical Allergy*, **7,** 109–115 (1977)

22 De LORENZO, R. J., FREEDMAN, S. D., YOKE, W. B. and MAURER, S. C. Stimulation of Ca^{2+} dependent neurotransmitter release and presynaptic nerve terminal protein phosphorylation by calmodulin and a calmodulin-like protein isolated from synaptic vesicles. *Proceedings of the National Academy of Sciences* (USA), **76,** 1838–1842 (1979)

23 DOBBINS, J. W., SHEAHAN, D. J. and BEHAR, J. Eosinophilic gastroenteritis with oesophageal involvement. *Gastroenterology*, **72,** 1312–1316 (1977)

24 DOLOVICH, J., HARGREAVE, F. E., CHALMERS, R., SHIER, K.-J., GAULDIE, J. and BIENENSTOCK, J. Late cutaneous allergic responses in isolated IgE-dependent reactions. *Journal of Allergy and Clinical Immunology*, **52,** 38–46 (1973)

25 DOLOVICH, J., PUNTHAKEE, N. D., MacMILLAN, A. B. and OSBALDESTON, G. J. Systemic mastocytosis: control of lifelong diarrhoea by ingested disodium cromoglycate. *Canadian Medical Association Journal*, **111,** 684–685 (1974)

26 FERGUSON, A. and PARROTT, D. Histopathology and time course of rejection of allografts of mouse small intestine. *Transplantation*, **15,** 546–554 (1973)

27 FRIER, S. and BERGER, H. Disodium cromoglycate in gastrointestinal protein intolerance. *Lancet*, **1,** 913–915 (1973)

28 GERRARD, J. W. Oral cromoglycate: its value in the treatment of adverse reactions to foods. *Annals of Allergy*, **42,** 135–138 (1979)

29 GLEICH, J. G., LOEGERING, D. A., KUEPPERS, F., BAJAJ, S. B. and MANN, K. G. Physiochemical and biological properties of the basic protein for guinea-pig eosinophil granules. *Journal of Experimental Medicine*, **140,** 313–322 (1974)

30 GOLDMAN, A. S., ANDERSON, D. W. Jr., SELLERS, W. A., SOPERSTEIN, S., KNIKER, W. T. and HALPERN, S. R. Milk allergy. I. Oral challenge with milk and isolated milk proteins in allergic children. *Pediatrics*, **32,** 425–443 (1963)

31 GRAY, I. and WALZER, M. Studies in mucous membrane hypersensitiveness; allergic reactions of the passively sensitised rectal mucous membrane. *American Journal of Digestive Diseases and Nutrition*, **4,** 707–712 (1938)

32 GRAY, I., HARTEN, M. and WALZER, M. Studies in mucous membrane hypersensitiveness; allergic reaction in the passively sensitised mucous membranes of the ileum and colon in humans. *Annals of Internal Medicine*, **13,** 2050–2056 (1940)

33 GRUSKAY, F. L. and COOKE, R. E. The gastrointestinal absorption of unaltered protein in normal infants and in infants recovering from diarrhoea. *Pediatrics*, **16,** 763–768 (1955)

34 HADDAD, Z. H., VERMA, S. and ZALRA, V. IgE antibodies to peptic and peptic-tryptic digests of β-lactoglobulin: significance in food hypersensitivity (abstract). *Journal of Allergy and Clinical Immunology*, **63,** 198 (1979)

35 HAMMER, B., ASHURST, P. and NAISH, J. Diseases associated with ulcerative colitis and Crohn's disease. *Gut*, **9,** 17–21 (1968)

36 HENDRICK, D. J., DAVIES, R. J., D'SOUZA, M. F. and PEPYS, J. An analysis of skin prick test reactions in 656 asthmatic patients. *Thorax*, **30,** 2–8 (1975)

37 HIRASHIMA, M., HONDA, M. and HAYASHI, H. The mediation of tissue eosinophilia in hypersensitivity reactions. II. Separation of a delayed eosinophil chemotactic factor from macrophage chemotactic factors. *Immunology*, **31,** 263–271 (1976)

38 HOGG, J. C. and HULBERT, W. Anatomic aspects of bronchial mucosal permeability. In *Airway Reactivity*, edited by F. E. Hargreave, 35–39. Ontario, Astra Pharmaceuticals Ltd. (1980)

39 HUBSCHER, T. Role of the eosinophil in the allergic reactions. II. Release of prostaglandins from human eosinophilic leukocytes. *Journal of Immunology*, **114,** 1389–1393 (1975)

40 INGELFINGER, F. J., LOWELL, F. C. and FRANKLIN, W. Medical progress: gastrointestinal allergy. *New England Journal of Medicine*, **241,** 303–308 (1949)

41 IYNGKARAN, N., ROBINSON, J. J., PRATHAR, K., SUMITHRAN, E. and YADAR, M. Cow's milk protein sensitive enteropathy. Combined clinical and biological criteria for diagnosis. *Archives of Diseases of Childhood*, **53,** 20–26 (1978)

42 ISHIZAKA, K., ISHIZAKA, T. and HORNBROOK, M. Physico-chemical properties of reaginic antibody. IV. Presence of a unique immunoglobulin as a carrier of reaginic reactivity. *Journal of Immunology*, **97,** 75–85 (1966)

43 JACKSON, P. G., LESSOF, M. Y., BAKER, R. W. R., FERRETT, J. and MacDONALD, D. M. Intestinal permeability in patients with eczema and food allergy. *Lancet*, **1,** 1285–1286 (1981)

44 JARRETT, E. E., JARRETT, W. F. and URQUHART, G. M. Quantitative studies in the kinetics of establishment and expulsion of intestinal nematode population in susceptible and immune hosts. *Nippostrongylus braziliensis* in the rat. *Parasitology*, **58,** 625–639 (1968)

45 KALINER, M. A. Mast cell-derived mediators and bronchial asthma. In *Airway Reactivity*, edited by F. E. Hargreave, 175–187. Ontario, Pharmaceuticals Canada Ltd. (1980)

46 KATZ, A. J., GOLDMAN, H. and GRAND, R. J. Gastric mucosal biopsy in eosinophilic (allergic) gastroenteritis. *Gastroenterology*, **73,** 705–709 (1977)

47 KAUFMAN, H. S. Allergy in the newborn. Skin test reactions confirmed by the Prausnitz-Kuestner test at birth. *Clinical Allergy*, **1,** 363–368 (1971)

48 KAY, A. B., STECHSCHULTE, D. J. and AUSTEN, K. F. An eosinophil leukocyte chemotactic factor of anaphylaxis. *Journal of Experimental Medicine*, **133,** 602–619 (1971)

49 KOCOSHIS, S. and GRYBOSKI, J. D. Use of cromolyn in combined gastrointestinal allergy. *Journal of the American Medical Association*, **242,** 1169–1172 (1979)

50 KUITUNEN, P., VISAKORPI, J. K. and SAVILAHTI, E. Malabsorption syndrome with cows' milk intolerance. Clinical findings and course in 54 cases. *Archives of Diseases of Childhood*, **50,** 351–356 (1975)

51 LANDRES, R. T., KUSTER, G. G. R. and STRUM, W. B. Eosinophilic esophagitis in a patient with vigorous achalasia. *Gastroenterology*, **74,** 1298–1301 (1978)

52 LESSOF, M. H., BUISSERET, P. D., MERRETT, T. G., MERRETT, J., WRAITH, D. G. and YOULTEN, L. J. F. Mechanisms involving prostaglandins in food intolerance. In *The Mast Cell*, edited by J. Pepys and A. M. Edwards, 406–410. Tunbridge Wells, Pitman Medical Publishing Co. Ltd. (1979)

53 LOVE, A. G. H. Mucosal histology and response to disodium cromoglycate in ulcerative colitis. In *The Mast Cell*, edited by J. Pepys and A. M. Edwards, 681. Tunbridge Wells, Pitman Medical Publishing Co. Ltd. (1979)

54 MACKIE, R. M. Intestinal permeability and atopic disease. *Lancet*, **II,** 155 (1981)

55 MALO, J. L., LONGBOTTOM, J. L., MITCHELL, J., HAWKINS, R. and PEPYS, J. Studies in chronic allergic broncho-pulmonary aspergillosis. Immunological findings. *Thorax*, **32,** 269–274 (1977)

56 MATOLEPSZY, J., KUCZYNSKA-SEKIETA, K. and CHACAJ, W. Five years of experience with Intal therapy in ulcerative colitis and pathogenic background of this therapy. In *The Mast Cell*, edited by J. Pepys and A. M. Edwards, 682–687. Tunbridge Wells, Pitman Medical Publishing Co. Ltd. (1979)

57 MANI, V. Sodium cromoglycate (Nalcrom) in the treatment of ulcerative colitis. In *The Mast Cell*, edited by J. Pepys and A. M. Edwards, 677–680. Tunbridge Wells, Pitman Medical Publishing Co. Ltd. (1979)

58 MAY, C. D., LEE, W. Y. and REMIGIO, L. Further studies of spontaneous histamine release from leukocytes of persons hypersensitive to food. (abstract) *Journal of Allergy and Clinical Immunology*, **61,** 157 (1978)

59 MILLER, D. L., HIRVONEN, T. and GITLIN, D. Synthesis of IgE by the human conceptus. *Journal of Allergy and Clinical Immunology*, **52,** 182–188 (1973)

60 MORRIS, T. and RHODES, J. Ulcerative colitis – is it an allergic disorder? In *The Mast Cell*, edited by J. Pepys and A. M. Edwards, 623–670. Tunbridge Wells, Pitman Medical Publishing Co. Ltd. (1979)

61 NEIJENS, H. J., DEGENHART, H. J., RATGEEP, R. and KERREBIJN, K. F. Spontaneous release of histamine in asthmatic children sensitive to nonspecific stimuli. In *The Mast Cell*, edited by J. Pepys and A. M. Edwards, 322–324. Tunbridge Wells, Pitman Medical Publishing Co. Ltd. (1979)

62 NELSON, T. L., KLEIN, G. L. and GALANT, S. P. Severe eosinophilic gastroenteritis successfully treated with an elemental diet. *Journal of Allergy and Clinical Immunology*, **63,** 198 (1979)

63 OTTOLENGHI, A. and BARNETT, H. D. The effect of drugs on the eosinophil leukocyte population of rat tissues. 1. Dexamethasone. *Journal of Pharmacology and Experimental Therapy*, **189,** 303–311 (1974)

64 PAGANELLI, R., LEVINSKY, R. J., BROSTOFF, J. and WRAITH, D. G. Immune complexes containing food proteins in normal and atopic subjects after oral challenge and effect of sodium cromoglycate on antigen absorption. *Lancet*, **1,** 1270–1272 (1979)

65 PARISH, W. E. Short-term anaphylactic IgG antibodies in human sera. *Lancet*, **2,** 591–592 (1970)

66 PATEL, K. R. Calcium antagonists in exercise-induced asthma. *British Medical Journal*, **282,** 932–933 (1981)

67 PEPYS, J. Hypersensitivity Diseases of the Lung due to Fungi and Organic Dusts. *Monograph 4.* Basle, Karger (1969)

68 PEPYS, J. Types of allergic reaction. *Clinical Allergy*, **3,** (Suppl.) 13–32 (1974)

69 PEPYS, J. Atopy. In *Clinical Aspects of Immunology*, edited by P. G. H. Gell, R. R. A. Coombs and P. J. Lachmann, 877–902. Oxford, Blackwell Scientific Publications (1975)

70 PEPYS, J. Clinical and therapeutic significance of patterns of allergic reactions of the lungs to extrinsic agents. *American Review of Respiratory Disease*, **116,** 573–588 (1977)

71 PEPYS, J. and HUTCHCROFT, B. J. Bronchial provocation tests in etiologic diagnosis and analysis of asthma. *American Review of Respiratory Disease*, **112,** 829–859 (1975)

72 PEPYS, J., PARISH, W. E., STENIUS-AARNIALA, B. and WIDE, L. Clinical corrections between long-term (IgE) and short-term (IgG) anaphylactic antibodies in atopic and 'non-atopic' subjects with respiratory allergic disease. *Clinical Allergy*, **9,** 645–658 (1979)

73 PEPYS, J., WELLS, I. D., D'SOUZA, M. F. and GREENBERG, M. Clinical and immunological responses to enzymes of *Bacillus subtilis* in factory workers and consumers. *Clinical Allergy*, **3,** (suppl.) 13–32 (1974)

74 PEPYS, M. B., DRUGUET, M., KLASS, H. J., DASH, A. C., MIRJAH, D. D. and PETRIE, A. Immunological studies in inflammatory bowel disease. In *Immunology of the Gut*. Ciba Foundation Symposium 46 (new series), North Holland, Elsevier/ Excerpta Medica (1977)

75 PIPER, P. J. and SEALE, J. P. Non-immunological release of slow-reacting substance from guinea-pig lungs. *British Journal of Pharmacology*, **67,** 67–72 (1979)

76 PRAUSNITZ, C. and KUESTNER, H. Studien uber die Ueberingfindlichkert. *Centralblatt fur Bakteriologie Parasitologie und Infektion*, **86,** 160 (1921)

77 RIDER, J. A., MOELLER, H. C., DEVEREAUX, R. G. and WRIGHT, R. R. The use of an intramucosal test to demonstrate food hypersensitivity in ulcerative colitis. *Acta Allergologica* (Kbh), **15,** (Suppl. 7) 486 (1960)

78 SALVAGGIO, J. E., CAVANAUGH, J. J. A., LOWELL, F. C. and LESKOWITZ, S. A comparison of the immunologic responses of normal and atopic individuals to intranasally administered antigen. *Journal of Allergy*, **35,** 62–69 (1964)

79 SANDER, D., N., BERGFELD, W. F. and KRAKAVER, R. S. Disodium cromoglycate therapy in mastocytosis. In *The Mast Cell*, edited by J. Pepys and A. M. Edwards, 591–596. Tunbridge Wells, Pitman Medical Publishing Co. Ltd. (1979)

80 SELBEKK, B. H. Mast-cell reactions in human jejunal mucosa. In *The Mast Cell*, edited by J. Pepys and A. M. Edwards, 710–715. Tunbridge Wells, Pitman Medical Publishing Co. Ltd. (1979)

81 SHINER, M. and SHMERLING, D. H. The immunopathology of coeliac disease. *Digestion*, **5,** 69–88 (1972)

82 SIDOROV, J. J. and MARCON, N. E. Long-term high-dosage disodium cromoglycate in ulcerative colitis (proctitis). In *The Mast Cell*, edited by J. Pepys and A. M. Edwards, 725–731. Tunbridge Wells, Pitman Medical Publishing Co. Ltd. (1979)

83 SOTER, N. A. The efficacy of the oral administration of disodium cromoglycate in systemic mastocytosis. In *The Mast Cell*, edited by J. Pepys and A. M. Edwards, 550–555. Tunbridge Wells, Pitman Medical Publishing Co. Ltd. (1979)

84 STENIUS, B., WIDE, K., SEYMOUR, W. M., HOLFORD-STREVENS, V. and PEPYS, J. Clinical significance of specific IgE to common allergens. *Clinical Allergy*, **1,** 37–55 (1971)

85 TADA, T. and ISHIZAKA, K. Distribution of gamma E-forming cells in lymphoid tissues of the human and monkey. *Journal of Immunology*, **104,** 377–387 (1970)

86 TAYLOR, B., NORMAN, A. P., ORGEL, H. A., STOKES, C. R., TUNER, M. W. and SOOTHILL, J. F. Transient IgA deficiency and the pathogenesis of infantile atopy. *Lancet*, **2,** 111–113 (1973)

87 THOMPSON, H. and BUCKMANN, P. Mast-cell population in rectal biopsies from patients with Crohn's disease. In *The Mast Cell*, edited by J. Pepys and A. M. Edwards, 697–701. Tunbridge Wells, Pitman Medical Publishing Co. Ltd. (1979)

88 VAZ, G. A., TAN, L. K. T. and GARRARD, J. W. Oral cromoglycate in treatment of adverse reactions to foods. *Lancet*, **1,** 1066–1068 (1978)

89 VISAKORPI, J. K. and IMMONEM, P. Intolerance to cows' milk and wheat gluten in the primary malabsorption syndrome in infancy. *Acta Paediatrica Scandinavica*, **56,** 49–56 (1967)

90 WARD, P. A. Chemotaxis of human eosinophils. *American Journal of Pathology*, **54,** 121–128 (1969)

91 WARREN, C. P. W., TAI, E. BATTEN, J. C., HUTCHCROFT, B. J. and PEPYS, J. Cystic fibrosis-immunological reactions to *A. fumigatus* and common allergens. *Clinical Allergy*, **5,** 1–12 (1975)

92 WASSERMAN, S. I. The mast cell and the inflammatory response. In *The Mast Cell*, edited by J. Pepys and A. M. Edwards, 9–20. Tunbridge Wells, Pitman Medical Publishing Co. Ltd. (1979)

93 WELSH, R. A. and GREER, J. C. Phagocytosis of mast cell granule by the eosinophilic leukocyte in the rat. *American Journal of Pathology*, **35,** 103–111 (1959)

94 WRAITH, D. G., YOUNG, G. V. W. and LEE, G. H. The management of food allergy with diet and Nalcrŏm. In *The Mast Cell*, edited by J. Pepys and A. M. Edwards, 443–449. Tunbridge Wells, Pitman Medical Publishing Co. Ltd. (1979)

14
Pathophysiology of hormonal diarrhea

R. Modigliani and J. J. Bernier

INTRODUCTION

Endocrine diarrhea results from the overproduction of a hormone (or a related neurotransmitter or paracrine messenger) by a tumor or hyperplasia of endocrine cells; it ceases when the anatomical lesion is eradicated and relapses with recurrence of tumor. Inappropriate secretion of a hormone can lead to diarrhea by several mechanisms:

(1) overproduction of upper digestive secretions which then overwhelm the reabsorptive capacity of the bowel;
(2) inhibition of upper digestive secretions leading to nutrient malabsorption;
(3) changes in small bowel motility;
(4) direct inhibition of water and ion absorption (or induction of secretion) by the intestine.

One approach to the mechanisms of endocrine diarrheas has been to test the effects of acute administration of the suspected hormones on intestinal function; this led to the discovery that many digestive 'hormones' inhibit intestinal absorption (or stimulate secretion) of fluid (*Table 14.1*). This approach, however, is not fully satisfactory because:

(1) the nature of the peptide responsible for the diarrhea is not always clear; availability of radioimmunoassays for an ever-increasing number of peptides has revealed that production of multiple hormones is the rule in endocrine diarrheas;
(2) the effects of chronic hormonal overload may be quite different from those of acute administration, as is clearly shown for glucagon[9, 31, 85].

Another approach has been to characterize directly the pathophysiological disorders in patients with endocrine diarrhea. In this research, the two variants of

Table 14.1 Hormones and related substances known to inhibit absorption (or promote secretion) of fluid by the intestine

	*Animals**	*Man*
Gastrin	+	+[70]
Secretin	+ or −	+[30]
Cholecystokinin	+ or −	+[67]
Glucagon	+	+[31]
Vasoactive intestinal peptide	+	+[47, 50]
Gastric inhibitory peptide	+	+[29]
Bombesin	+[38]	NT†
Thyrocalcitonin	+	+[26, 27]
Serotonin	+	NT†
Substance P	+[39]	NT†
Neurotensin	+	NT†
Prostaglandins	+	+[66]

* reference in 69 unless otherwise stated.
† NT: not tested.

the intestinal perfusion method have been useful: the slow marker perfusion technique[96] allows measurement of the spontaneous intraluminal flow rate of fluid and solutes, in fasting and post-prandial periods, and at one or several levels of the small intestine. Differences in flow rates measured at two sites give the net movement (absorption or secretion) occurring between these two points. Transcolonic net movement can be deduced from flow rates in the terminal ileum and the stool output. The second technique, rapid perfusion of artificial solutions[71], is best suited to explore specific mechanisms of intestinal transport, such as absorption against a concentration gradient or glucose-stimulated sodium transport. The following chapter will be devoted to the contribution of these methods to the understanding of endocrine diarrheas, as seen in Zollinger-Ellison syndrome, endocrine cholera, medullary carcinoma of the thyroid, carcinoid syndrome and miscellaneous other conditions.

ZOLLINGER-ELLISON SYNDROME (ZES) AND MASTOCYTOSIS

The primary pathophysiological abnormality responsible for diarrhea in ZES is overproduction of gastrin which stimulates gastric acid secretion so that large volumes of acid enter the duodenum. It is also generally believed[79] that absorption of this fluid by the small intestine is impaired by a low intraluminal pH, villous atrophy, inflammatory changes in the proximal small bowel and increased blood levels of gastrin[70] and thyrocalcitonin[26, 27]. In order to establish the roles of these abnormalities in ZES diarrhea directly, we studied four patients with this syndrome by the slow marker perfusion technique[80].

Upper digestive secretions

The spontaneous flow rate at the angle of Treitz was greatly increased, reaching 14.3–23.6/24 h (i.e. three to five times the upper limit of normal); it was estimated that a major part (55–67 per cent) of this fluid originated from the biliary-pancreaticoduodenal secretions. Gastric aspiration reduced flow rates at the angle of Treitz by 60–90 per cent, suggesting that a large part of the secretions were due to entry of gastric juice into the duodenum. Furthermore, when gastric aspirates were replaced by instillation of equal volumes of neutral saline into the duodenum, flow remained within the normal range at the duodenojejunal junction. This finding emphasises the prominent role of the acid (rather than volume) in promoting the outflow of alkaline duodenal secretion.

Small intestine

Comparison of fluid flow at the angle of Treitz with that in the terminal ileum shows that 57–74 per cent of the fluid entering the jejunum is reabsorbed by the small intestine. This proportion is even higher than that measured when duodenal flow rates identical to those seen in ZES are produced artificially in normal subjects by infusing isotonic saline into the stomach[76]. Thus, contrary to what was anticipated, the small intestine reabsorbs greater than normal amounts of water and electrolytes in ZES. Furthermore it could be shown in two patients that the contribution of the proximal jejunum to this reabsorption was important: 28 per cent of fluid passing the ligament of Treitz had already disappeared 30 cm distal to this point.

Large intestine

Comparison of flows in the distal ileum with stool volumes indicated that the colon further reabsorbed fluid, which resulted in an overall intestinal reabsorption of 98–99 per cent of the volume calculated to enter the jejunum. Actual amounts of fluid reabsorbed by the colon are large but do not exceed the maximal reabsorptive capacity of this organ as established in normal subjects by Debongnie and Phillips[15].

It can be concluded that in ZES, gastric acid hypersecretion induces a copious alkaline secretion into the duodenal lumen leading to very high flows of fluid at the angle of Treitz. The small intestine and the colon reabsorb a high percentage of this fluid overload.

Mastocytosis

The mechanism of diarrhea associated with mastocytosis is usually believed to be similar to that of ZES, even though gastric hypersecretion is induced by overproduction of histamine rather than gastrin[24]. We had the opportunity to study a patient with systemic mastocytosis, massive secretory diarrhea (1500 ml/day which persisted during fasting) and basal gastric hypersecretion of 35 mM/h. Cimetidine (2400 mg/24 h) and ranitidine (300–900 mg/24 h), which controlled gastric hyperacidity, failed to improve the diarrhea. The patient had increased prostaglandin D_2 excretion in the urine, and the stool output decreased by 50 per cent when aspirin was given. This case suggests that gastric hyperacidity is not the main mechanism of diarrhea in systemic mastocytosis, and that prostaglandin overproduction might be an important factor.

ENDOCRINE CHOLERA

Endocrine cholera seems a more appropriate term than does WDHA syndrome (watery diarrhea, hypokalemia and achlorhydria) or 'pancreatic cholera', since achlorhydria is inconstant[79] and the tumor may be extrapancreatic[94]. Copious watery diarrhea is the main symptom of this disease which may be caused by a pancreatic endocrine tumor (benign or malignant), islet cell hyperplasia or a ganglioneuroma (or ganglioneuroblastoma); the association of endocrine cholera with bronchial carcinoma has been reported in one instance[88].

Humoral mediator(s) of endocrine cholera (EC)

Whereas gastrin is clearly the hormonal mediator of ZES, the nature of the humoral factor(s) responsible for diarrhea in EC remains uncertain[5, 23, 34]. There is strong evidence to incriminate VIP as the main, if not the sole, mediator, at least when a tumor is present. The arguments supporting this view are as follows:

(1) serum VIP is elevated in the majority of patients with tumors (*Table 14.2*);
(2) blood levels of VIP usually parallel the clinical activity of the disease after surgery or chemotherapy[2, 19, 37, 40, 92];
(3) the biological actions of VIP (induction of intestinal secretion and diarrhea[14, 47, 48, 50, 73, 91] inhibition of gastric secretion, vasodilatation, gallbladder relaxation and hypercalcemia[19, 87]), are consistent with the main manifestations of EC[95] (profuse diarrhea, hypochlorhydria, flushing, distended gallbladder and hypercalcemia); and
(4) high VIP levels are not found in other humoral diarrheas[5].

Table 14.2 Serum vasoactive intestinal peptide levels in endocrine cholera

Tumoral EC	Increased serum VIP
Islet cell tumor[2, 5, 11, 18, 28, 32, 39, 51, 53, 57, 60, 62, 72, 77, 81, 84, 86, 89, 93]	73/83 (88%)
Neural crest tumor[5, 7, 20, 37, 41, 53, 68, 83]	14/14 (100%)
Non-tumoral EC	
Islet cell hyperplasia[5, 18, 42, 53, 84, 88, 90, 93]	6/33 (18%)

The figures are only approximate because some patients are mentioned in more than one publication.

The reasons why the role of VIP still remains controversial are many.

(1) Errors in VIP radioimmunoassay account for reports of improvement of diarrhea despite stable plasma VIP[39,40], and of elevated VIP in laxative induced diarrhea[53].
(2) Some pathophysiological features of EC do not fit with established biological actions of VIP: firstly, VIP is thought to induce intestinal secretion by stimulating mucosal adenylate cyclase[91]. However, diarrhea occurs at plasma levels (70 pmol/l)[73] much lower than those necessary to stimulate cyclase *in vitro* (100 nmol/l)[44]; moreover normal mucosal levels of cAMP have been reported in EC patients[39, 53, 62, 90]. Secondly, whereas VIP has been clearly shown to inhibit absorption (or induce secretion) of water and ions in both the small *and* large intestine in animal[48, 91] and in man[14, 47, 50], colonic function has been shown to be normal in most patients with EC (*see below*). However, this might represent a difference between the acute and chronic effects of VIP.
(3) EC tumors may produce other mediators (prostaglandins[55], TCT[55, 75, 82], GIP[42], PP[55], neurotensin[28], enkephalin[28]) some of which are secretory agents. These other agents have been recognized in addition to VIP or, exceptionally, as the sole recognizable hormone[36, 61, 75].

Finally, patients with EC and islet cell hyperplasia (without a tumor) should be considered separately because only a minority of them have elevated circulating levels of VIP (*Table 14.2*). Some patients produce one or several recognized humoral agents[42, 93], but in a few cases no mediator at all can be detected. It, should be borne in mind that the diagnosis of islet cell hyperplasia is difficult and requires quantitative morphometric histology; furthermore, surreptitious laxative abuse which closely mimicks EC may be extremely difficult to rule out and has been reported to be associated with islet cell hyperplasia[58].

Pathophysiology of diarrhea

EC diarrhea is usually profuse, reaching several liters per day, persists on fasting and leads to dehydration, hypokalemia and acidosis[95]. The osmolality of fecal fluid is 280–300 mmol/l and can be accounted for essentially by the concentrations of sodium, potassium and anions[51, 53, 62]. The stool pH is frequently alkaline[62]. The mechanisms of the diarrhea of EC is not fully elucidated because (a) EC is rare, the patients are acutely ill and difficult to study; and (b) the pathophysiology may vary from case to case, as suggested by the variability of the hormonal profile discussed above. The role of upper digestive secretions, or impaired absorption in the small intestine or colon in the genesis of diarrhea will be discussed.

Upper digestive secretions

The abnormalities in EC are diminished basal and stimulated gastric acid output[6], distended gallbladder containing bile with high bicarbonate and low bile salt concentrations[81], and normal production of pancreatic juice in response to exogenous hormone[81] and to a meal[62]. Obviously, minor abnormalities of these functions are not diarrheogenic. However, in one patient[89] whose tumor produced secretin (in addition to VIP, serotonin, entero- and pancreatoglucagon) pancreatic hypersecretion (very high basal duodenal fluid and bicarbonate output, not increased by exogenous secretin) played an important role in the pathogenesis of the diarrhea. Diarrhea was controlled by duodenal aspiration alone.

Small intestine

The duodenum is difficult to study but is probably the site of water and ion malabsorption (or secretion): in the absence of increased pancreatico-biliary secretions, supranormal fluid output has been measured[53, 72, 81] at the angle of Treitz. The jejuno-ileum is in a secretory state, as shown by the increase of fasting flow from the proximal jejunum down to the terminal ileum[78, 81]. Segmental perfusion of test solutions demonstrates secretion of water and sodium into the jejunum,[53, 81] especially when a plasma-like electrolyte solution is used[51, 62, 63]. Contradictory results have been reported for the jejunal absorption of non-electrolytes and their effect on sodium transport. We found in two patients (with increased serum levels of VIP, TCT and PGs) an abolition of glucose- and leucine-stimulated sodium transport although absorption of the sugar and amino acid were normal[72, 81]. This is consistent with the fact that in one of these patients, oral glucose (150 g per day) did not reduce stool volume[81]. Measurement of unidirectional sodium fluxes showed that glucose stimulated the lumen-to-plasma flux of sodium, but also induced an abnormal increase in the reverse flux[72]. Exactly opposite results have been found by others[53] in three patients (with high VIP but normal PGs and TCT levels): glucose stimulated sodium transport normally but was itself malabsorbed. It is of interest that glucose malabsorption persisted in one patient despite extirpation of the tumor and a return to normal water and ion absorption and serum VIP levels[53]. In the only patient in which GIP was the single detectable hormone, the jejunum secreted sodium and water abnormally[42]. Ileal absorption measured by the segmental perfusion technique was found to be normal except in one patient who malabsorbed sodium and chloride from a 50 mmol sodium chloride solution[53], and another subject who malabsorbed potassium[81].

Colon

Clearly the colon does not secrete fluid in endocrine cholera. Comparison of ileal to fecal outputs showed that in two out of four patients[72, 86] the colon reabsorbed large amounts of fluid and sodium[72]. In these cases, colonic absorption reached 6.5 liters per day, a figure close to the maximal reabsorptive capacity of the human colon[15]. One of these patients had a temporary ileostomy: the excluded colon did not secrete fluid and, in fact, reabsorbed ileostomy fluid which was introduced into the caecum[81]. In two other cases however the colonic reabsorptive function was impaired. Fluid was not absorbed in one case[72] and absorption was well below the maximal capacity of the colon in the other[86]. There is some clinical evidence that diarrhea in EC is increased when dehydration is corrected by intravenous saline[2]. Finally, the colon is the source of the massive fecal excretion of potassium seen in all patients[72,81].

It can be concluded that in EC, despite its rarity and the fragmentary and somewhat contradictory nature of results, pancreatico-biliary secretions do not contribute to diarrhea, the small intestine is in a secretory state and is the source of the diarrhea, and that the colon reabsorbs variable amounts of fluid and sodium but secretes large quantities of potassium.

Treatment of EC diarrhea

About half EC patients have metastasis at diagnosis[46] and response to chemotherapy is inconstant[62] and sometimes short-lived. Symptomatic treatment of diarrhea is of major importance in these patients, since the malignancy is usually quite indolent. *Table 14.3* lists the drugs reported to reduce fecal losses in EC and gives their proposed mode of action. It should be noted that, except for steroids, efficacy of these drugs is largely anecdotal; it is also likely that negative therapeutic attempts are under-reported.

Table 14.3 Symptomatic treatment of diarrhea in endocrine cholera

Drug	*References reporting reduction of diarrhea*	*Changes in serum VIP*	*Other proposed modes of action*
Glucorticoids	2, 11, 25, 51, 57, 65	inconstant decrease	Stimulation of intestinal absorption of water and salt[4, 10] Decrease in serum TCT[51]
Lithium	77	stable	Decrease in hormone-induced adenylcyclase activation*
Nicotinic acid	42	not done†	Decrease in hormone-induced adenylcyclase activation*
Somatostatin	57, 59, 86	decrease	Inhibition of VIP-induced intestinal secretion[8] Inhibition of upper digestive secretions[1]
Metoclopramide	60	slight decrease§	
Indomethacin	36	not done**	Inhibition of prostaglandin synthesis

* This proposed mode of action does not fit with the normal jejunal mucosa adenylcyclase found in endocrine cholera (EC) patients

† The only mediator of diarrhea which could be detected was gastric inhibitory polypeptide (GIP); changes in its plasma concentration during nicotinic acid therapy were not reported.

§ Whereas plasma total vasoactive intestinal polypeptide (VIP) decreased very slightly on metoclopramide, there was a change in the chromatographic profile with a dramatic fall in peak four (corresponding to biologicaly active, 28 aminoacids VIP) and an increase in peak three (presumed to be biologically inactive).

** Prostaglandins were the only mediator of diarrhea detected in this case.

MEDULLARY CARCINOMA OF THE THYROID

About 30 per cent of patients with medullary carcinoma of the thyroid (MCT) develop diarrhea[97]. The nature of the diarrheogenic principle in this disease is not clear. Thyrocalcitonin (TCT) has a clear cut secretory effect on the human jejunum and ileum[26, 27] in acute experiments but its effect on the colon is unknown. Plasma from one patient with MCT and severe diarrhea was shown to inhibit small intestinal fluid absorption in dogs; this effect was abolished when calcitonin was removed from the plasma and restored on restitution of comparable hormone levels with pure TCT[12]. In this case however the technique used to remove TCT from the plasma was clearly non-selective, and it remains to be explained why diarrhea occurs in only one third of patients with MCT whereas TCT is invariably raised in this condition. Prostaglandins (PG) have also been suggested as mediators of diarrhea in MCT[98]; however several patients with high plasma PG levels and no diarrhea have been reported[35]. Conversely, diarrhea may occur despite normal blood PG and inhibition of prostaglandin synthesis may fail to control this symptom[12, 33]. Therefore it remains possible that MCT diarrhea is mediated by another, still unknown, substance.

Pathophysiology of diarrhea

Clinical evidence suggests an important role of decreased transit time in the mechanism of this diarrhea[3]. However direct investigations of diarrhea in this disease is limited to three cases. These have shown normal jejunal absorption of water and ions in two patients; ileal function was also normal in one of these cases (J. C. Rambaud, unpublished data) but in the other an inability to absorb sodium and chloride against a concentration gradient, and abnormal mucosal permeability were reported[33]. The absorptive capacity of the colon may be impaired. In two patients with copious diarrhea, the flow rate in the distal ileum was normal in one case (J. C. Rambaud, unpublished data) and increased in the other one[12].

CARCINOID SYNDROME

It is usually accepted that serotonin produced by carcinoid tumors is involved in the pathophysiology of diarrhea[79]. Thus, patients with carcinoid diarrhea have increased levels of urinary 5HIAA and/or blood serotonin; blockers of synthesis or action usually control the diarrhea; and serotonin reproduces, in normal man, the changes in bowel motility observed in carcinoid patients. Both acute[43] and chronic[17] administration of serotonin induces a net secretion of fluid by the rabbit small intestine. However increased production of serotonin is not invariably associated with diarrhea in patients with carcinoid tumors. Other humoral agents[79] such as 5-hydroxytryptophan, kallikrein, calcitonin, histamine and prostaglandin are occasionally produced in excess and may act synergistically with serotonin to produce diarrhea.

The exact disorder in intestinal handling of water and ions responsible for carcinoid diarrhea is incompletely understood. Jejunal and colonic secretion (or malabsorption) of fluid and electrolytes has been found in some patients who have undergone perfusion experiments[13]. Somatostatin infusion improves the diarrhea[13, 16] and the jejunal dysfunction. There is clinical evidence for a rapid transit time in carcinoid diarrhea[79] probably due to an increased propulsive activity in the small intestine. Codeine has been shown to reduce stool volume and to normalize intestinal motility[79]. Whether this drug acts directly by stimulation of intestinal absorption or through its action on motility, or both, is unknown.

MISCELLANEOUS ENDOCRINE DIARRHEAS

Diarrhea can also be seen in other endocrine diseases though less frequently and usually not as a prominent symptom.

Out of the six patients with somatostatinoma[21, 22, 45, 52, 54, 74] four had steatorrhea[21, 52, 54, 74] and three had diarrhea[21, 52, 54]. Steatorrhea is probably due to pancreatic enzyme deficiency[21]; sugar and aminoacid malabsorption as evidenced by the D-xylose test[21] or intestinal perfusion study[52] may reflect a direct effect of somatostatin on nutrient absorption[49]. Diarrhea is more likely secondary to nutrient malabsorption than to a direct effect of somatostatin, since this peptide does not change water and ion absorption by normal small intestine and inhibits fluid secretion in both experimental[8] and clinical situations[13, 16, 86].

Diarrhea occurs in 15 percent of patients with *pancreatic glucagonoma*[56] but its mechanism is unknown. Pancreatic exocrine function has been found greatly reduced in one patient with a tumor in the head of the gland[63].

The incidence of diarrhea in hyperthyroidism is of 10 percent at least[64]. Its pathophysiology remains obscure but decreased transit time is probably one of the main mechanisms[64].

References

1 ARNOLD, R. and LANKISCH, P. G. Somatostatin and the gastrointestinal tract. *Clinics in Gastroenterology*, **9,** 733–753 (1980)

2 BARRACLOUGH, M. A. and BLOOM, S. R. Vipoma of the pancreas. Observations on the diarrhea and circulatory disturbances. *Archives of Internal Medicine*, **139,** 467–471 (1979)

3 BERNIER, J. J., RAMBAUD, J. C., CATTAN, D. and PROST, A. Diarrhoea associated with medullary carcinoma of the thyroid. *Gut*, **10,** 980–985 (1969)

4 BINDER, H. J. Effect of dexamethasone on electrolyte transport in the large intestine of the rat. *Gastroenterology*, **75,** 212–217 (1978)

5 BLOOM, S. R. Vasoactive intestinal peptide, the major mediator of the WDHA (pancreatic cholera) syndrome: value of measurement in diagnosis and treatment. *American Journal of Digestive Diseases*, **23,** 373–376 (1978)

6 BLOOM, S. R., LONG, R. G., BRYANT, M. G., MITCHELL, S. J. and POLAK, J. M. Clinical biochemical and pathological studies on 62 vipomas. *Gastroenterology*, **78,** 1143 (1980) (abstract)

7 CARSON, D. J., GLASGOW, J. F. T. and ARDILL, J. Watery diarrhea and elevated vasoactive intestinal polypeptide associated with a massive neurofibroma in early childhood. *Journal of the Royal Society of Medicine*, **73,** 69–72 (1980)

8 CARTER, R. F., BITAR, K. N., ZFASS, A. M. and MAKHLOUF, G. M. Inhibition of VIP-stimulated secretion and cyclic AMP production by somatostatin in the rat. *Gastroenterology*, **74,** 726–730 (1978)

9 CASPARY, W. F. and LUCKE, H. Intestinal adaptation in response to chronic glucagon administration. In *Intestinal Ion Transport*, edited by J. W. L. Robinson. 345–352. Lancaster, MTP Press Ltd (1976)

10 CHARNEY, A. N., KINSEY, M. D., MYERS, L., GIANNELLA, R. A. and GOTS, R. E. Na^+-K^+-activated adenosine triphosphatase and intestinal electrolyte transport. Effect of adrenal steroids. *Journal of Clinical Investigation*, **56,** 653–660 (1975)

11 COOPERMAN, A. V., DESANTIS, D., WINKELMAN, E., FARMES, R., EVERSMAN, J. and SAĪD, S. Watery diarrhea syndrome: two unusual cases and further evidence that VIP is a humoral mediator. *Annals of Surgery*, **187,** 325–328 (1978)

12 COX, T. M., FAGAN, E. A., HILLYARD, C. J., ALLISON, D. J. and CHADWICK, V. S. Role of calcitonin in diarrhoea associated with medullary carcinoma of the thyroid. *Gut*, **20,** 629–633 (1979)

13 DAVIS, G. R., CAMP, R. C., RASKIN, P. and KREJS, G. J. Effect of somatostatin infusion on jejunal water and electrolyte transport in a patient with secretory diarrhea due to malignant carcinoid syndrome. *Gastroenterology*, **78,** 346–349 (1980)

14 DAVIS, G. R., SANTA ANNA, C. A., MORAWSKI, S. G. and FORDTRAN, J. S. Effect of vasoactive intestinal polypeptide on active and passive transport in the human jejunum. *Journal of Clinical Investigation*, **67,** 1687–1694 (1981)

15 DEBONGNIE, J. C. and PHILLIPS, S. F. Capacity of the human colon to absorb fluid. *Gastroenterology*, **74,** 698–703 (1978)

16 DHARMASATHAPHORN, K., SHERWIN, R. S., CATALAND, S., JAFFE, B. and DOBBINS, J. Somatostatin inhibits diarrhea in the carcinoid syndrome. *Annals of Internal Medicine*, **92,** 68–69 (1980)

17 DONOWITZ, M. and CHARNEY, A. N. Effect of chronic elevation of blood serotonin on intestinal transport. *Gastroenterology*, **70,** 880 (1976) (abstract)

18 EBEID, A. M., MURRAY, P. D. and FISHER, J. E. Vasoactive intestinal peptide and the watery diarrhea syndrome. *Annals of Surgery*, **187,** 411–416 (1978)

19 FAHRENKRUG, J. Vasoactive intestinal peptide. *Clinics in Gastroenterology*, **9,** 633–643 (1980)

20 FONTAINE, J. L., GIRARDET, J. P., BATAILLE, D., LAGARDÈRE, B. and LEMERLE, J. Sympathome et diarrhée par hypersécrétion de 'Vasoactive intestinal peptide'. A propos d'une nouvelle observation. *Archives Française de Pédiatrie*, **34,** 577–578 (1977) (letter)

21 GALMICHE, J. P., CHAYVIALLE, P. M., DUBOIS, P. M., DAVID, L., DESCOS, F., PAULIN, C., DUCASTELLE, T., COLIN, R. and GEFFROY, Y. Calcitonin-producing pancreatic somatostatinoma. *Gastroenterology*, **78,** 1577–1583 (1980)

22 GANDA, O. P., WEIR, G. C., SOELNER, J. S, LEGG, M. A., CHICK, W. L., PATEL, Y. C., EBEID, A. M., GARBAY, K. H. and REICHLIN, S. Somatostatinoma: a somatostatin-containing tumor of the endocrine pancreas. *New England Journal of Medicine*, **296,** 963–967 (1977)

23 GARDNER, J. D. Plasma VIP in patients with watery diarrhea syndrome. *American Journal of Digestive Diseases*, **23,** 370–373 (1978)

24 GARDNER, J. D. Pathogenesis of secretory diarrhea. In *Secretory Diarrhea*, edited by M. Field, J. S. Fordtran and S. G. Schultz, 153–158. American Physiological Society, Baltimore, Waverly Press Inc. (1980)

25 GRAHAM, D. Y., JOHNSON, C. D., BENTLIF, P. S. and KELSEY, J. R. Islet cell carcinoma, pancreatic cholera and vasoactive intestinal peptide. *Annals of Internal Medicine*, **83,** 782–785 (1975)

26 GRAY, T. K., BIEBERDORF, F. A. and FORDTRAN, J. S. Thyrocalcitonin and the jejunal absorption of calcium, water and electrolytes in normal subjects. *Journal of Clinical Investigation*, **52,** 3084–3088 (1973)

27 GRAY, T. K., BRANNAN, P., JUAN, D., MORAWSKI, G. and FORDTRAN, J. S. Ion transport changes during calcitonin-induced intestinal secretion in man. *Gastroenterology*, **71,** 392–398 (1976)

28 GUTNIAK, M., ROSENQUIST, U., GRIMELIUS, L., LUNDBERG, J. M., HÖKFELT, T., ROKAEUS, A., ROSELL, S., LUNDQUIST, G., FAHRENKRUG, J., SUNDBLED, R. and GUTNIAK, E. Report on a patient with watery diarrhoea syndrome caused by a pancreatic tumour containing neurotensin, enkephalin and calcitonin. *Acta Medica Scandinavica*, **208,** 95–100 (1980)

29 HELMAN, C. A. and BARBEZAT, G. O. The effect of gastric inhibitory polypeptide on human jejunal water and electrolyte transport. *Gastroenterology*, **72,** 376–379 (1977)

30 HICKS, T. and TURNBERG, L. A. The influence of secretin on ion transport in the human jejunum. *Gut*, **14,** 485–490 (1973)

31 HICKS, T. and TURNBERG, L. A. Influence of glucagon on the human jejunum. *Gastroenterology*, **67,** 1114–1118 (1974)

32 HUTCHEON, D. F., BAYLESS, T. M., CAMERON, J. L. and BAYLIN, S. B. Hormone-mediated watery diarrhea in a family with multiple endocrine neoplasms. *Annals of Internal Medicine*, **90,** 932–934 (1979)

33 ISAACS, P., WHITTAKER, S. M. and TURNBERG, L. A. Diarrhea associated with medullary carcinoma of the thyroid. Studies of intestinal function in a patient. *Gastroenterology*, **67,** 521–526 (1974)

34 JAFFE, B. M. To be or not to VIP. *Gastroenterology*, **76,** 417–420 (1979)

35 JAFFE, B. M. and CONDON, S. Prostaglandins E and F in endocrine diarrheogenic syndromes. *Annals of Surgery*, **184,** 516–524 (1976)

36 JAFFE, B. M., KOPEN, D. F., DESCHRYVER-KECSKEMETI, K., GINGERICH, R. L. and GREIDER, M. Indomethacin-responsive pancreatic cholera. *New England Journal of Medicine*, **297,** 817–821 (1977)

37 JANSEN-GOEMANS, A. and ENGELHARDT, J. Intractable diarrhea in a boy with vasoactive intestinal peptide-producing ganglioneuroblastoma. *Pediatrics*, **590,** 710–716 (1977)

38 KACHUR, J. F., MILLER, R. J., FIELD, M. and RIVIER, J. Possible role of substance P. bombesin and neurotensin in the regulation of ileal electrolyte transport. *Gastroenterology*, **80,** 1186 (1981) (abstract)

39 KAHN, C. R., LEVY, A. G., GARDNER, J. D., MILLER, J. V., GORDON, P. and SCHEIN, P. S. Pancreatic cholera: beneficial effects of treatment with streptozotocin. *New England Journal of Medicine*, **292,** 941–945 (1975)

40 KAHN, C. R., LEVY, A. G., GARDNER, J. D. and SCHEIN, P. S. Treatment of pancreatic cholera. *New England Journal of Medicine*, **293,** 198 (1975) (letter)

41 KAPLAN, S. J., HOLLBROOK, C. T., McDANIEL, H. G., BUNTAIN, W. L. and CRIST, W. M. Vasoactive intestinal peptide secreting tumors of childhood. *American Journal of Diseases of Childhood*, **134,** 21–24 (1980)

42 KIDD, G. S., DONOWITZ, M., O'DORISIO, T., CATALAND, S. and NEWMAN, F. Mild chronic watery diarrhea-hypokalemia syndrome associated with pancreatic islet cell hyperplasia. Elevated plasma and tissue levels of gastric inhibitory polypeptide and successful management with nicotinic acid. *American Journal of Medicine*, **66,** 883–888 (1979)

43 KISLOFF, B. and MOORE, E, W. Effect of serotonin on water and electrolyte transport in the *in vivo* rabbit small intestine. *Gastroenterology*, **71,** 1033–1038 (1976)

44 KLAEVEMAN, H. J., CONLON, T. P., LEVY, A. G. and GARDNER, J. D. Effects of gastrointestinal hormones on adenylate cyclase activity in human jejunal mucosa. *Gastroenterology*, **68,** 667–675 (1975)

45 KOVACS, K., HORWATH, E., EZRIN, C., SEPP, H. and ELKAN, I. Immunoreactive somatostatin in pancreatic islet-cell carcinoma accompanied by ectopic ACTH syndrome. *Lancet*, **1,** 1365–1366 (1977) (letter)

46 KRAFT, A. R., TOMPKINS, R. K. and ZOLLINGER, R. M. Recognition and management of the diarrheal syndrome caused by non-β islet cell tumors of the pancreas. *American Journal of Surgery*, **119,** 163–170 (1970)

47 KREJS, G. J. Effect of VIP infusion on water and ion transport in the human large intestine. *Gastroenterology*, **78,** 1200 (1980) (abstract)

48 KREJS, G. H., BARKLEY, R. M., READ, N. W. and FORDTRAN, J. S. Intestinal secretion induced by vasoactive intestinal polypeptide. A comparison with cholera toxin in the canine jejunum *in vivo*. *Journal of Clinical Investigation*, **61,** 1337–1345 (1978)

49 KREJS, G. J., BROWNE, R. and RASKIN, P. S. Effect of intravenous somatostatin on jejunal absorption of glucose, amino acids, water and electrolytes. *Gastroenterology*, **78,** 26–31 (1980)

50 KREJS, G. J. and FORDTRAN, J. S. Effect of VIP infusion on water and ion transport in the human jejunum. *Gastroenterology*, **78,** 722–727 (1980)

51 KREJS, G. J., HENDLER, R. S. and FORDTRAN, J. S. Diagnostic and pathophysiologic studies in patients with chronic diarrhea. In *Secretory Diarrhea*, edited by M. Field, J. S. Fordtran and S. G. Schultz, 141–151. American Physiological Society, Baltimore, Waverly Press Inc (1980)

52 KREJS, G. J., ORCI, L., CONLON, J. M., RAVAZZOLA, M., DAVIS, G. R., RASKIN, P., COLLINS, S. M., McCARTHY, D. M., BAETENS, D., RUBENSTEIN, A., ALDOR, T. A. M. and UNGER, R. H. Somatostatinoma syndrome. Biochemical morphologic and clinical features. *New England Journal of Medicine*, **301,** 285–292 (1979)

53 KREJS, G. J., WALSH, J. H., MORAWSKI, B. A. and FORDTRAN, J. S. Intractable diarrhea. Intestinal perfusion studies and plasma VIP concentrations in patients with pancreatic cholera syndrome and surreptitious ingestion of laxatives and diuretics. *American Journal of Digestive Diseases*, **22,** 280–292 (1977)

54 LARSSON, I. I., HIRSCH, M. A., HOLST, J. J., INGEMANSSON, S., KÜHL, C., LINDKAER JENSEN, S., LUNDQUIST, G., REHFELD, J. F. and SCHWARTZ, T. W. Pancreatic somatostatinoma: clinical features and physiological implications. *Lancet*, **1,** 666–668 (1977)

55 LARSSON, L. I., SCHWARTZ, T., LUNDQVIST, G., CHANCE, R. E., SUNDLER, F., REHFELD, J. F., GRIMELIUS, I., FAHRENKRUG, J., SCHAFFALITZKY DE MUCKADELL, O. B. and MOON, N. Occurrence of human pancreatic polypeptide in pancreatic endocrine tumors. *American Journal of Pathology*, **85,** 675–684 (1976)

56 LEICHTER, S. B. Clinical and metabolic aspects of glucagonoma. *Medicine*, **59,** 103–113 (1980)

57 LENNON, J., BLOOM, S. R. and SIRCUS, W. Studies on blood levels of vasoactive intestinal peptide (VIP) and pancreatic polypeptide (PP) and their relation to clinical behavior in a case of Verner-Morrison syndrome. *Italian Journal of Gastroenterology*, **18,** 104–106 (1978)

58 LESNA, M., HAMLYN, A. M., VENABLES, C. W. and RECORD, C. O. Chronic laxative abuse associated with pancreatic islet cell hyperplasia. *Gut*, **18,** 1032–1035 (1977)

59 LONG, R. G., BARNES, A. J., ADRIAN, T. E., MALLINSON, C. N., BROWN, M. R., VALE, W., RINER, J. E., CHRISTOFIDES, N. D. and BLOOM, S. R. Suppression of pancreatic endocrine tumour secretion by long-acting somatostatin analogue. *Lancet*, **2,** 764–767 (1979)

60 LONG, R. G., BRYANT, M. G., YVILLE, P. M., POLAK, J. M. and BLOOM, S. R. Mixed pancreatic apudoma with symptoms of excess vasoactive intestinal polypeptide and insulin: improvement of diarrhea with metoclopramide. *Gut*, **22,** 505–511 (1981)

61 LUNDQVIST, G., KRAUSE, U., LARSSON, L. I., GRIMELIUS, L., SCHAFFALITZKY DE MUCKADELL, O. B., FAHRENKRUG, J., JOHNSON, M. and CHANCE, R. E. A pancreatic-polypeptide-producing tumour associated with the WDHA syndrome. *Scandinavian Journal of Gastroenterology*, **13,** 715–718 (1978)

62 McGILL, D. B., MILLER, L. J., CARNEY, J. A., PHILLIPS, S. F., GO, V. L. W. and SCHUTT, A. J. Hormonal diarrhea due to pancreatic tumor. *Gastroenterology*, **79,** 571–582 (1980)

63 MALLINSON, C. M., BLOOM, S. R., WARIN, A. P., SALMON, P. R. and COX, B. A glucagonoma syndrome. *Lancet*, **2,** 1–5 (1974)

64 MARÉCHAUD, R., RAMBAUD, J. C. and MATUCHANSKY, C. Manifestations intestinales des affections thyroidiennes. Aspects cliniques et physiopathologiques actuels. *Gastroentérologie Clinque et Biologique*, **4,** 899–910 (1980)

65 MARKS, I. N., BANK, S. and LOUW, J. H. Islet cell tumor of the pancreas with reversible watery diarrhea and achlorhydria. *Gastroenterology*, **52,** 695–708 (1967)

66 MATUCHANSKY, C. and BERNIER, J. J. Effect of prostaglandin E_1 on glucose, water and electrolyte absorption in the human jejunum. *Gastroenterology*, **64,** 1111 –1118 (1973)

67 MATUCHANSKY, C., HUET, P. M., MARY, J. Y., RAMBAUD, J. C. and BERNIER, J. J. Effects of cholecystokinin and metoclopramide on jejunal movements of water and electrolytes and on transit time of luminal fluid in man. *European Journal of Clinical Investigation*, **2,** 169–175 (1972)

68 MITCHELL, C. H., SINATRA, F. R., CROST, F. W., GRIFFIN, R. and SUNSHINE, P. Intractable watery diarrhea, ganglioneuroblastoma and vasoactive intestinal peptide. *Journal of Pediatrics*, **89,** 593–595 (1976)

69 MODIGLIANI, R., BERNIER, J. J., MATUCHANSKY, C. and RAMBAUD, J. C. Intestinal water and electrolyte transport in man under the effect of exogenous hormones of the gut and prostaglandins and in patients with endocrine tumors of the pancreas. In

Progress in Gastroenterology, volume 3, edited by G. B. J. Glass, 285–319. New York, Grune and Stratton (1977)

70 MODIGLIANI, R., MARY, J. Y. and BERNIER, J. J. Effects of synthetic human gastrin I upon movements of water, electrolytes and glucose across the human small intestine. *Gastroenterology*, **71,** 978–984 (1976)

71 MODIGLIANI, R., RAMBAUD, J. C. and BERNIER, J. J. The method of intraluminal perfusion of the human small intestine. I. Principle and technique. *Digestion*, **9,** 176–192 (1973)

72 MODIGLIANI, R., RAMBAUD, J. C., MATUCHANSKY, C. and BERNIER, J. J. Hormones, intestinal secretion and diarrhea: human studies. In *Frontiers of Knowledge in the Diarrheal Diseases*, edited by H. D. Janowitz and D. B. Sachar, 289–302. Upper Montclair New Jersey, Project in Health Inc. (1979)

73 MODLIN, I. M., BLOOM, S. R. and MITCHELL, S. J. Experimental evidence for vasoactive intestinal peptide as the cause of the watery diarrhea syndrome. *Gastroenterology*, **75,** 1051–1054 (1978)

74 De NUTTE, N., SOMERS, C., CEPTS, W., JACOBS, M. and PIPELEERS, D. Pancreatic hormone release in tumour-associated hypersomatostatinemia. *Diabetologia*, **15,** 227 (1978) (abstract)

75 OBERG, K., LÖÖF, L., BOSTRÖM, H., GRIMELIUS, L., FAHRENKRUG, J. and LUNDQVIST, G. Hypersecretion of calcitonin in patients with the Verner-Morrison syndrome. *Scandinavian Journal of Gastroenterology*, **16,** 135–144 (1981)

76 PALMA, R., VIDON, N. and BERNIER, J. J. Maximal capacity for fluid absorption in human bowel. *Digestive Diseases and Sciences*, **26,** 929–934 (1981)

77 PANDOL, S. J., KORMAN, L. Y., McCARTHY, D. M. and GARDNER, J. D. Beneficial effect of oral lithium carbonate in the treatment of pancreatic cholera syndrome. *New England Journal of Medicine*, **302,** 1403–1404 (1980)

78 PHILLIPS, S. F., DEVROEDE, G. J. Functions of the large intestine. *International Review of Physiology. Gastrointestinal Physiology (III)*, **19,** 263–290 (1979)

79 RAMBAUD, J. C. and MATUCHANSKY, C. Diarrhea and digestive endocrine tumors. *Clinics in Gastroenterology*, **3,** 657–670 (1974)

80 RAMBAUD, J. C., MODIGLIANI, R., EMONTS, P., MATUCHANSKY, C., VIDON, N., BESTERMAN, H. and BERNIER, J. J. Fluid secretions in the duodenum and intestinal handling of water and electrolytes in the Zollinger-Ellison syndrome. *American Journal of Digestive Diseases*, **23,** 1089–1097 (1978)

81 RAMBAUD, J. C., MODIGLIANI, R., MATUCHANSKY, C., BLOOM, S., SAÏD, S. I., PESSAYRE, D. and BERNIER, J. J. Pancreatic cholera: studies on tumoral secretions and pathophysiology of diarrhea. *Gastroenterology*, **69,** 110–122 (1975)

82 RAMBAUD, J. C., NISARD, A., MODIGLIANI, R., CALMETTE, C., MOUKTAR, M. S., HILL, P. A. and BESTERMAN, H. Hypercalcitoninaemia in vipomas. *Lancet*, **1,** 220 (1978) (letter)

83 RICOUR, C., DUHAMEL, J. F., LESEC, G. and SCHWEISGUTH, O. Diarrhée cholériforme dans un cas de ganglioneuroblastome. Mise en évidence d'un taux plasmatique élevé de 'vasoactive intestinal peptide' (VIP). *Archives Françaises de Pédiatrie*, **34,** 552–555 (1977)

84 ROMINGER, J., ESCOFFERY, R., CHEY, W. Y., MENGY, R. and LOCALIO, A. Observations on watery diarrhea syndrome associated with apudoma. *Gastroenterology*, **70,** 1246 (1980) (abstract)

85 RUDO, N. D. and ROSENBERG, I. H. Chronic glucagon administration enhances intestinal transport in the rat. *Proceedings of the Society for Experimental Biology and Medicine*, **142,** 521–525 (1973)

86 RUSKONÉ, A., RENÉ, E., CHAYVIALLE, J. A., BONIN, B., PIGNAL, F., KREMER, M., BONFILS, S. and RAMBAUD, J. C. Effects of somatostatin on diarrhea and on small intestinal water and electrolyte transport in a patient with pancreatic cholera. *Digestive Diseases and Sciences*, **27,** 459–466 (1982)

87 SAÏD, S. I. Vasoactive intestinal peptide (VIP): current status. In *Gastrointestinal Hormones*, edited by J. C. Thomson, 591–597. Austin, University of Texas Press (1975)

88 SAÏD, S. I. and FALOONA, G. R. Elevated plasma and tissue levels of vasoactive intestinal peptide in the watery diarrhea syndrome due to pancreatic, bronchogenic and other tumors. *New England Journal of Medicine*, **293,** 155–160 (1975)

89 SCHMITT, M. G., SOERGEL, K. H., HENSLEY, G. T. and CHEY, W. Y. Watery diarrhea associated with pancreatic islet cell carcinoma. *Gastroenterology*, **69,** 206–216 (1975)

90 SCHWARTZ, S. E., FITZGERALD, M. A., LEVINE, R. A. and SCHWARTZEL, E. H. Intestinal cyclic nucleotides in 'pancreatic cholera': evidence against a second messenger role in intestinal secretion. *Gastroenterology*, **70,** 936 (1976) (abstract)

91 SCHWARTZ, C. J., KIMBERG, D. V., SHEERIN, H. E., FIELD, M. and SAÏD, S. I. Vasoactive intestinal peptide stimulation of adenylate cyclase and active electrolyte secretion in intestinal mucosa. *Journal of Clinical Investigation*, **54,** 536–544 (1974)

92 SIEGEL, S. R. and MUGGIA, F. M. Treatment of 'pancreatic cholera'. *New England Journal of Medicine*, **293,** 198 (1975) (letter)

93 SOERGEL, K. H., BJORK, J. T. and WOOD, C. M. The WDHA syndrome: no correlation between clinical course, plasma hormone level and small intestinal function. In *Diarrhea in Disorders of Intestinal Transport*, edited by H. Ruppin, W. Domschke and K. H. Soergel, 133–139. Stuttgart, Georg Thieme Verlag (1981)

94 TRUMP, D. L., LIVINGSTON, J. N. and BAYLIN, S. B. Watery diarrhea syndrome in an adult with ganglioneuroma-pheochromocytoma. Identification of vasoactive intestinal peptide, calcitonin and catecholamines and assessment of their biologic activity. *Cancer*, **40,** 1526–1532 (1977)

95 VERNER, J. V. and MORRISON, A. N. Non-B islet tumours and the syndrome of watery diarrhoea, hypokalaemia and hypochlorhydria. *Clinics in Gastroenterology*, **3,** 595–607 (1974)

96 WHALEN, G. E., HARRIS, J. A., GEENEN, J. E. and SOERGEL, K. H. Sodium and water absorption from the human small intestine. The accuracy of the perfusion method. *Gastroenterology*, **51,** 975–984 (1966)

97 WILLIAMS, E. D. Diarrhoea and thyroid carcinoma. *Proceedings of the Royal Society of Medicine*, **59,** 602–603 (1966)

98 WILLIAMS, E. D., KARIM, S. M. M. and SANDLER, M. Prostaglandin secretion by medullary carcinoma of the thyroid. A possible cause of the associated diarrhoea. *Lancet*, **1,** 22–23 (1968)

15
Motility disorders in small bowel diseases

G. Vantrappen and J. Janssens

Disordered transit of bowel contents occurs in many gastrointestinal diseases, yet the relation between motility and disease is still unclear for several reasons.

(1) Although the relation between electrical activity and contraction of smooth muscle has been extensively studied the relationship between muscle contraction and propulsion of intraluminal contents is less well understood.
(2) Until recently small intestinal motor activity was described in terms of numbers and types of contraction waves or a 'motility index', but motility patterns were not recognized. The interdigestive myoelectric complex or migrating motor complex (MMC) was identified in dogs in 1969[39] and has since been found in most animal species including man; its characteristics and the control mechanism have been studied extensively[48].
(3) The relation between motility and other gastrointestinal functions, such as absorption and secretion, is also incompletely understood. Only recently it was proven that secretion as well as absorption are closely related to the different phases of the MMC[11, 32, 45].

DISORDERS OF THE MIGRATING MOTOR COMPLEX (MMC) OF THE SMALL INTESTINE

The MMC has four phases[8, 42] which follow each other and recycle continuously as long as they are not interrupted by feeding. During phase one the bowel is quiescent. Phase two is characterized by irregular motor activity which becomes more intense near the end of this phase. The contractions of phase two are sometimes organised in a pattern consisting of clusters of a few contractions alternating with short periods of quiescence. This pattern has been called 'minute rhythm'[17] or 'burst-activity'[43, 44]. Some bursts occur simultaneously at adjacent levels of small bowel, others progress distally over a distance of 50 cm and more. Sometimes a single progressive contraction sweeps down the small bowel at high speed (the progression velocity of the slow waves); it is called the peristaltic rush[16].

The function of these different motor patterns during phase two and their relation to propulsion has not been established. Phase three, also called the activity front, is the most characteristic part of the MMC cycle. It consists of an uninterrupted burst of contractions occurring at the maximal contraction frequency. The activity front is followed by a fourth phase of rapidly declining motor activity, which in turn is followed by phase one of a new cycle. The cycle duration in man is variable but is on average 1.5 to 2 hours[42]. Every phase migrates downward; therefore every phase is always present somewhere in the small intestine.

Bacterial overgrowth

Simultaneous manometric and radiocinematographic studies have shown that the contraction waves of the activity front are highly propulsive in both dogs[9] and man[42]. They clear the bowel of all injected contrast material completely and quickly. Vantrappen *et al.* speculated that if the function of the MMC is to keep the bowel clean, absence of MMC's might result in stasis of food remnants, secretions and desquamated cells, thus creating an ideal culture medium for the development of small bowel bacterial overgrowth[42]. To test this hypothesis they examined the interdigestive motor activity of the small bowel in 18 patients with a positive $^{14}CO_2$ bile acid breath test (12 patients with small intestinal bacterial overgrowth and six with ileal malabsorption for bile acids), in nine patients with various gastrointestinal disorders but a normal $^{14}CO_2$ breath test and in a control group of 18 normal subjects. All normal subjects and all but five patients had normal MMC's with normal activity fronts. In four patients the activity front was absent and in one it was greatly disordered. All five patients had bacterial overgrowth of the small bowel: one of these had systemic sclerosis, one had Crohn's disease without obstruction, another had had a total gastrectomy and two had no demonstrable lesion. The authors concluded that absence of the activity front of the MMC can produce small intestinal bacterial overgrowth. That absence of the activity front induces small intestinal bacterial overgrowth was recently proven experimentally by Scott and Cahall[36]. These authors treated rats with morphine or phenylephrine and cultured segments of the small bowel and its contents for aerobic and anaerobic bacteria. Opposite to its effect on the small bowel of man, morphine eliminated the activity front in rats and phenylephrine in the doses administered had the same effect. If the activity front was absent for more than 6 to 15 hours, the rats developed small intestinal bacterial overgrowth. If the rats were killed after the drugs had been stopped and the activity front had been allowed to reoccur, bacterial overgrowth was no longer present.

Postoperative ileus

This is a condition in which there is apparently no or only minimal propulsion. Catchpole and Duthie studied the gastroduodenal MMC in postoperative patients (five patients with truncal vagotomy and pyloroplasty, three patients with Billroth I partial gastrectomy, and three patients with other surgical procedures[4]). Phase three activity reappeared in the duodenum within two hours of abdominal closure. The cycle duration was shorter than in non-operated patients and initially only phases one and three were present. Gastric MMC's reappeared after 10 to 15 hours but were not well coordinated with those of the duodenum. These studies confirm in man the results obtained in dogs by Smith *et al.*[37] These authors studied the effect of laparotomy with rubbing of the small bowel and exposing it to air on the MMC activity and on the transport of plastic spheres. They found that the operative procedures promptly inhibited the MMC in the stomach and in the small intestine Phase three reappeared at scattered sites along the small bowel on the first (sometimes on the second) day and in the stomach on the second postoperative day, but the phase three activity remained segmental without aboral progression. Only after three to seven days the preoperative pattern was re-established. A mean of 65 hours was required for the plastic spheres to leave the stomach and a mean of 23 hours to travel from the duodenum in the colon. Anesthesia alone inhibited the MMC pattern, but the inhibition was mostly confined to the anesthesia period itself. Adrenergic blocking agents were able to prevent the prolonged postoperative abolishment of phase three in the stomach but not in the small intestine.

Other abnormalities in disease

Malagelada *et al.* studied the MMC in patients with diabetic and postvagotomy gastroparesis[23]. The MMC was absent in the stomach but normal in the duodenum and the small bowel. Studies of Sarr *et al.* indicated that the various phases of the MMC have a marked effect on intestinal transit and absorption[32]. However, up to now it is not known whether motility disturbances other than the absence of MMC activity fronts contribute to the pathogenesis of some ill-defined conditions of malabsorption.

Feeding interrupts the migrating motor complex and changes the interdigestive pattern into a pattern of digestive activity[8,42]. The mechanism that induces the change from the fasted into the fed pattern is multifactorial and humoral as well as nervous mechanisms are involved[10,41]. The interruption of the MMC by food must be a very important mechanism preventing the digested food products from being swept away by the activity front. However, no disease states have been described thus far in man in which the disruption of the MMC by food is lacking.

Recently Foster *et al.* described a high frequency wave form which appeared in the proximal jejunum of four patients with various gastrointestinal diseases (two patients with postvagotomy diarrhea, one diabetic with gastric stasis and one patient with unexplained abdominal pain)[18]. The abnormal motor pattern, called Q-complex, was characterized by discrete bursts of regular pressure waves of high amplitude. The bursts lasted for 18 to 72 seconds. The frequency of the contractions during the burst was higher (15–18/min) than usually recorded in the jejunum. Q-complexes occurred at irregular intervals during which the intestine was quiescent or showed normal phase two activity. In one patient the occurrence of Q-complexes was associated with mesogastric pain. The significance of this Q-complex is not yet clear.

MOTILITY PATTERNS IN DIARRHEA

Abnormal bowel motility is probably the most frequently suspected but the least understood cause of diarrhea. Abnormal motility could result in diarrhea if it would decrease mucosal absorption because of inadequate mixing or because of shortened mucosal contact time. However few studies have tried to correlate muscular contractions with flow. Using mechanical models to describe the effect of contractions of the circular or the longitudinal muscle layer on intestinal flow, Christensen *et al.*[6] showed that longitudinal contractions produce an exchange of fluid between the core and the periphery of the conduit but minimal propulsion, whereas contractions of the circular muscle induce much less exchange between core and periphery but produce considerable longitudinal displacement or propulsion. Nevertheless since the recognition of the MMC motility pattern, many investigators have looked for other motility patterns that could be diarrheagenic.

Type II peristalsis

Code described a powerful peristaltic contraction in the canine small bowel that replaced the activity front and progressed to the terminal ileum[7]. This motor pattern was called type II peristalsis (in contrast to the type I peristaltic contractions of the activity front of the MMC). Characteristic for this type II peristalsis was the finding that pacesetter potentials (slow waves) became smaller, their frequency slower; later, slow waves disappeared (for a cycle or two) and the recording was occupied by a sequence of action potentials. The propagation velocity of the type II peristaltic pattern was slower than the propagation of the individual pacesetter potentials. On fluoroscopy type II peristaltic contractions were highly propulsive.

'Pseudofronts'

Marlett and Code identified in the small bowel of dogs with celiac and superior mesenteric ganglionectomy an abnormal electrical pattern which they called a pseudofront[24]. It consisted of a series of peristaltic contractions extending over 1/4 to 1/2 of the length of the small bowel, identical to the activity front except that it did not migrate. The pseudofront may be a diarrheagenic motor pattern as all the dogs developed diarrhea after this kind of operation. A similar pattern has been observed in dogs after the intravenous administration of CCK (4 μg/kg)[40].

Migrating action potential complex (MAPC) and repetitive bursts of action potentials (RBAP)

Mathias *et al.* studied the myoelectrical pattern of the rabbit ileum in response to diarrheagenic bacteria and their toxins. These authors noted in rabbit ileal loops exposed to live *Vibro cholerae* or to cholera enterotoxin the occurrence of an abnormal electrical pattern they called the migrating action potential complex (MAPC)[26]. It is a burst of intense spiking activity of 2–5 seconds or longer, that obliterates the lumen, progresses over a distance of at least 2.5 cm and propells the intraluminal contents in an aboral direction. Although no change in slow wave frequency was noted, some distortion in slow wave configuration was observed just before the onset of the MACC activity. The number of MAPC's varied widely with a mean frequency of 7.1 per hour. That this MAPC pattern was not merely a consequence of the increased intraluminal fluid content was suggested by the fact that the MAPC activity began four hours after loop inoculation, a time period beyond the well-known intestinal secretory effect of cholera enterotoxin. Moreover it could not be reproduced by constant infusion of 0.9 per cent NaCl. In a further study Mathias *et al.* showed that the MAPC activity may be due to prostaglandin release, as indomethacin abolished MAPC activity and intraluminal infusion of prostaglandin F2α (2 μg/kg/min) was able to induce similar MAPC's[25]. The occurrence of MAPC activity can be induced in rabbit ileal loops by several strains of *Salmonella typhimurium*[47]. It can be induced also by live toxigenic *E. coli* or its filtrate, the effect being mediated by the heat-labile enterotoxin[2].

Burns *et al.* studied the effect of invasive strains of *E. coli* on the myoelectrical activity of the small intestine of New Zealand white rabbits[3]. They found two distinct complex patterns: repetitive bursts of action potentials (RBAPs) occurring predominantly in the infected ligated ileal loop and MAPC activity occurring predominantly in the uninfected small bowel orad to the ligated ileal loop. The authors concluded that MAPC activity was characteristic of 'non-invasion' and that RBAPs correlated with enterocyte injury. RBAPs and MAPC activity have also been described after *Shigella dysenteriae* I enterotoxin[27], *Clostridium perfringens* A enterotoxin and *Clostridium difficile* enterotoxin[20]. Both MAPC and RBAP activity have several characteristics in common to what Code described as type II peristalsis in dogs[7].

These studies indicate that, at least in animals, specific motor patterns can be induced by diarrheagenic bacteria and their toxins and may contribute to the diarrhea in these diseases. Unfortunately analogous studies have not been performed in man.

Laxatives

Several investigators have examined the effect of laxatives on small intestinal motility. Mathias *et al.* studied the effect of castor oil and its active component, ricinoleic acid, on rabbit ileal loops. They found an abnormal electrical pattern that was similar to the electrical activity they had seen previously after cholera toxin (MAPC-activity)[28]. When ricinoleic acid was perfused intraluminally in the first section of the duodenum, the abnormal pattern was observed in the jejunum and the ileum but not in the duodenum. Atchison *et al.* studied the effect of castor oil on the electrical activity of the small bowel of the fasted conscious dog[1]. They found a novel pattern of spiking activity consisting of short repetitive bursts of spike potentials which migrated the length of the recording site; phase three activity of the MMC was no longer present. This pattern seems most similar to Code's type II peristalsis or RBAP activity. Quinidine sulphate produces diarrhea in dogs and induces abnormally long activity fronts[7].

The effect of castor oil on the MMC of healthy subjects was examined by Vantrappen *et al.*[43, 44]. Castor oil was administered in doses (30 to 100 ml) which induced at least one urgent bowel movement during the recording period. Castor oil significantly reduced the number of activity fronts in the upper small intestine but normal fronts persisted. The incidence of contraction bursts as well as the duration of the 'minute rhythm' during phase two were significantly reduced, but the total number of phase two contractions was not affected. Thus, in contrast to the dog[1] castor oil in man did not disrupt the MMC completely, did not induce a novel pattern, but produced some degree of disorganization of various interdigestive motility patterns. It must be noted that the dose of castor oil used in man was lower than that used in dogs, and that in the human studies the motor activity was only monitored in the upper small intestine.

MOTILITY PATTERNS IN CHRONIC IDIOPATHIC INTESTINAL PSEUDO-OBSTRUCTION

Intestinal pseudo-obstruction is a clinical syndrome, characterized by signs of intestinal obstruction but without a demonstrable organic occlusion. A number of diseases including scleroderma, muscular dystrophies, amyloidosis, myxoedema, diabetes mellitus etc., may give rise to pseudo-obstruction. When no apparent cause is found the disease is called chronic idiopathic intestinal pseudo-obstruction (CIIP). As the intestinal motor function is regulated by the interactions of smooth muscle with nervous and hormonal mechanisms of control, CIIP may occur if any of these systems fails. And indeed, in the majority of patients with CIIP distinctive abnormalities can be found either in the smooth muscle or in the myenteric plexus.

CIIP may occur sporadically or as a familial entity. Familial visceral myopathy (or 'hereditary hollow visceral myopathy') is characterized by thinning and degeneration of the smooth muscle[34, 35]. The affected muscle cells show a variety of abnormalities including cell fragmentation and collagen deposition around degenerating cells giving the muscle a honeycombed appearance called 'vacuolar degeneration'; interestingly in most cases the longitudinal muscle coat seems to be more affected than the circular layer. The disease not only involves the small bowel, but the oesophagus, the colon, the urinary bladder and even the muscle of the iris may also be affected. The disease seems to be a pure smooth muscle disorder not mediated by inflammatory cells, vasculitis or neural disease.

In familial visceral neuropathy (with neuronal intranuclear inclusions) the most prominent lesion is a significant reduction in the number of neurons in the nerve plexuses, 30 per cent of which contain mildly eosinophilic material in the nuclei not resembling any known viral inclusion[33]. The disease is not limited to the bowel as the same type of neuronal inclusion can be found in the brain, spinal cord, peripheral nerves and the autonomic nervous system. Thus the myenteric plexus is affected only as part of a broader neurological illness. Familial visceral myopathy and familial visceral neuropathy are hereditary diseases. However, some cases of visceral myopathy have been described without any apparent familial involvement. There are also degenerative disorders of the myenteric plexus, which are not familial, do not involve other areas of the nervous system and have no intranuclear neuronal inclusions. Other cases of CIIP have no apparent lesions in either the muscle layer or nerves.

Faulk *et al.* studied duodenal motility in a family affected by hereditary visceral myopathy[14]. They found a low frequency and amplitude of the duodenal contractions. Drugs such as edrophonium, bethanechol, neostigmine, and CCK-octapeptide induced contractions, indicating that the resting muscle was sensitive to such excitatory agents. Lewis *et al.* studied a 35 year old female with familial CIIP[22]. Duodenal slow waves occurred at a normal rate but were seen only in the presence of spike activity. One activity front of an MMC was seen. Injection of bethanechol and edrophonium induced marked contractile activity. At laparotomy bipolar electrodes were implanted subserosally[31]. Immediately postoperatively the jejunal slow wave frequency was very low (4.75 cycles/min) and highly irregular but its frequency and regularity increased over the next hour. Thereafter all slow wave activity disappeared except during the occurrence of an activity front. Electrical stimulation at a time slow waves were absent was unable to restore the slow wave rhythm; stimulation at a time slow waves were present resulted in a decrease of the slow wave frequency (probably because it was already maximal). The frequency of the MMC cycle was increased with a mean cycle duration of 34.7 min. Meperidine and small doses of PGF 2α initiated an activity front. Morphine, pentagastrin and larger doses of PGF 2α initiated slow waves and spike activity simultaneously at all electrodes. Feeding induced a fed pattern of activity. *In vitro* studies on strips of longitudinal and circular smooth muscle removed during laparotomy showed only quantitative differences with normal smooth muscle. The authors concluded that the motor abnormalities in this patient were probably due to hyperpolarization of the intestinal smooth muscle. Sullivan *et al.* studied gastrointestinal myoelectrical activity in four sporadic cases of CIIP[38]. A full thickness small bowel biopsy in these patients showed normal smooth muscle, normal ganglion cells in the myenteric plexus, but no special staining techniques for nerve tissue were performed. The slow wave activity was normal and secretin stimulated spiking activity and contractions. However, basal duodenal spiking activity was markedly increased as compared to normals (suggesting lack of inhibitory control from myenteric ganglia), and the contraction response of the small bowel to distension (which is probably neurally mediated) was abnormal. The authors proposed that the primary dysfunction was neural. Waterfall *et al.* investigated the small intestinal electrical activity in a child with CIIP[46]. The frequency gradient of the slow waves in the proximal small bowel was normal. In the mid-jejunum, however, this gradient was inversed, corresponding to the radiological finding of both orad and caudad moving contractions. Prolonged bursts of spike potentials throughout the slow wave cycle were present on many slow waves in the mid-jejunum. A neurogenic rather than a myogenic abnormality was suggested.

SCLERODERMA

The small bowel is involved in 20 to 60 per cent of patients with systemic sclerosis. Scleroderma is often associated with hypomotility and stasis of intestinal contents resulting in bacterial overgrowth. In some cases the motility disturbances are so severe that they cause chronic intestinal pseudo-obstruction. The pathogenesis of the small bowel motility disturbances in scleroderma was studied by Di Marino *et al.*[12] Slow wave frequency and progression and resting spiking activity were normal but, in contrast to controls, patients with scleroderma did not react to distension of the duodenum by an increase in the amount of spiking activity. Stimulation with secretin or pentagastrin increased duodenal spiking activity in some patients only. The group showing a normal response to hormonal stimuli had a shorter duration of the disease and a defect in neural activation seemed most likely. In those who failed to respond to hormones, the smooth muscle appeared to be unable to contract although still capable to generate slow waves. Thus both neural and smooth muscular abnormalities contribute to the hypomotility in scleroderma patients.

DYSTROPHIA MYOTONICA

Dystrophia myotonica is a chronic familial condition, characterized by myotonia and wasting of skeletal muscle. Involvement of gastrointestinal smooth muscle may impair oesophageal peristalsis and gastric emptying and produce a disordered pattern of defecation and colonic dilatation. Small bowel dilatation and prolonged transit time have been described and the condition may give rise to pseudo-obstruction. Lewis and Daniel[21] reported reduced amplitudes of contractions in stomach and duodenum, normal MMC's and the anticipated response to feeding. The maximum rate of contraction was sometimes clearly above the normal maximal rate (3.8 c/min in the stomach and 18.5 c/min in the duodenum). These maximum rates occurred independently of the rates at adjacent sites. The authors concluded that phase locking must be absent during these periods of more rapidly oscillating slow waves.

DIABETES MELLITUS

Although diabetic diarrhea is an established entity, its pathogenesis has been studied only sporadically. Older studies using balloon kymography have shown reduced motility of the small bowel in diabetics with autonomic neuropathy as compared with normal controls[29]. In a recent study in patients with gastroparesis diabeticorum, Malagelada *et al.* found that the activity front of the migrating motor complex was absent in the stomach but normal in the duodenum[23]. The small intestine motor disturbances and the diarrhea in diabetics have commonly been attributed to visceral neuropathy, because of the frequent coexistence with symptoms of generalized autonomic dysfunction, and also because similar intermittent diarrhea is found after vagotomy and use of ganglionic blocking agents.

THYROID DISORDERS

Gastric emptying and intestinal transit are rapid in animals and in man with thyroid hyperfunction, the hypermotility subsiding after treatment[19, 30]. On the other hand hypothyroidism is associated with constipation and is a well known cause of chronic intestinal pseudo-obstruction.

The underlying mechanisms for altered intestinal motility are unknown. Vagotomy does not block the increased motor activity in hyperthyroidism[15] and the possible effect on motility of the altered catecholamine metabolism in hyperthyroid patients has not been well studied. The effect of thyroid disease on the slow waves of the small intestine may well be important. The frequency of the duodenal slow waves is substantially increased in hyperthyroid patients and the duodenal frequency may persist to levels of 160 cm or more from the incisors[5]. Such phase locking over a long segment of small bowel may increase propulsion and transit. In hypothyroid patients both the duodenal slow wave frequency and the duodenal contraction rate are lower than in controls[13].

References

1 ATCHISON, W. D., STEWART, J. J. and BASS, P. A unique distribution of laxative induced spike potentials from the small intestine of the dog. *American Journal of Digestive Diseases*, **23,** 513–520 (1978)

2 BURNS, T. W., MATHIAS, J. R., CARLSON, G. M., MARTIN, J. I. and SHIELDS, R. P. Effect of toxigenic *Escherichia coli* on myoelectric activity of small intestine. *American Journal of Physiology*, **235,** E311–315 (1978)

3 BURNS, T. W., MATHIAS, J. R., MARTIN, J. L., CARLSON, G. M. and SHIELDS, R. P. Alteration of myoelectric activity of small intestine by invasive *Escherichia coli. American Journal of Physiology*, **238,** G57–G62 (1980)

4 CATCHPOLE, B. N. and DUTHIE, H. L. Postoperative gastrointestinal complexes. In *Gastrointestinal Motility in Health and Disease* (Proceedings of the 6th International Symposium on Gastrointestinal Motility), edited by H. L. Duthie, 33–41. Lancaster, MTP Press Ltd. (1978)

5 CHRISTENSEN, J. The controls of the gastrointestinal movements. *New England Journal of Medicine*, **285,** 85–98 (1971)

6 CHRISTENSEN, J. and MACAGNO, E. O. Small intestinal motility: the problem of relating contractions to flow. In *Frontiers of Knowledge in the Diarrheal Diseases*, edited by H. D. Janowitz and D. B. Sachar, 195–210. Upper Montclair, NJ, Projects in Health Inc. (1979)

7 CODE, C. F. Diarrheogenic motor and electrical patterns of the bowel. In *Frontiers of Knowledge in the Diarrheal Diseases*, edited by H. D. Janowitz and D. B. Sachar, 227–241. Upper Montclair, NJ, Projects in Health Inc. (1979)

8 CODE, C. F. and MARLETT, J. A. The interdigestive myoelectric complex of the stomach and small bowel of dogs. *Journal of Physiology* (London), **246,** 289–309 (1975)

9 CODE, C. F. and SCHLEGEL, J. F. The gastrointestinal interdigestive housekeeper: motor correlates of the interdigestive myoelectric complex of the dog. In *Proceedings of the Fourth International Symposium as Gastrointestinal Motility*,

edited by E. E. Daniel, J. A. L. Gilbert, B. Schofield, T. K. Schmitka and G. Scott, 631–634. Banff, Canada, Vancouver Mitchell Press Ltd. (1974)

10 DIAMANT, N. E., HALL, K., MUI, H. and El-SHARKAWY, T. Y. Vagal control of the feeding motor pattern in the lower esophageal sphincter, stomach and upper small intestine of dog. In *Gastrointestinal Motility*, edited by J. Christensen, 365–370. New York, Raven Press (1980)

11 DI MAGNO, E. P., HENDRICKS, J. C., GO., V. L. W. and DOZOIS, R. R. Relationships among canine fasting pancreatic and biliary secretions, pancreatic duct pressure, and duodenal phase III motor activity. Boldyreff revisited. *Digestive Diseases and Sciences*, **24,** 689–693 (1979)

12 DI MARINO, A. J., CARLSON, G., HYERS, A., SCHUMACHER, H. R. and COHEN, S. Duodenal myoelectric activity in scleroderma. Abnormal responses to mechanical and hormonal stimuli. *New England Journal of Medicine*, **289,** 1220–1223 (1973)

13 DURET, R. L. and BASTENIE, P. A. Intestinal disorders in hypothyroidism. Clinical and manometric study. *American Journal of Digestive Diseases*, **16,** 723–727 (1971)

14 FAULK, D. L., ANURAS, S., GARDNER, G. D., MITROS, F. A., SUMMERS, R. W. and CHRISTENSEN, J. A familial visceral myopathy. *Annals of Internal Medicine*, **89,** 600–606 (1978)

15 FETTER, D., BARRON, L. and CARLSON, A. J. The effect of induced hyperthyroidism on the gastrointestinal motility of vagotomized dogs. *American Journal of Physiology*, **101,** 605–611 (1932)

16 FLECKENSTEIN, P. Migrating electrical spike activity in the fasting human small intestine. *American Journal of Digestive Diseases*, **23,** 769–775 (1978)

17 FLECKENSTEIN, P. and ØIGAARD, A. Electrical spike activity in the human small intestine. *American Journal of Digestive Diseases*, **23,** 776–780 (1978)

18 FOSTER, G. E., ARDEN-JONES, J. R., BEATTIC, A. L. and HARDCASTLE, J. D. Introducing the Q-complex. An abnormal jejunal motility pattern. *Zeitschrift für Gastroenterologie*, **29,** 409–410 (1981)

19 JOHANSSON, H. Gastrointestinal function related to thyroid activity. *Acta Chirurgica Scandinavia*, **359,** (Suppl.) 1–88 (1966)

20 JUSTUS, P. B., MATHIAS, J. R., CARLSON, G. H., MARTIN, J. L., FORMAL, S. and SHIELDS, R. P. The myoelectric activity of the small intestine in response to *Clostridium perfringens* A enterotoxin and *Clostridium difficile* culture filtrate. In *Gastrointestinal Motility*, edited by J. Christensen, 379–386. New York, Raven Press (1980)

21 LEWIS, T. D. and DANIEL, E. E. Gastroduodenal motility in a case of dystrophia myotonica. *Gastroenterology*, **81,** 145–149 (1981)

22 LEWIS, T. D., DANIEL, E. E., SARNA, S. K., WATERFALL, W. E. and MARZIO, L. Idiopathic intestinal pseudo-obstruction. Report of a case, with intraluminal studies of mechanical and electrical activity, and response to drugs. *Gastroenterology*, **74,** 107–111 (1978)

23 MALAGELADA, J. R., REES, N. D. W., MAZOTTA, L. J. and GO, V. L. W. Gastric motor abnormalities in diabetic and postvagotomy gastroparesis: effect of metoclopramide and bethanechol. *Gastroenterology*, **78,** 286–293 (1980)

24 MARLETT, J. A. and CODE, C. F. Effects of celiac and superior mesenteric ganglionectomy on interdigestive myoelectric complex in dogs. *American Journal of Physiology*, **237,** E432–E436 (1979)

25 MATHIAS, J. R, CARLSON, G. M., BERTIGER, G., MARTIN, J. G. and COHEN, S. Migrating action potential complex of cholera: a possible prostaglandin-induced response. *American Journal of Physiology*, **232,** E529–E534 (1977)

26 MATHIAS, J. R., CARLSON, G. M., DI MARINO, A. J., BERTIGER, G., MORTON, M. E. and COHEN, S. Intestinal myoelectric activity in response to live *Vibrio cholerae* and Cholera enterotoxin. *Journal of Clinical Investigation*, **58,** 91–96 (1976)

27 MATHIAS, J. R., CARLSON, G. M., MARTIN, J. L., SHIELDS, R. P. and FORMAL, S. *Shigella dysenteriae* I enterotoxin: proposed role in pathogenesis of shigellosis. *American Journal of Physiology*, **239,** G382–386 (1980)

28 MATHIAS, J. R., MARTIN, J. L., BURNS, T. W., CARLSON, G. H. and SHIELDS, R. P. Ricinoleic acid effects on the electrical activity of the small intestine in rabbits. *Journal of Clinical Investigation*, **61,** 640–644 (1978)

29 McNALLY, E. F., REINHARD, A. E. and SCHWARTZ, P. E. Small bowel motility in diabetics. *American Journal of Digestive Diseases*, **14,** 163–169 (1969)

30 NEPORENT, M. I. and SPESIVTZWA, V. G. Motor function of gastrointestinal tract before and after I_{131} therapy in patients with thyrotoxicosis. *Federation Proceedings,* (Suppl.), T1177–T1180 (1963)

31 SARNA, S. K., DANIEL, E. E., WATERFALL, W. E., LEWIS, T. D. and MARZIO, L. Postoperative gastrointestinal electrical and mechanical activities in a patient with idiopathic intestinal pseudo-obstruction. *Gastroenterology*, **74,** 112–120 (1978)

32 SARR, M. G., KELLY, K. A. and PHILLIPS, S. F. Canine jejunum absorption and transit during interdigestive and digestive motor states. *American Journal of Physiology*, **289,** G167–G172 (1980)

33 SCHUFFLER, H. D., BIRD, T. D., SUMI, S. M. and COOK, A. A familial neuronal disease presenting as intestinal pseudo-obstruction. *Gastroenterology*, **75,** 889–898 (1978)

34 SCHUFFLER, H. D., LOWE, H. C. and BILL, A. H. Studies of idiopathic intestinal pseudo-obstruction. 1. Hereditary hollow visceral myopathy. Clinical and pathological studies. *Gastroenterology*, **73,** 339–344 (1977)

35 SCHUFFLER, H. D. and POPE, C. F. Studies on idiopathic intestinal pseudo-obstruction 2. Hereditary hollow visceral myopathy: family studies. *Gastroenterology*, **73,** 339–344 (1977)

36 SCOTT, L. D. and CAHALL, D. L. Influence of the interdigestive myoelectric complex on enteric flora in the rat. *Gastroenterology* (in press)

37 SMITH, J., KELLY, K. A. and WEINSHILBOUM, R. M. Pathophysiology of postoperative ileus. *Archives of Surgery*, **112,** 203–209 (1977)

38 SULLIVAN, M. A., SNAPE, W. J., MATARAZZO, S. A., PETROKUBI, R. J., JEFFRIES, G. and COHEN, S. Gastrointestinal myoelectrical activity in idiopathic intestinal pseudo-obstruction. *New England Journal of Medicine*, **297,** 233–238 (1977)

39 SZURSZEWSKI, J. H. A migrating electric complex of the canine small intestine. *American Journal of Physiology*, **217,** 1757–1763 (1969)

40 TAN, L. and CODE, C. F. The effects of cholecystokinin (CCK) on the canine gastrointestinal (GI) tract at different phases of the interdigestive myoelectric complex (IDMEC). *Physiologist*, **17,** 341 (1974)

41 THOMAS, P. A. and KELLY, K. A. Hormonal control of interdigestive cycles of canine proximal stomach. *American Journal of Physiology*, **237,** E192–E197 (1979)

42 VANTRAPPEN, G., JANSSENS, J., HELLEMANS, J. and GHOOS, Y. The interdigestive motor complex of normal subjects and patients with bacterial overgrowth of the small intestine. *Journal of Clinical Investigation*, **69,** 1158–1166 (1977)

43 VANTRAPPEN, G., JANSSENS, J., HELLEMANS, J. and PEETERS, T. The interdigestive motor activity of the bowel in man in normal and pathological conditions. In *Frontiers of Knowledge in the Diarrheal Diseases*, edited by H. D. Janowitz and D. B. Sachar, 243–252. Upper Montclair, NJ, Projects in Health Inc. (1979)

44 VANTRAPPEN, G., JANSSENS, J. and PEETERS, T. The migrating motor complex. *Medical Clinics of North America*, **65,** 1311–1329 (1981)

45 VANTRAPPEN, G., PEETERS T. L. and JANSSENS, J. The secretory component of the interdigestive migrating motor complex in man. *Scandinavian Journal of Gastroenterology*, **14,** 663–667 (1979)

46 WATERFALL, W. E, CAMERON, G. S., SARNA, S. K., LEWIS, T. D. and DANIEL, E. E. Disorganised electrical activity in a child with idiopathic intestinal pseudo-obstruction. *Gut*, **22,** 77–83 (1981)

47 WEISBERG, P. B., CARLSON, G. H. and COHEN, S. Effect of *Salmonella typhimurium* on myoelectrical activity in the rabbit ileum. *Gastroenterology*, **74,** 47–51 (1978)

48 WINGATE, D. L. Backwards and forwards with the migrating complex. *Digestive Diseases and Sciences*, **26,** 641–666 (1981)

16
Surgical aspects of small bowel motility

John H. Pemberton and Keith A. Kelly

Every operation on the small intestine alters small intestinal motility and transit to some extent. The alterations sometimes impair function and lead to symptoms. The aim of this chapter is to describe the motor alterations which follow small bowel operations and to present some current and new methods of treatment for dealing with symptoms when they appear.

POSTOPERATIVE ILEUS

Postoperative ileus is characterized by a lack of propulsive gastrointestinal contractions. The small bowel dilates. Secretions, debris and gas accumulate within its lumen. The abdomen distends, bowel movements cease, and nausea and vomiting ensue. Ileus follows almost every operation during which the abdomen is opened and the intestines handled. In general, the longer the operation and the more the handling, the greater the ileus.

A major motor abnormality present in ileus is the abolition of the cyclical interdigestive myoelectric complexes (IMC), those contractile complexes that move periodically down the gastrointestinal tract during fasting. In health, the complexes sweep the tract clean of debris, gas and indigestible ingesta during the interdigestive period (*see* Chapter 7). In ileus, the complexes are absent (*Figure 16.1*)[21], and interdigestive enteric content accumulates. Abolition of the complexes may be secondary to an enhanced release of norepinephrine from enteric neurons activated reflexly by the operative trauma[7]. The norepinephrine probably inhibits the complexes by hyperpolarizing the enteric smooth muscle cells and by decreasing the release of acetylcholine from enteric neurons. The inhibition occurs not only in the small bowel, but also in the stomach and colon[24]. Two to five days usually elapse before the augmented release of norepinephrine subsides, the complexes return, and intestinal contractions resume.

Treatment of postoperative ileus consists of nil per os, nasogastric suction, and administration of parenteral nutrition. Sympatholytic and parasympathomimetic

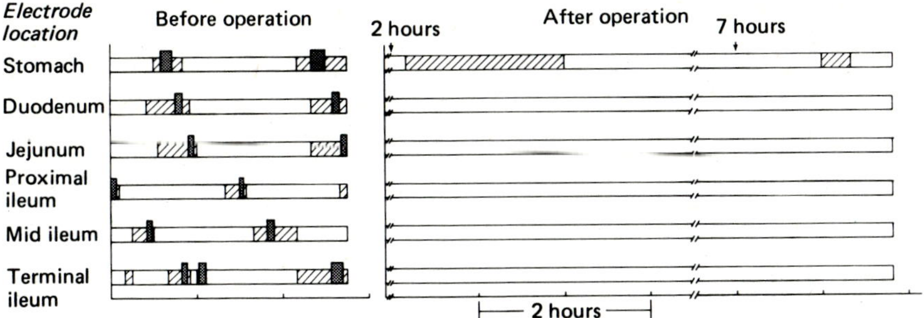

Figure 16.1 Diagrams of occurrence of phases of canine interdigestive myoelectric complexes before and after celiotomy and handling of small intestine (□) phase 1; (▨) phase 2 and 4; (▦) phase 3. (From Smith *et al.*[21], courtesy of the Editor and Publishers, *Archives of Surgery*)

agents, together with sympathetic blockers, have also been used in an attempt to hasten the return of motility,[4] but these treatments have risks that may outweigh their benefits.

INTESTINAL TRANSECTION

Incisions and partial transections of the enteric wall do not greatly alter the pattern of intestinal motility. However, complete transections do disturb both the frequency of intestinal contractions and their pattern of aboral propagation.

In health, intestinal contractions are controlled by cyclic changes in electrical potential, the pacesetter potentials, generated by the tunica muscularis of the small bowel (*see* Chapter 7). A site in the proximal duodenum generates the pacesetter potentials at the fastest rate and acts as the small intestinal pacemaker[12]. The cycles propagate distally from the pacemaker to the remaining small bowel, phasing the onset of contractions as they go. The system behaves like a series of bidirectionally coupled relaxation oscillators, the high-frequency duodenal oscillator driving a chain of distal oscillators of progressively declining frequency[19].

Transverse transections uncouple the chain of oscillators at the operative site and block distal propagation of the pacesetter potentials. A new pacemaker arises distal to the transections which also sends pacesetter potentials distally, but it oscillates at a slower frequency. Thus, transection decreases the maximum frequency of contractions in the distal bowel and abolishes propagation of contractions across the operative incision. These changes may lead to symptoms, but as yet no clear-cut pathophysiological abnormalities have been identified. In fact, small intestinal transit is not altered by transection and reanastomosis[3].

Transection also blocks propagation of interdigestive myoelectric complexes across the line of division, at least temporarily. Such blockage could lead to accumulation of interdigestive intestinal content in the bowel proximal to the cut, but appropriate tests have not as yet been done.

INTESTINAL RESECTION

Duodenum

Resection of the proximal duodenum removes the dominant pacemaker of the small intestine, and likely decreases the frequency of contraction in the distal bowel. However, because the decrease in frequency is probably small, no major changes in distal motility and transit have been reported.

Resection or bypass of the entire duodenum removes receptors sensitive to the acid, osmolarity, fatty acids and tryptophan in chyme. These receptors exert a negative feedback on gastric emptying via neural and hormonal pathways. More rapid gastric emptying ensues after duodenal resection, which, in turn, results in distention, contractions and rapid transit through the small intestine. A complex of symptoms called the 'dumping syndrome' results. In addition, a gastroenterostomy is required after duodenal resection to restore enteric continuity. Gastroenterostomy predisposes to enterogastric reflux, stomal ulceration, and obstruction of the afferent or efferent stomal limbs. Moreover, defective fat absorption has been noted after gastroenterostomy, possibly because of loss of the coordinated appearance of chyme, bile and pancreatic juice in the duodenum.

Jejunum

After partial jejunal resection and anastomosis, a decrease in contractile frequency distal to the resection and a block in propagation of pacesetter potentials across the anastomosis occur, changes similar to those following transverse transection alone. These changes have only a minor effect on function. For example, transit after such resections is unchanged from control[3]. However, total or near total jejunal resection causes 'intestinal hurry'. The rapid transit may lead to malabsorption, diarrhea, weight loss and fluid and electrolyte imbalance.

Ileum

Partial ileal resection, unlike partial jejunal resection, results in a 2- to 3-fold speeding of intestinal transit[3]. Moreover, extensive ileal resections are less well tolerated than extensive jejunal resections. The ileum is the site of absorption of bile salts and vitamin B_{12}, and so both are malabsorbed after ileal resections. Furthermore, less hyperplasia of villi occurs in the jejunum after large ileal resections than occurs in the ileum after large jejunal resections, a factor contributing to the more prominent malabsorption after ileal resections.

INTESTINAL BYPASS

Some operations designed to combat morbid obesity involve bypassing large segments of jejuno-ileum, leaving only 20 cm of proximal jejunum and 10 cm of distal ileum in enteric continuity. The proximal end of the excluded segment is usually closed, while the distal end is anastomosed to the colon. Rapid transit of ingested food through the incontinuity segments and loss of absorbing surface leads to weight loss. Some adaptation of the incontinuity segments does occur over the first and second postoperative year. The segments dilate and elongate, and their mucosa becomes hyperplastic. These adaptive changes may lessen diarrhea in some patients and even halt weight loss. More often, however, rapid transit and diarrhea continue.

The motility of the bypassed bowel has not been carefully studied. The lumen of the bypassed segment becomes smaller and its wall thins, but changes in its motor patterns have not been documented.

ILEOSTOMY

Brooke ileostomy

Type I contractions (amplitude, 5 to 15 cm water; duration, 5 sec), type III contractions (amplitude, 5 to 30 cm water; duration, 1 to 3 min), and interdigestive myoelectric complexes (IMC) are present in the ileum of patients with Brooke ileostomy[1,5], just as in the ileum in health. Type IV waves (amplitude, 10 to 60 cm water; duration, about 1 min) may also be found after ileostomy, but only when the stoma is obstructed[13]. The mean time between ingestion and appearance of a test meal in the terminal ileum is slower in ileostomy patients (127 min) than in controls (30–60 min) (unpublished observations). The slower transit may be because fewer action potentials and contractions are present in the ileum of ileostomy patients than in controls[22].

Continent ileostomy

The continent ileostomy (Kock pouch), that ileostomy which has a valved, ileal reservoir constructed just proximal to the stoma, preserves ileal motility well. Ileal pacesetter potentials are generated by the pouch at a frequency of about 9/min[1]. Action potentials, sometimes superimposed on the pacesetter potentials, trigger contractions. Interdigestive myoelectric complexes are also detected at their usual frequency of about 1 complex/2 h. However, the incisions and techniques of construction of the pouch and the obstruction to pouch outflow created by the pouch's valve result in marked dilatation of the pouch. The pouch accommodates much larger volumes of ileal content than does the ileum of a Brooke ileostomy patient, and yet intrapouch pressure remains low (*Figure 16.2*). Nonetheless, with distention of the pouch to volumes of 100–300 ml, large amplitude, type IV

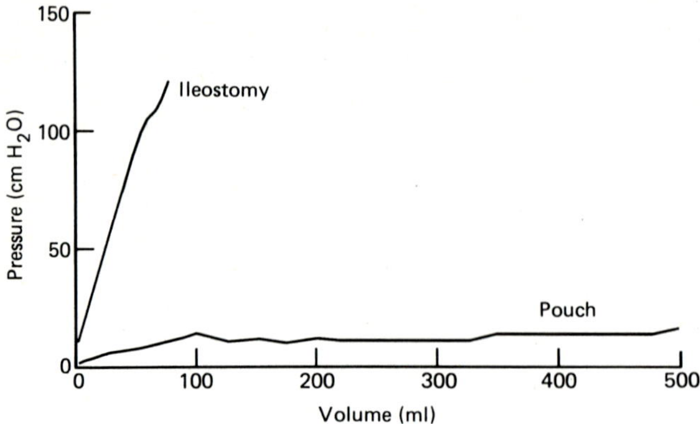

Figure 16.2 Effect of a pre-stomal ileal pouch on canine terminal ileal pressure-volume curves after ileostomy. (From Pemberton[18], courtesy of the Editor and Publishers, *Surgery*)

contractions do appear[1]. Such contractions, no doubt, threaten the integrity of the pouch. Frequent intubations of the pouch will prevent overdistension and, thus, the appearance of type IV contractions.

Ileostomy obstructing device

An ileostomy can also be made continent using an indwelling stomal occluding device[18]. The technique employs chronic, intermittent, stomal obstruction to achieve gradual dilatation of the terminal ileum, increased ileal capacity, and ultimately continence. Ileal accommodation is greatly enhanced (*Figure 16.3*). However, in experiments in dogs, few other changes in intestinal motility have been detected[18]. For example, barium sulfate passed from the stomach to the distal ileum of dogs undergoing chronic intermittent stomal obstruction in about 2.5 h, a value similar to that of controls. Similar experiments in man have shown similar adaptation (unpublished observations).

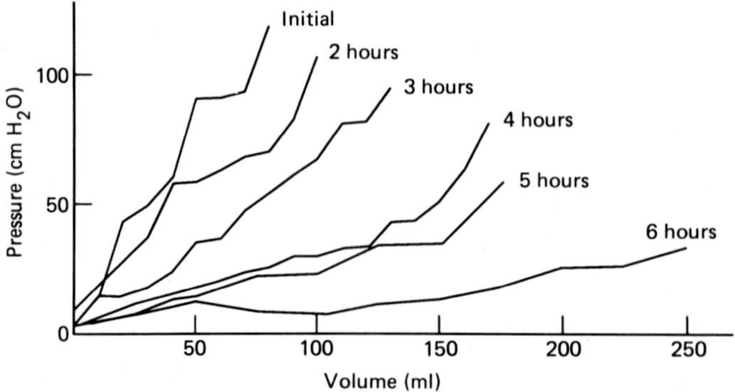

Figure 16.3 Effect of lengthening the period of chronic intermittent ileostomy occlusion on terminal ileal pressure-volume curves in a dog.

Ileal-anal anastomosis

Ileal-anal anastomosis also achieves fecal continence after resection of the large intestine. The rationale of this procedure is similar to that of the ileostomy obstructing device, except that the patient's own anal sphincter provides the intermittent obstruction instead of the device. Type I and type IV ileal contractions are present after ileal-anal anastomosis (unpublished observations). The type IV contractions may stress the ability of the sphincter to resist forward fecal flow. Thus, construction of an ileal pouch just proximal to the anastomosis[17] to minimize the increases in pressure created by such contractions could enhance ileal accommodation, decrease intraluminal pressure during filling, and aid continence. Further work is needed.

INTESTINAL DENERVATION

Vagotomy

Truncal vagotomy impairs the temporal regularity and decreases the frequency of phase III of the interdigestive myoelectric complex (IMC) in dogs[15]. Moreover, feeding does not consistently interrupt the IMC after the vagotomy. The failure of interruption may be due to loss of direct neural inhibition of IMCs or to decreased postprandial release of gastrin after vagotomy[23]. In health, gastrin interrupts the IMC. These findings have clinical implications. If feeding does not always abolish the IMC in man after vagotomy, the intense contractions of phase III of the IMC may be present postprandially. The rapid intestinal transit and diarrhea sometimes encountered after vagotomy may be due to the inappropriate persistence of the IMC.

Recently, a new form of vagotomy, proximal gastric vagotomy, has been introduced as a less disabling alternative to truncal vagotomy in the surgical treatment of peptic ulcer. Indeed, after proximal gastric vagotomy, which preserves vagal innervation to the small intestine, small bowel motility is preserved and postvagotomy diarrhea nearly prevented[14].

Transplantation

A more complete external denervation than that produced by vagotomy results from transplantation of the small intestine. Such transplantations can either be *in situ* or at heterotopic locations in the alimentary tract. An example of the latter is the use of free jejunal autotransplants to replace the cervical esophagus in patients with extensive laryngeal cancers[16]. Tests performed to evaluate the motor activity of such heterotopic jejunal transplants showed that pacesetter potentials were present in the transplants at the expected jejunal frequency of 9 to 10/min. Action potentials, hence contractions, were also recorded with the pacesetter potentials, and bursts of interdigestive contractions similar to those recorded in intact human and canine small bowel were found. Interestingly, upon instillation of food directly into the stomach, the interdigestive bursts were abolished in the autograft, thus implying an important role for hormonal inhibition of postprandial myoelectric activity.

In contrast, autotransplantation of canine jejunoileum[20] has shown that the interdigestive myoelectric complexes (IMCs) were present in the autotransplant, but their period was shorter than in the innervated duodenum. Temporal association between IMCs in the intact and the transplanted segments was lost, and feeding did not interrupt the IMCs in the autotransplants. These data thus suggest an important role for extrinsic nerves in preserving the orderly aboral migration of the IMCs and in postprandial inhibition of fasting electrical activity.

These observations suggest that clinical application of small intestinal transplantation would be associated with some motor abnormalities. Indeed, nearly all of our dogs developed diarrhea for 2 to 6 weeks after operation. However, the motor changes tended to resolve and the diarrhea to subside, so that by 6 weeks our animals returned to apparent good health. Moreover, they remained in good health for the ensuing 6 to 12 months, the duration of their follow-up. Thus, if the rejection of transplanted small intestinal homografts could be prevented, the motor and absorptive functions of the transplanted bowel should provide satisfactory enteric function.

PROCEDURES TO MODIFY TRANSIT

Reversed segments

Reversed intestinal segments have been used to slow gastric emptying in patients with the postgastrectomy dumping syndrome or to slow intestinal transit in patients with postvagotomy diarrhea or the diarrhea after intestinal resection. The segments retain their oral-aboral polarity after reversal and so drive content orally or at least slow aboral transit when they are in position. Intestinal propulsion proximal to the reversed segment remains unchanged from controls, while distally propulsion is accelerated[10]. Segmenting (non-propulsive) activity is also increased distally.

Alterations in intestinal motility and transit, such as those produced by reversing intestinal segments, likely alter intestinal absorption. In fasted dogs with luminally isolated, but extrinsically innervated small intestinal loops, absorption of glucose and electrolytes from the loops is greater during periods of slow transit through the loops than during periods of rapid transit. In contrast, slowing of transit achieved by chronic progressive obstruction does not alter absorption of glucose, water or electrolytes in ileostomy dogs[18]. This latter finding may be due to a resulting bacterial overgrowth that may negate any potential benefit of slowed transit. In germ-free dogs, segments of ileum continued to absorb water and electrolytes during periods of obstruction[11].

Intestinal pacing

Intestinal pacing has an advantage over the reversed intestinal segment as a means of modifying intestinal transit. Reversed segments create a permanent functional obstruction to aboral flow, whereas intestinal pacing provides a temporary obstruction that can be turned on or off at will.

The pacesetter potentials of canine small bowel can be entrained or captured by pacing the bowel electrically using implanted electrodes[2]. Over the proximal 10 to 30 percent of small bowel, the pacesetter potentials are driven to more rapid frequencies when the frequency of stimulation is either as fast as or faster than the frequency of the natural pacemaker. The pacesetter potentials of bowel distal to the proximal frequency plateau, however, cannot be so driven. The bowel must first be transected to decrease the frequency of the pacesetter potentials, after which they can then be paced.

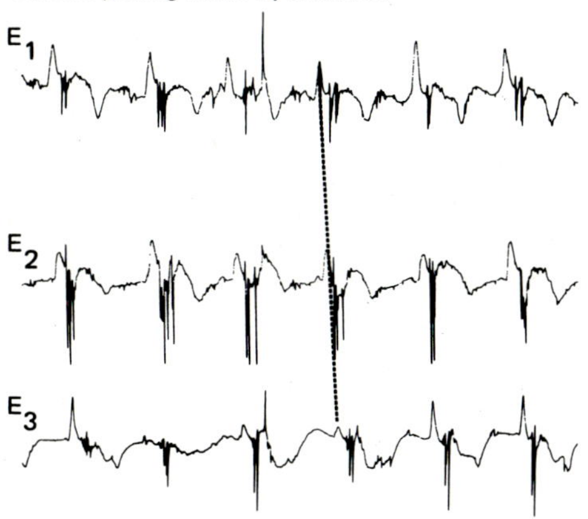

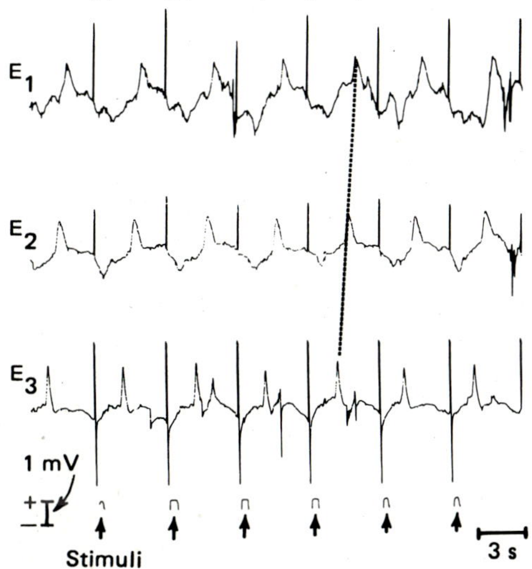

Figure 16.4 Effect of electrical pacing on canine small intestinal pacesetter potentials. E_1, E_2 and E_3 are electrodes placed sequentially 10 cm apart on the mid-duodenum. Stimuli (4 mA, 50 ms) are given at a distal duodenal site. (From Gladen and Kelly[8], courtesy of the Editor and Publishers, *Surgery*)

During pacing, not only are pacesetter potentials entrained, but the direction of their propagation is reversed in the bowel oral to the pacing site (*Figure 16.4*). Reversing the direction of propagation of the pacesetter potentials reverses the direction of propagation of contractions, and hence slows or reverses transit of bowel content. Moreover, retrograde pacing increases small intestinal absorption of simple crystalloid solutions in control dogs[6] and in dogs with the 'short bowel' syndrome[8], and decreases weight loss in the latter dogs[9].

The clinical application of gastrointestinal pacing awaits further refinement of equipment and application. Possible future uses include retrograde pacing of the proximal small bowel in patients with the postgastrectomy dumping syndrome, retrograde pacing of the distal small bowel in patients with postvagotomy diarrhea or the short bowel syndrome, and forward pacing of the bowel in patients with ileus caused by abnormal patterns of pacesetter potentials.

References

1 AKWARI, O. E., KELLY, K. A. and PHILLIPS, S. F. Myoelectric and motor patterns of continent pouch and conventional ileostomy. *Surgery, Gynecology and Obstetrics*, **150,** 363–371 (1980)

2 AKWARI, O. E., KELLY, K. A., STEINBACH, J. H. and CODE, C. F. Electric pacing of intact and transected canine small intestine and its computer model. *American Journal of Physiology*, **299,** 1188–1197 (1975)

3 BOOTH, C. C., EVANS, K. T., MENYIES, T. and STREET, D. F. Intestinal hypertrophy following partial resection of the small bowel in the rat. *British Journal of Surgery*, **46,** 403–410 (1959)

4 CATCHPOLE, B. N. Ileus: use of sympathetic blocking agents in its treatment. *Surgery*, **66,** 811–820 (1969)

5 CODE, C. F., ROGERS, A. G., SCHLEGEL, J., HIGHTOWER, N. C. and BARGEN, J. A. Motility patterns in the terminal ileum: studies on two patients with ulcerative colitis and iliac stomas. *Gastroenterology*, **32,** 651–665 (1957)

6 COLLIN, J., KELLY, K. A. and PHILLIPS, S.F. Increased canine jejunal absorption of water, glucose and sodium with intestinal pacing. *American Journal of Digestive Diseases*, **23,** 1121–1124 (1978)

7 DUBOIS, H., WEISE, V. K. and KOPIN, I. J. Postoperative ileus in the rat: physiology, etiology and treatment. *Annals of Surgery*, **178,** 781–786 (1973)

8 GLADEN, H. E. and KELLY, K. A. Enhancing absorption in the canine short bowel syndrome by intestinal pacing. *Surgery*, **88,** 281–286 (1980)

9 GLADEN, H. E. and KELLY, K. A. Electrical pacing for short bowel syndrome. *Surgery, Gynecology and Obstetrics*, **153,** 697–700 (1981)

10 GUSTAVSON, S. Transport of small bowel contents after interposition of an antiperistaltic jejunal segment in the rat. *European Surgical Research*, **11,** 381–393 (1979)

11 HENEGHAN, J. B., ROBINSON, J. W. L., MENGE, H. and WINISTORFER, B. Intestinal absorption in germ free dogs. *European Journal of Clinical Investigation*, **11,** 285–290 (1981)

12 HERMON-TAYLOR, J. and CODE, C. F. Localization of the duodenal pacemaker and its role in the organization of duodenal myoelectric activity. *Gut*, **12,** 40–47 (1971)

13 INGLEFINGER, F. J. and ABBOTT, W. D. Intubation studies of the human small intestine. XX. The diagnostic significance of motor disturbances. *American Journal of Digestive Diseases*, **7,** 468–474 (1940)

14 JOHNSTON, D. and GOLIGHER, J. C. Selective, highly selective, or truncal vagotomy? In 1976 – a clinical appraisal. *Surgical Clinics of North America*, **56,** 1313–1334 (1976)

15 MARIK, F. and CODE, C. F. Control of the interdigestive myoelectric activity in dogs by the vagus nerves and pentagastrin. *Gastroenterology*, **69,** 387–395 (1975)

16 MEYERS, W. C., SEIGLER, H. F., HANKS, J. B., THOMPSON, W. M., POSTLETHWAIT, R., JONES, S. R., AKWARI, O. E. and COLE, T. B. Postoperative function of 'free' jejunal transplants for replacement of the cervical esophagus. *Annals of Surgery*, **192,** 439–450 (1981)

17 NICHOLLS, R. J., BELLIVEAU, P., NEILL, M., WILKS, M. and TABAQCHALI, S. Restorative proctocolectomy with ileal reservoir: a pathophysiological assessment. *Gut*, **22,** 462–468 (1981)

18 PEMBERTON, J. H., KELLY, K. A. and PHILLIPS, S. F. Achieving ileostomy continence with an indwelling stomal device. *Surgery*, **90,** 336–343 (1981)

19 SARNA, S. K., DANIEL, E. E. and KINGMA, G. J. Simulation of slow-wave electrical activity of small intestine. *American Journal of Physiology*, **221,** 166–175 (1971)

20 SARR, M. G. and KELLY, K. A. Myoelectric activity of the autotransplanted canine jejunoileum. *Gastroenterology*, **81,** 303–310 (1981)

21 SMITH, J., KELLY, K. A. and WEINSHILBAUM, R. M. Pathophysiology of postoperative ileus. *Archives of Surgery*, **112,** 203–209 (1977)

22 WATERFALL, W. E., BROWN, B. H., DUTHIE, H. L. and WHITTAKER, G. E. The effects of humoral agents on the myoelectrical activity of the terminal ileum. *Gut*, **13,** 528–534 (1972)

23 WEISBRODT, N. W., COPELAND, E. M., MOORE, E. P., KEARLEY, R. R. and JOHNSON, L. R. Effect of vagotomy on electrical activity of the small intestine of the dog. *American Journal of Physiology*, **228,** 650–654 (1975)

24 WOODS, J. H., ERICKSON, L. W., CONDON, R. E., SCHULTE, W. J. and SILLIN, L. R. Postoperative ileus: a colonic problem? *Surgery*, **84,** 527–533 (1978)

17

Infectious agents and inducers of cytotoxicity in Crohn's disease and ulcerative colitis

Gary Gitnick

Crohn *et al.*[18] were first to propose that infectious agents might be causative factors in Crohn's disease (CD), and earlier Bargen[2] had postulated an infectious cause for ulcerative colitis (UC). Further impetus to pursue research in this area was provided by the reports of Mitchell and Rees[43] and Cave *et al.*[13] that small (less than 220 nm) transmissible agents from human tissues induced changes similar to inflammatory bowel disease in mice and rabbits. Farmer *et al.*[25] reported early virological studies.

SPONTANEOUS INFLAMMATORY BOWEL DISEASE IN ANIMALS

Inflammatory bowel diseases similar to those seen in humans have been described in a number of species. In some cases the cause can be traced to viruses[34], in others to bacteria[3] and in still others to a combination of viruses with bacterial flora[52].

Among the best described is feline infectious peritonitis (FIP), a transmissible disease of cats caused by a coronavirus, a pleomorphic RNA virus which is 75 nm in diameter with radiating spike-like projections of its outer envelope[32, 71]. The virus is heat and ether labile and phenol resistant. The progressive, non-responsive, febrile peritonitis caused by this agent was first reported in 1953, and the virus has subsequently been identified as the FIP virus. The peritonitis is serofibrinous, accompanied by large volumes of transudate and characterized by miliary granulomas of the serosal surfaces of viscera, particularly the liver and intestines. In recent years it has been recognized that the virus can affect other systems, and produce granulomatous disease of the lungs, central nervous system, eyes, kidneys, liver or visceral lymph nodes. In this infection, differences in the immune state of the host can result in markedly different disease manifestations[33].

There are other veterinary diseases which affect the colon and/or small intestine and produce diseases that resemble the inflammatory bowel diseases of man. Many of the causative organisms have not been described or even sought in human diseases. Among these widely different veterinary pathogens are: the soil algae, *Prototheca*, which causes an inflammatory bowel disease of the large and small intestine of dogs complete with extracolonic manifestations such as arthritis, iritis, and dermatitis[70]; an *anaerobe*, a species of the genus *Clostridium*, which produces an ulcerative enteritis of birds[5], the parvoviruses, including the small, DNA cryptotrophic virus which causes feline infectious enteritis; an anaerobic spirochete which interacts with one or more Gram-negative obligate anaerobes to produce an ulcerative colitis of swine[41]; and the *Mycobacterium johne* which produces granulomatous inflammation of the intestine in ruminants[48]. Some other interesting diseases that are probably caused by an infectious agent because of favorable responses to antibiotics include canine colitis, which histologically bears a strong resemblance to human ulcerative colitis[69], and canine granulomatous enteritis which resembles Crohn's disease including the presence of granulomas and giant cells[63].

ANIMAL TRANSMISSION STUDIES

In 1935, Mones and Sanjuan[44] inoculated crude filtrates obtained from the intestinal tissue of patients with inflammatory bowel diseases into rabbits, causing changes similar to those found in UC (*Table 17.1*). Mitchell and Rees[43] transmitted

Table 17.1 Animal transmission studies

Year	Study	Finding
1935	Mones and Sanjuan[44]	Transmitted ulcerative colitis to rabbits
1970	Mitchell and Rees[43]	Transmitted granulomas to mouse foot pads
1973	Bolton *et al.*[7]	No transmission to mouse foot pads
1973	Cave *et al.*[13]	Transmitted granulomas to rabbit ileum
1976	Cave *et al.*[11]	Transmitted ulceration to rabbit colon mucosa
1976 1977	Taub *et al*[65] and Donnelly *et al.*[21]	Control tissues produce granulomas in mouse foot pads
1980	Das *et al.*[19]	CD filtrates produced lymphomas and splenic antigen in athymic mice
1980	Gitnick *et al.*[27]	No transmission to rabbit ileum/colon
1981	Cohen *et al.*[16]	Transmitted granulomas to rabbit ileum

granulomas to the foot pads of mice inoculated with filtrates prepared from CD tissue, but others failed to reproduce this work[7,66]. Cave *et al.*[13] then reported their ability to inoculate rabbits intraserosally with tissue from patients with CD or UC and transmit inflammatory changes suggestive of organ specific inflammatory bowel disease. Simonowitz *et al.*[60], in attempting to confirm this work, were not able to transmit granulomas but observed an inflammatory process in the bowel wall of rabbits inoculated with CD material. We have been unable to confirm this work[39].

Transmission in mice

Mitchell and Rees (1970)[43] reported that they were able to induce granulomas in the foot pads of CBA mice by injecting tissue from a patient with CD, but not by using control tissue. These granulomas evolved slowly over three months to two years and were present in normal and immunodeficient CBA mice. These findings were partially confirmed by Taub *et al.*[66], but not by Bolton *et al.*[7] or Heatley *et al.*[31] using different strains of mice. Subsequently, Mitchell and Rees extended their experiments and reported second generation passage of the histological changes. Pretreatment of the homogenates by filtration, autoclaving, irradiation and freezing, has shown that the transmissible material passes a 220 nm filter and withstands freezing, but is destroyed by autoclaving and irradiation. Cave *et al.*[12] demonstrated similar findings in both normal and immunodeficient CBA mice and A_2G inbred mice. Frozen and 220 nm filtrates were both effective at inducing granulomas given intraperitoneally or via the foot pads. Both Mitchell and Rees[43] and Cave *et al.*[12] reported systemic spread of the granulomatous process to the intestine. This occurred late, at least nine months after injection. Taub *et al.*[66] suggested that the process is non-specific since some of their controls induced similar changes. However, with control inocula these changes occurred early at 25 days and had disappeared in 150 days. Thus, this inflammatory reaction is temporally different and may have a different cause[41]. Cohen *et al.*[15] reported C57B10/J and Balb/C mice were more susceptible to the granuloma inciting agent in CD tissues than were CBA mice. He also noted transient granulomas in his control mice, but by 12 months only the CD mice showed persistence of the granulomatous reaction.

Cave *et al.*[12] also noted that A_2G mice injected with UC tissues developed slowly evolving granulomas that could not be differentiated histologically from those induced by CD tissues. The inciting factor passed a 0.2 μ filter and withstood freezing. The transmissible agents for CD and UC have been found in ileum, colon and mesenteric lymph nodes. On passage, the agent for CD has been demonstrated in ileum, lymph nodes, foot pads, liver and spleen.

Das *et al.*[20] reported that 9 of 96 athymic mice inoculated with tissue filtrates from the intestine of CD patients developed lymphomas which contained an antigen that by an immunofluorescence test reacted specifically with an antibody in CD sera but not with UC sera and a few other control sera. Particles resembling C Type murine viruses were found in the lymphomas. The number of disease control tissues and sera tested were small. Until this work is successfully repeated in other laboratories and the number of disease control tissues and sera expanded, its significance is uncertain.

Transmission in rabbits

Cave *et al.*[10, 11, 13] employed the New Zealand white rabbit as an experimental animal because it is large enough to withstand serial biopsy of the intestine. In the initial study, frozen CD tissue homogenates induced slowly evolving granulomas in the ileum, colon, mesenteric lymph nodes and liver of some of the recipient rabbits. Control tissues did not incite any changes over the same 9 month period of observation. Subsequently, a larger study, using fresh CD tissue (6 patients), UC tissue (2 patients) and 5 with other diseases was initiated[10]. In this study cell-free filtrates (220 nm) induced a granulomatous response over 3 to 24 months in some of the recipient animals. Control animals were consistently negative. The rabbits injected with UC homogenates developed slowly evolving round cell infiltrates[11]. This was predominantly mucosal in distribution, localized to the cecum and colon, but with rectal sparing. Successful passage of tissues from both the initial CD and UC rabbits followed direct injection of the bowel or intravenous injection using crude homogenates or cell-free filtrates. The latter route of injection revealed intestinal selectivity of the histological changes, which were similar to those in the first generation of animals. Furthermore, five of the CD donors were common to both the mouse and rabbit studies, and three of these induced lesions in both species.

Simonowitz *et al.*[60] were able to induce a chronic inflammatory response in the colon, ileum and cecum of New Zealand White rabbits. Lesions took 12 months to evolve and were demonstrably different from control animals. The investigators concluded that they had not transmitted chronic Crohn's disease, but they could not exclude the presence of a transmissible agent. Donnelly *et al.*[21] again using New Zealand white rabbits, induced a local inflammatory response with both CD and control tissue homogenates using a coarse homogenate. The response in an additional group of animals was abolished by preincubation of the homogenate with ampicillin. Orr[46] reported negative results with transmission to New Zealand white rabbits as did Heatley *et al.*[31] The latter group were also unsuccessful using Sprague Dawley rats and guinea pigs.

ISOLATION OF ORGANISMS

The search for an infectious cause of Crohn's disease and ulcerative colitis extends back more than 50 years. Agents that have been considered as possibly causative have included the tubercle bacillus, *Shigella*, *E. histolytica*, and lymphopathia venereum virus. In recents years other bacterial causes of diarrhea have been described. These include *Yersinia pseudotuberculosis*, *Campylobacter fetus ss jejuni*, *Aeronomas hydrophila* and *Clostridium difficile*. More recently, interest has focused on anaerobic organisms including the *Eubacteria* and *Peptostreptococcus* (strains ME47, ME46 and C18), cell wall-defective *Pseudomonas*-like bacteria, *Escherichia coli*, mycobacteria and *Mycoplasma*.

Because of the histological and radiographical similarities between intestinal tuberculosis and Crohn's disease, investigations were recently undertaken seeking acid fast organisms in the mesenteric lymph nodes of inflammatory bowel disease patients[61]. Forty-two of 76 mesenteric lymph nodes from Crohn's disease patients and 14 of 27 mesenteric lymph nodes from ulcerative colitis patients as well as 3 of 41 lymph nodes from patients with other diseases yielded acid fast organisms 6 to 18 months after the cultures were first taken. The acid fast organism described by these investigations is exceedingly slow-growing. These same investigators described the isolation of *Mycobacterium kansasii* from one Crohn's disease patient[9]. However, they have not been able at the time of their recent report to identify the acid-fast mycobacteria being reproducibly cultivated in patients with Crohn's disease and ulcerative colitis. In addition, a Gram-positive *Coryneform* organism was isolated or detected in up to 32 per cent of the 76 Crohn's disease specimens and in up to 11 per cent of the 27 ulcerative colitis specimens as well as in 7 per cent of the control specimens[73]. Eubacteria and peptostreptococci have been found in the faecal flora of patients with Crohn's disease[68]. Others have described the detection of specific IgE antibody to *E. coli* 0127B8 in the sera of patients with Crohn's disease and ulcerative colitis but not in control sera[56]. Unfortunately, the number of patients studied is small in this serological survey.

The picture was further complicated when Parent and Mitchell[47] reported that cell wall-defective *Pseudomonas*-like bacteria could be isolated from each of nine CD patients and from none of nine UC patients nor from others with non-inflammatory gastrointestinal diseases. Although these studies used a small number of patients and did not include other inflammatory illnesses such as diverticulitis, ischemic bowel disease, and appendicitis, they have raised the implication that cell wall-defective *Pseudomonas*-like bacteria may play a role in the pathogenesis of CD. Serological studies performed by Whorwell *et al.*[74] did not reveal antibodies to certain cell wall-defective bacteria in inflammatory bowel disease patients.

The possible role of *Cl. difficile* in inflammatory bowel disease was originally reported by LaMont and Trnka[38]. These investigators found *Cl. difficile* toxin in stools during symptomatic relapse in six patients including five with UC and one with CD. Three of these six patients had recently received sulfasalazine therapy while three others had no recent documented exposure to antimicrobial agents. Three of the six patients demonstrated prompt improvement with vancomycin therapy which has now become the treatment of choice in patients with *Cl. difficile*-induced diarrhea or colitis. A more recent report by these investigators indicated that *Cl. difficile* toxin was detected in the stools of patients with inflammatory bowel disease in 10 of 26 relapses[67]. Bolten *et al.*[6] also performed the tissue culture assay for this toxin in inflammatory bowel disease patients. These investigators found positive results in four of 17 UC patients and one of seven with CD; two of the five patients with positive assays had received sulfasalazine and four improved when treated with vancomycin or metronidazole.

The combined experience from these two groups is provocative in suggesting that *Cl. difficile* may play a role in some relapses of both CD and UC. This has important implications regarding the diagnosis and treatment of these patients. It should be emphasized that the issue here concerns the mechanism of relapse and there is little evidence that *Cl. difficile* is responsible for the underlying disease. Previous studies indicate that patients with *Cl. difficile*-induced colitis are not subject to relapsing disease (unless treated with vancomycin); furthermore, inflammatory bowel disease patients with *Cl. difficile* toxin also suffer subsequent relapses in which this toxin is not detected[42].

While these interesting transmission studies were being undertaken, we were seeking agents in tissue filtrates from patients with CD and UC[25] (*Table 17.2*). We

Table 17.2 Studies of viruses and cytotoxins in Crohn's disease and ulcerative colitis

Study	Findings
1962 Schnierson *et al.*[57]	No viruses found in UC or CD
1973 Farmer *et al.*[25]	No specific viral serology in CD, CMV superinfection in UC
1975 Aronson *et al.*[1]	Small RNA virus in CD using WI-38 tissue cultures
1976 Gitnick *et al.*[26]	Development of sensitive tissue culture systems for CD CPE and EM studies
1976 Korsmeyer *et al.*[35]	Anti-RNA antibodies in IBD patients and relatives but not in matched controls
1977 Strickland *et al.*[64]	Lymphocytotoxic antibodies in IBD patients and spouses but not in matched controls
1977 Whorwell *et al.*[75]	Isolation of reovirus-like agent in CD
1977 Reimann[50]	EM of virus-like particles in CD
1977 Cooper *et al.*[17]	CMV in UC toxic megacolon
1979 Greenberg *et al.*[29]	*Mycoplasma hyorhinas* and SV40 found in Aronson, *et al.* materials
1980 Phillpotts *et al.*[49]	? Tissue factors in CD using WI-38 but no CPE in rabbit ileum or avian tissue culture
1980 Gitnick *et al.*[27]	Confirmed UC and CD CPE in each tissue culture system
1982 McLaren and Gitnick[40]	Heat labile cytotoxin in CD; Heat stable cytotoxin in UC and colon CA; heat labile cytotoxin in UC and colon CA

CA = carcinoma.
CD = Crohn's disease.
CMV = cytomegalovirus.
CPE = cytopathic effect.
EM = electron microscopy.
IBD = inflammatory bowel disease.
UC = ulcerative colitis.

reported a statistically significant serological association of cytomegalovirus with UC. The failure of these studies to demonstrate an association between cytomegalovirus and CD was confirmed by the investigations of Roche and Huang[51], who used hybridization techniques; these investigations, however, did not evaluate the already established association of cytomegalovirus and UC.

CYTOTOXICITY INDUCING AGENTS

Aronson *et al.*[1] reported that biopsies of CD tissue and tissue from some other intestinal disorders produce a cytopathic effect on early passage human diploid lung fibroblasts (WI-38). This effect could be passaged. Subsequent characterization suggests that the agents were small RNA viruses that were acid and ether stable, heat stable at 60°C for one hour and labile in the presence of magnesium chloride. The agents were found to be pathogenic for newborn CBA mice. Beeken *et al.*[4] extended these observations. Gitnick *et al.*[26] using a different technology, which included homogenization and filtration through a 0.2 μm filter, showed that a cytopathic substance could be isolated from CD tissues and another material could be isolated from UC tissues (*Table 17.3*). Both were shown to produce cytopathic effect in a rabbit ileal cell line and subsequently were shown to destroy resistance inducing factor free chick embryo fibroblasts and Peking duck embryo fibroblasts. Neutralization tests employing human sera as well as guinea pig immune sera have suggested that these agents are not immunologically identical.

Preliminary electron microscopic evidence also suggested differing morphologies. The fact that the cytopathic inducers could be serially passaged made it conceivable that these are either living, replicating agents of a size consistent with a virus or highly concentrated toxic materials. Whorwell *et al.*[75] suggested that the agents were rotaviruses; however, this was refuted serologically with temporally matched control sera. Phillpotts *et al.*[49] using different methods than those previously reported, suggested that the cytopathic change was induced by low and middle molecular weight non-viable tissue factors. The nature of these factors was not identified. They did not attempt exact reproduction of the previous reports by using the same techniques used by others.

Table 17.3 (CPE) Cytopathic effect inducers in gastrointestinal disease

	Total number	*Positive CPE*
Crohn's disease		
Ileitis	36	35
Colitis	27	27
Ileocolitis	7	7
Ulcerative colitis		
Backwash ileitis	2	2
Colon	27	27
Colon carcinoma*	27	27
Radiation enteritis	5	2
Necrotizing enterocolitis	1	1
Colonic polyps – benign	2	0
Familial polyposis – benign	2	1
Volvulus	1	0
Hirschsprung's disease	2	0
Diverticulitis	23	1
Normal ileum	5	0
Normal colon	1	0

*Grossly normal intestinal tissue studied.

One group of investigators recently reported that the cytopathic effects described by us were more common in control tissues and were not passageable[45]. Unfortunately these investigators failed to adhere to the guidelines published in previous reports[26, 28]. The effect which they describe is suggestive of non-specific tissue degeneration which we have often seen. The problems with this recent report are the following. (1) The tissue inoculum which was used consisted of a crude homogenate of rectal biopsies obtained at sigmoidoscopy. We found that such mucosal specimens will only produce non-specific degeneration. They are too small to undergo the processing procedures described by us and in fact these investigators did not undertake these processing procedures. We have only used full thickness surgical specimens of sufficient size to insure that the final product will have been washed, minced, suspended, centrifuged and the supernatant passed through a 0.2 μm filter. (2) These investigators used tissue culture systems which have been found to be insensitive to the cytopathic effect we describe. They did not utilize the two tissue culture systems which have been found to be exquisitely sensitive to cytotoxins, RIFF free chick embryo tissue culture and rabbit ileum tissue culture. (3) Finally, the medium used and the conditions of incubation differed from those reported by us. Future investigators should strive to avoid such pitfalls. To accomplish this, exchanges of material as well as exchanges of information and careful adherence to already published methods must be encouraged.

Greenberg *et al.*[29] reported finding a *Mycoplasma hyorhinis* contaminating some of the cultures used by Aronson *et al.*[1], but were unable to find *Mycoplasma* in the cultures reported by Gitnick *et al.*[26]. Reimann[50] presented electron microscopic evidence of virus-like particles in CD tissue and Dourmashkin *et al.*[22] described a possible precursor to the aphthoid ulcer and myxovirus-like budding from the surface of epithelial cells.

Mechanisms of tissue damage

Studies by Strickland *et al.*[64] have identified high levels of antibodies to synthetic double-stranded RNA and lymphocytotoxic antibodies in the sera of patients with either CD or UC and their unaffected spouses. These studies also revealed high levels of circulating interferon in patients with inflammatory bowel disease. Cellular mechanisms of tissue damage in inflammatory bowel disease are suggested by several studies which have investigated the *in vitro* cytotoxic effect of inflammatory bowel disease peripheral blood lymphocytes to colon epithelial cells in short-term culture[59]. The cell responsible for this effect is reported to have the characteristics of a K-cell[62]. Recent studies of circulating non-specific K-cell activity in inflammatory bowel disease have yielded conflicting results. Increased K-cell activity in CD using a plaque assay was reported by Eckhardt *et al.*[23]. In contrast, Britton *et al.*[8], using an antibody dependent cellular cytotoxicity assay with a mouse lymphoma line as a non-specific target, reported insignificant differences between peripheral blood lymphocytes from CD and normal subjects. The possible role of K-cells in the bowel damage of inflammatory bowel disease has been further clouded by reports that this cell is absent in lymphoid populations derived from the intestine, both in inflammatory bowel disease and in control subjects. The study by Britton *et al.*[8] clearly showed enhanced K-cell activity in mesenteric lymph node cells from patients with CD when compared to disease control mesenteric node cells. Recent work by Shorter *et al.*[14] indicates that a major reason for the apparent lack of K-cell activity reported by other investigators in intestinally derived lymphoid cells is selective deflection of this subpopulation during the prolonged (18 hour) process of lymphoid cell isolation from the gut.

Effector lymphocytes that are responsible for *in vitro* cytotoxicity against virus infected target cells in humans may include both T-cells[36, 37, 53] and K-cells[30, 55, 58, 72]. Further, interferon has been shown to substantially enhance spontaneous cell-mediated cytotoxicity activity against virus infected targets[54]. In addition to being potentially important mechanisms of resistance to recovery from viral infection, such reactions may also be important in the genesis of chronic tissue damage. For example, the development of chronic hepatitis in patients with hepatitis B infection has been linked to such cytotoxic effects[24]. Similar mechanisms could be postulated as contributing to the chronic intestinal damage in inflammatory bowel disease.

Role of infectious agents in cytotoxicity

Thus, transmissible cytopathic agents have been described in CD and UC[28]. Although several laboratories have reported the existence of such agents, others have been unable to isolate them. Many problems have existed in extending the initial reports. Among these have been the inability to cultivate the cytopathic materials to high enough titer to allow proper characterization. The low titer of the cytopathic materials also precluded obtaining adequate electron microscopic photographs of these putative agents. One group recently suggested that the transmissible materials could not be found in tissue culture utilizing modifications of tissue culture systems initially reported; when other systems were used, however, a cytopathic toxic factor could be identified[45]. Subsequently we reported that following inoculation of tissue culture with filtrates from CD and UC 0.2 μm filtrates, a transient cytopathic effect could be seen in rabbit ileum tissue culture. After this, the tissue culture system recovered and then a definite and extensive cytopathic effect developed. In contrast, in chick embryo tissue culture within 48 hours of inoculation extensive cytopathic effect developed leading to destruction of the cell sheath and no late cytopathic effect inducer could be demonstrated[39, 40]. We further reported that the factor responsible for the cytopathic effect in rabbit ileum tissue culture and the early severe cytopathic effect in chick embryo tissue culture was a non-viable toxin unrelated to *Cl. difficile* or other clostridial toxins and unrelated to *E. coli* toxin.

Progress in the control of Crohn's disease and ulcerative colitis is unlikely until a better understanding of the pathogenesis of these diseases is achieved. In our ongoing studies seeking the role, if any, of infectious agents in the pathogenesis of CD and UC, we have recently described the presence of cytotoxins capable of destroying colon, ileal and chick embryo cells while sparing 16 other tissue culture systems[40]. These cytotoxins may be of bacterial, viral or tissue origin. If these cytotoxic substances were of tissue origin, the narrow range of cell cytotoxicity would be difficult to explain. The selective cytotoxicity for colon, ileum and chick embryo cells, while sparing other tissue culture systems, would not be characteristic of a general cell toxin. They are not immunologically related to, nor do they have, the physical and chemical properties of *Cl. difficile* or *E. coli* toxins.

Figure 17.1 Pathogenesis of ulcerative colitis or Crohn's disease; hypothesis

Inciting agent
Virus or viral product
Bacteria or bacterial product
Environmental toxin
and/or
Food antigen
↓
Susceptible host
↓
Immune mediation
↓
Cytotoxin effector
↓
Cell destruction

The inducers of cytopathology which have now been partially characterized and isolated from CD, UC and some control specimens may represent the effector system responsible for the final development of tissue destruction in these diseases. This hypothesis is based on the reproducible finding of these cytopathic inducers in patients with these illnesses and the unique ability of these cytotoxins to destroy only a narrow range of host cells. This range includes colon, ileum or chick embryo cells but excludes most other human animal tissue systems. The finding of this narrow range of cytotoxicity suggests the possibility that these inducers of cytotoxicity may represent one step in the pathway which leads to tissue destruction in these illnesses. One hypothesis for the development of UC or CD is outlined in *Figure 17.1*. It is conceivable that the large and small intestine may react in only a limited number of ways to a variety of insults. A number of inciting agents or combinations of inciting agents may initiate the processes leading to these diseases. These inciting agents may include viruses or viral products, bacteria or bacterial products such as endotoxins, environmental toxins and/or food antigens. In a susceptible host, these may stimulate immune mediation possibly leading to the process which eventually produces a cytotoxin that in turn produces cell destruction. Alternatively, these cytotoxins may have no pathogenic role in spite of their limited range of cytotoxicity.

CONCLUSIONS

Many bacterial organisms have now been found in increased quantities or prevalence in Crohn's disease and/or ulcerative colitis, none of which has been shown to fulfil Koch's postulates. The finding of an unusual bacterial flora does not imply causation. It may represent a secondary phenomenon related to the inflammatory process rather than a primary phenomenon which causes the condition. Unfortunately, many of the microbial studies have confined exploration to patients with Crohn's disease or ulcerative colitis but have not included a search with equal vigor in patient's with a variety of other bowel diseases such as diverticulitis, ischemic colitis, radiation enteritis, and various malignant processes. Cultured specimens have not been shown to reproduce disease in animal hosts. Until Koch's postulates are fulfilled, these unusual bacterial populations must be considered probable epiphenomena rather than causative agents when considered singly.

The possibility of a viral cause of Crohn's disease or ulcerative colitis has fascinated many investigators. The interesting finding of lymphocytotoxic antibodies in the family and household contacts of Crohn's disease patients, the studies demonstrating the presence of a 'transmissible' agent and the cytopathic changes seen following inoculation of tissue cultures with Crohn's disease or ulcerative colitis tissues all suggested a viral cause for these diseases. Furthermore, the occasional development of ulcerative colitis or Crohn's disease among husbands and wives suggested an infectious basis. However, similar though not necessarily identical, cytopathic effects are seen in approximately 20 per cent of non-inflammatory bowel disease intestinal tissues evaluated. Although these effects appear to be due to differing substances, the presence of such changes in control materials raises important questions about the significance of the cytopathic findings in Crohn's disease and ulcerative colitis tissue even though the differences in frequencies are great (95 per cent vs 20 per cent). Many investigators have been unable to confirm the results of the laboratories reporting cytopathic changes. Viral particles have not been identified reproducibly in spite of many attempts at electron microscopic evaluation. Koch's postulates have not been successfully fulfilled. All of these points cast doubt on the likelihood that a conventional virus produces either of these diseases. Nevertheless, the possibility of an unusual microbial or viral infection remains real.

VERIFICATION OF DATA AND UNANSWERED QUESTIONS

The history of infectious agents in the inflammatory bowel diseases is clear. Although this report documents existing knowledge, important problems still exist. Some of these include:

(1) studies of viral transmission to animals, such as athymic mice, isolation of viruses, and isolation of cell wall-defective bacteria are reported in the literature, but lack confirmation. It is essential that the existing literature be either confirmed or negated so that a data base can be established from which all investigators can work;

(2) if viruses do indeed exist, they have been cultivated to titers too low to allow proper characterization. Efforts must be undertaken to boost titers and to provide sufficient antigen to allow laboratories to evaluate and characterize the isolated agents;

(3) the role of infectious agents in these diseases must be defined. If the role is to be a causative one, Koch's postulates should be fulfilled. The cytopathic agents and the cell wall-defective bacteria now described in inflammatory bowel diseases are at least as likely to be present as superinfections rather than as

causative agents. Care must be taken so that enthusiasm over the description of the flora of the intestinal tract does not overcome the relevance of Koch's postulates in science. Furthermore, the possible interaction of infectious agents with immune parameters needs close attention. If Koch's postulates are not fulfilled, the presence of these agents should be better explained. Do they have a role in altering motility or secretion, thereby joining in the responsibility for the development of diarrhea? Do they play a role in the eventual development of malignancies? Do they alter metabolic products and, in turn, affect the physiology of the intestine? These questions merit further investigation.

SUGGESTIONS FOR FUTURE PROGRESS

The histopathology and course of Crohn's disease and ulcerative colitis are compatible with the interaction of infectious agents in the development of an immunologically mediated disease among patients with a genetic predisposition. The recent demonstration of specific cellular cytotoxins uniquely capable of destroying intestinal tissue while sparing other tissues raises a concept which requires further investigation. Constituents of the endogenous bacterial or viral flora, bacterial products such as endotoxins and lipopolysaccharides, viral cell wall material, and defective interfering viral particles working singly or in combination need to be considered as possible initiating agents in the long process eventually leading to these disease states. At the very least, these concepts merit further cooperative, collaborative examination among groups combining the interests of virologists, bacteriologists, biochemists, immunologists and geneticists. This type of collaborative approach may eventually unravel the mysteries of causation. It is incumbent on current and future investigators, manuscript reviewers, and journal editors to insist on certain basic criteria which will help to form a data base that can be relied upon in the coming years without requiring unnecessary repetition because of inadequate documentation in earlier studies. Thus, the patient population studies need to be carefully characterized.

(1) When dealing with ulcerative colitis, patients should be described as having proctitis, left-sided colitis, or pancolitis. Patients with Crohn's disease need to be identified as having colitis, ilecolitis, ileitis, or proximal disease.
(2) The treatment history of patients needs to be clearly defined. Prior treatment with corticosteroids, the dosages utilized and the periods in which corticosteroids were given need to be described. The utilization of other immunosuppressives such as azathioprine and 6-mercaptopurine should be documented.
(3) Investigators must strive to adequately control their studies. Appropriate disease controls as well as normal controls must be included in future programs.
(4) Specimens must be evaluated under code in order to avoid, to as great an extent as possible, any prejudice in assessing assay systems. Provocative studies need to be rapidly repeated by independent groups.

Funding agencies must be encouraged to support programs aimed at confirming or negating potentially important studies. Without confirmation, unnecessary extensions of inadequate data may be undertaken. Regular communication among investigators in this field should be fostered. Symposia, regular informal meetings, newsletters, and exchanges of investigators and materials should be encouraged.

References

1 ARONSON, M. D., PHILLIPS, C. A., BEEKEN, W. L. *et al.* Isolation and characterization of a viral agent from intestinal tissue of patients with Crohn's disease and other chronic intestinal disorders. *Progress in Medical Virology*, **21,** 165–176 (1975)

2 BARGEN, J. A. Experimental studies on the etiology of chronic ulcerative colitis. *Journal of the American Medical Association*, **83,** 332 (1924)

3 BARTHOLD, S. E., COLEMAN, G. L., BHATT, P. N. *et al.* The etiology of transmissible murine colonic hyperplasia. *Laboratory Animal Science*, **26,** 889–894 (1976)

4 BEEKEN, W. L., MITCHELL, D. N. and CAVE, D. R. Evidence for a transmissible agent in Crohn's disease. A new sensitive system. *Clinics in Gastroenterology*, **5,** 289–302 (1976)

5 BERKHOFF, G. A. and CAMPBELL, S. G. Etiology and pathogenesis of ulcerative enteritis ('Quail Disease'), isolation of the causative anaerobe. *Avian Diseases*, **18,** 186 (1974)

6 BOLTEN, R. P., SHERIFF, R. J. and READ, A. E. *Clostridium difficile* associated diarrhea: a role in inflammatory bowel disease? *Lancet*, **1,** 383–384 (1980)

7 BOLTON, P. M., OWEN, E., HEATLEY, R. V. *et al.* Negative findings in laboratory animals for a transmissible agent in Crohn's disease. *Lancet*, **2,** 1122–1124 (1973)

8 BRITTON, S., EKLUNG, A. E. and BIRD, A. G. Appearance of Killer (K) cells in the mesenteric lymph nodes in Crohn's disease. *Gastroenterology*, **75,** 218–220 (1978)

9 BURNHAM, W. R., LENNARD-JONES, J. E., STANFORD, J. L. and BIRD, R. G. Mycobacteria as a possible cause of inflammatory bowel disease. *Lancet*, **2,** 693–696 (1978)

10 CAVE, D. R., MITCHELL, D. N. and BROOKE, B. N. Experimental animal studies of the etiology and pathogenesis of Crohn's disease. *Gastroenterology*, **69,** 618–624 (1975)

11 CAVE, D. R., MITCHELL, D. N. and BROOKE, B. N. Evidence of an agent transmissible from ulcerative colitis tissue. *Lancet*, **1,** 1311 (1976)

12 CAVE, D. R., MITCHELL, D. N. and BROOKE, B. N. Induction of granulomas in mice by Crohn's disease tissues. *Gastroenterology*, **75,** 632–637 (1978)

13 CAVE, D. R., MITCHELL, D. N., KANE, S. P. *et al.* Further animal evidence of a transmissible agent in Crohn's disease. *Lancet*, **2,** 1120–1122 (1973)

14 SHORTER, R. G., CHIBA, M., THAYER, W. *et al.* Cytotoxic studies in human colonic intra-epithelial and lamina propria lymphocytes. *Gastroenterology*, **78,** 1259 (1980)

15 COHEN, Z., COOKE, M. G. and FESTENSTEIN, H. The transmission of human Crohn's disease in inbred strains of mice. *Annals of Royal College of Physicians and Surgeons of Canada*, **11,** 51 (1978)

16 COHEN, Z., LEUNG, M. K., JIRSCH, D. *et al.* Transmission of IBD homogenates in inbred mice and rabbits. In *Recent Advances in Crohn's Disease*, edited by A. S. Pena, I. T. Weterman, C. C. Booth and W. Strober, 259–265. The Hague, Martinus Nijhoff Publishers (1981)

17 COOPER, H. S., RAFFENSPERGER, E. C. and JONAS, L. Cytomegalovirus inclusions in patients with ulcerative colitis and toxic dilation requiring colonic resection. *Gastroenterology*, **72,** 1253–1256 (1977)

18 CROHN, B. B., GINSBERG, L. and OPPENHEIMER, G. D. Regional ileitis, a pathologic and clinical entity. *Journal of the American Medical Association*, **99,** 1323 (1932)

19 DAS, K. M., VALENZUELA, I. and MORECKI, R. Crohn disease lymph node homogenates produce murine lymphoma in athymic mice. *Proceedings of the National Academy of Sciences of the USA*, **77,** 588–592 (1980)

20 DAS, K. M., WILLIAMS, S. E., VALENZUELA, I. and BAUM, S. G. Induction of lymphoma in athymic (nu/nu) mice by Crohn's disease tissue filtrates: A model for the study of Crohn's disease. In *Recent Advances in Crohn's Disease*, edited by A. S. Pena, I. T. Weterman, C. C. Booth and W. Strober, 266–271. The Hague: Martinus Nijhoff Publishers (1981)

21 DONNELLY, B. J., DELANEY, P. V. and HEALY, T. M. Evidence for a transmissible factor in Crohn's disease. *Gut*, **18,** 360–363 (1977)

22 DOURMASHKIN, R. R., O'MORAINE, C. and LEVI, A. S. Electron microscopic evidence for epithelial damage in the pathogenesis of Crohn's disease. *Gut*, **20,** A932 (1979)

23 ECKHARDT, R. , KOOS, P., DIER, C. H. *et al.* K lymphocytes (killer cells) in Crohn's disease and acute virus B hepatitis. *Gut*, **18,** 1010–1016 (1977)

24 EDGINGTON, T. S. and CHISARI, F. V. Immune responses to hepatitis B virus coded and induced antigens in chronic active hepatitis. In *Immune Reactions in Liver Disease*, edited by A. L. W. F. Eddleston, J. C. P. Weber and R. Williams, 44. New York: Focal Press (1979)

25 FARMER, G. W., VINCENT, M. M., FUCCILLO, D. A., BARBOSA, L. H., RITMAN, S., SEVER, J. L. and GITNICK, G. L. Viral investigations in ulcerative colitis and regional enteritis. *Gastroenterology*, **65,** 8–18 (1973)

26 GITNICK, G. L., ARTHUR, M. M. and SHIBATA, I. Cultivation of viral agents from Crohn's disease: a new sensitive system. *Lancet*, **2,** 215–217 (1976)

27 GITNICK, G. L., CAVE, D. and KIRSNER, J. *et al.* (IBD Research Group). Infectious agents in inflammatory bowel disease (IBD): status report. *Gastroenterology*, **78,** 1185 (1980)

28 GITNICK, G. L., ROSEN, V. J., ARTHUR, M. H. and HERTWECK, S. A. Evidence for the isolation of a new virus from ulcerative colitis patients: comparison with virus derived from Crohn's disease. *Digestive Diseases and Sciences*, **24,** 609–619 (1979)

29 GREENBERG, H. B., GEBHARD, R. L., McCLAIN, C. J. *et al.* Antibodies to viral gastroenteritis viruses in Crohn's disease. *Gastroenterology*, **76,** 349 (1979)

30 HARFAST, B., ANDERSSON, T. and PERLMANN, P. Human lymphocyte cytotoxicity against mumps virus-infected target cells. Requirement for non-T cells. *Journal of Immunology*, **114,** 1820 (1975)

31 HEATLEY, R. V., BOLTON, P. M., OWEN, E. *et al.*A search for a transmissible agent in Crohn's disease. *Gut*, **16,** 528–532 (1975)

32 HOSHINO, Y. and SCOTT, F. W. Brief communications: replication of feline infectious peritonitis virus in organ cultures of feline tissue. *Cornell Veterinarian*, **68,** 411–417 (1978)

33 JOHNSON, R. H. Feline panleucopaenia virus – *in vitro* comparison of strains with a mink enteritis virus. *Journal of Small Animal Practice*, **8,** 319 (1967)

34 JONSSON, L. and MARTINSSON, K. Regional ileitis in pigs. *Acta Veterinaria Scandinavica*, **17,** 223–232 (1976)

35 KORSMEYER, S. J. WILLIAMS, R. C., Jnr., WILSON, I. D. *et al.* Lymphocytotoxic and RNA antibodies in inflammatory bowel disease: comparative study in patients and their families. *Annals of the New York Academy of Sciences*, **278,** 574–585 (1976)

36 KRETH, W. H., KACKELL, M. Y. and TERR MEULEN, V. Demonstration of *in vitro* lymphocyte-mediated cytoxicity against measles virus in SSPE. *Journal of Immunology*, **114,** 1042 (1975)

37 LABOWSKI, R. J., EDELMAN, R., RUSTIGIAN, R. *et al.* Studies of cell-mediated immunity to measles virus by *in vitro* lymphocyte-mediated cytotoxicity. *Journal of Infectious Diseases*, **129,** 233–239 (1974)

38 LaMONT, J. T. and TRNKA, Y Therapeutic implications of *Clostridium difficile* toxin during relapse of chronic inflammatory bowel disease. *Lancet*, **1,** 381–383 (1980)

39 McLAREN, L., BARTLETT, J. and GITNICK, G. Infectious agents in inflammatory bowel disease: collaborative studies. *Gastroenterology*, **80,** 1228 (1981)

40 McLAREN, L. and GITNICK, G. Ulcerative colitis and Crohn's disease tissue cytotoxins. *Gastroenterology*, **82,** 1381–1388 (1982)

41 MEYER, R., SIMON, J. and BYERLY, M. C. A. The etiology of swine dysentery. III. The role of selected Gram-negative obligate anaerobes. *Veterinary Pathology*, **12,** 46 (1975)

42 MEYERS, S., MAYER, L., BUTTONE, E. *et al.* Occurrence of *Clostridium difficile* toxin during the course of inflammatory bowel disease. *Gastroenterology*, **80,** 697–700 (1981)

43 MITCHELL, D. N. and REES, R. J. W. Agent transmissible from Crohn's disease tissue. *Lancet*, **2,** 168–171 (1970)

44 MONES, F. G. and SANJUAN, P. *Salvat Editores*, S. A. Barcelona 41 Colle de Mallarca 49 (1935)

45 MORAIN, C. O., PRESTAGE, H., HARRISON, P., LEVI, A. J. and TYRRELL, D. A. Cytopathic effects in cultures inoculated with material from Crohn's disease. *Gut*, **22,** 823–826 (1981)

46 ORR, M. M. Experimental intestinal granulomas. *Proceedings of the Royal Society of Medicine*, **68,** 34 (1975)

47 PARENT, K. and MITCHELL, P. D. Bacterial variants: etiologic agent in Crohn's disease? *Gastroenterology*, **71,** 365–368 (1976)

48 PATTERSON, D. S. P. and BERRETT, S. Malabsorption in Johne's disease in cattle. *Journal of Medical Microbiology*, **2,** 237 (1969)

49 PHILLPOTTS, R. J., HERMON-TAYLOR, J., TEICH, N. M. *et al.* A search for persistent virus infection in Crohn's disease. *Gut*, **21,** 202–207 (1980)

50 REIMANN, J. F. Further electron microscopic evidence of virus-like particles in Crohn's disease. *Acta Hepatogastroenterologia*, **24,** 116 (1977)

51 ROCHE, J. K. and HUANG, E. S. Viral DNA in inflammatory bowel disease: CMV-bearing cells as a target for immune-mediated enterocytolysis. *Gastroenterology*, **72,** 228–233 (1977)

52 ROHOVSKY, M. W. and GRIESEMER, R. A. Experimental feline infectious enteritis in germ free cat. *Pathologia Veterinaria*, **4,** 391–410 (1967)

53 ROLA-PLESCZYNSKI, M., HURTADO, R. C., WOODY, J. N. *et al.* Identification of the cell population involved in viral-specific cell-mediated cytotoxicity in man: evidence for T cell specificity. *Journal of Immunology*, **115,** 239 (1975)

54 SANTOLI, D., TRINCHIERI, G. and KAPROWSKI, H. Cell-mediated cytotoxicity against virus-infected target cells in humans. II. Interferon induction and activation of natural killer cells. *Journal of Immunology*, **121,** 532 (1978)

55 SANTOLI, D., TRINCHIERI, G. and LIEF, F. S. I. Characterization of the effector lymphocyte. *Journal of Immunology*, **121,** 526 (1978)

56 SEWELL, H. F., BASU, M. K., THOMPSON, R. A., FLACK, V. and ASQUITH, P. Specific immunoglobulin E antibody to *E. coli* 0127 B8 in sera of patients with inflammatory bowel disease. In *Recent Advances in Crohn's Disease*, edited by A. S. Pena, I. T. Weterman, C. C. Booth and W. Strober, 309–311. The Hague: Martinus Nijhoff Publishers (1981)

57 SCHNEIRSON, S. S., GARLOCK, J. H., SHORE, B. *et al.* Studies on the viral etiology of regional enteritis and ulcerative colitis: a negative report. *American Journal of Digestive Diseases*, **7,** 839–843 (1962)

58 SHORE, S. L., BLACK, C. M., MELEWICZ, P. M. *et al.* Antibody-dependent cell-mediated cytotoxicity to target cells infected with type 1 and type 2 herpes simplex virus. *Journal of Immunology*, **116,** 194 (1976)

59 SHORTER, R. G., HUIZENGA, K. and SPENCER, R. J. A working hypothesis for the etiology and pathogenesis of nonspecific inflammatory bowel disease. *American Journal of Digestive Diseases*, **17,** 1024 (1972)

60 SIMONOWITZ, D., BLOCK, G. E., RIDELL, R. H. *et al.* The production of an unusual tissue reaction in rabbit bowel injected with Crohn's disease homogenates. *Surgery*, **82,** 211–218 (1977)

61 STANFORD, J. L. Acid fast organisms in Crohn's disease and ulcerative colitis. In *Recent Advances in Crohn's Disease*, edited by A. S. Pena, I. T. Weterman, C. C. Booth and W. Strober, 274–278. The Hague: Martinus Nijhoff Publishers (1981)

62 STOBO, J. D., TOMASI, T. B., HUIZENGA, K. A. *et al. In vitro* studies of inflammatory bowel disease. *Gastroenterology*, **70,** 171 (1976)

63 STRANDE, A., SOMMERS, S. C. and PETRAK, M. Regional enterocolitis in cocker spaniel dogs. *Archives of Pathology*, **57,** 357 (1954)

64 STRICKLAND, R. G., MILLER, W. C., VOLPICELLI, N. A. *et al.* Lymphocytotoxic antibodies in patients with inflammatory bowel disease and their spouses – evidence for a transmissible agent. *Clinical and Experimental Immunology*, **30,** 188–192 (1977)

65 TAUB, R. N., SACHAR, D., JANOWITZ, H. *et al.* Induction of granulomas in mice by inoculation of tissue homogenates from patients with inflammatory bowel disease and sarcoidosis. *Annals of the New York Academy of Sciences*, **278,** 560–564 (1976)

66 TAUB, R. N. and SILTZBACK, L. E. Proceedings of the VI International Conference on Sarcoidosis, 1122–1124. University of Tokyo Press (1974)

67 TRNKA, Y. M. and LaMONT, J. T. Association of *Clostridium difficile* toxin with symptomatic relapse of chronic inflammatory bowel disease. *Gastroenterology*, **80,** 693–696 (1980)

68 Van De MERWE, J. P. A possible role of *Eubacterium* and *Peptostreptococcus* species in the aetiology of Crohn's disease. In *Recent Advances in Crohn's Disease*, edited by A. S. Pena, I. T. Weterman, C. C. Booth and W. Strober, 291–296. The Hague: Martinus Nijhoff Publishers (1981)

69 Van KRUININGEN, H. J. Canine colitis comparable to regional enteritis and mucosal colitis in man. *Gastroenterology*, **62,** 1128 (1972)

70 Van KRUININGEN, H. J. Protothecal enterocolitis in a dog. *American Veterinary Medical Association Journal*, **157,** 56 (1979)

71 WARD, J. M. Morphogenesis of a virus in cats with experimental feline infectious peritonitis. *Virology*, **41,** 191–914 (1970)

72 WATSON, D. W., QUIGLEY, A. and BOLT, R. J. Effect of lymphocytes from patients with ulcerative colitis on human adult colon epithelial cells. *Gastroenterology*, **51,** 985 (1966)

73 WHITE, S. A. Investigation into the identity of acid fast organisms isolated from Crohn's disease and ulcerative colitis. In *Recent Advances in Crohn's Disease*, edited by A. S. Pena, I. T. Weterman, C. C. Booth and W. Strober, 278–282. The Hague: Martinus Nijhoff Publishers (1981)

74 WHORWELL, P. J., BEEKEN, W. L., DAVIDSON, I. W. and WRIGHT, R. Search by immunofluorescence for antigens of rotavirus, *Pseudomonas maltophilia* and *Mycobacterium kansasii* in Crohn's disease. *Lancet*, **2,** 697–698 (1978)

75 WHORWELL, P. J., BEEKEN, W. L., PHILLIPS, C. A. *et al.*Isolation of reovirus-like agents from patients with Crohn's disease. *Lancet*, **1,** 1169–1171 (1977)

18
Spectrum of infectious agents in acute diarrhoea

Ruth F. Bishop

INTRODUCTION

'A reliable set of bowels is worth more
to a man than any quantity of brains'
Henry Wheeler Shaw[38].

Although intended to express the 19th century upper class preoccupation with flatulence, dyspepsia and constipation, this quotation can still be ruefully appreciated today. Acute diarrhoea is second only to the common cold in causing ill-health throughout life. It is a serious threat to life in young children and in the elderly, and a cause of physical and social distress in older children and healthy adults.

During the past decade there has been a renaissance of interest in the aetiology and pathophysiology of acute diarrhoea, and in the mechanisms of immunity of the gut. Progress is reviewed comprehensively in recent publications[12, 15, 22, 26, 36]. Advances in understanding have buoyed hopes that worldwide control of disease and death due to acute diarrhoea is now a realistic aim.

ENTERIC PATHOGENS – ASSAULT APPROACHES

Acute infectious diarrhoea is the consequence of injury to the gut either by toxins present 'externally' to the gut, or 'internally' after invasion of the gut mucosa. The injury, however inflicted, upsets the finely tuned balance between absorption and secretion across the gut mucosa so that there is net accumulation of fluid in the gut lumen. Injury to the upper gut is usually accompanied by bowel actions that are copious and watery. Injury to the ileum and large intestine may not produce copious diarrhoea, but the increased likelihood of invasion and inflammation is associated with greater abdominal pain and passage of blood and mucus.

Non-invasive ('external') infections

Many micro-organisms causing acute diarrhoea do so through their capacity to form exotoxins during multiplication outside the gut mucosa. These exotoxins can be formed in food and then ingested, or formed at the luminal surface of the gut after colonization of the lumen or adherence to epithelial cells. These exotoxins are either enterotoxins or cytotoxins. An enterotoxin is defined as a heat labile or heat stable exotoxin that alters the biochemical functions of the gut epithelial cell without causing demonstrable histopathological changes. A cytotoxin disrupts the structural integrity of the epithelial cell membranes. This may incidentally lead to invasion of the gut wall with considerable inflammation and necrotic change in the surrounding mucosa.

Pre-formed toxins in food

Ingestion of food containing large numbers of micro-organisms need not, *per se*, result in clinical illness, but will certainly do so if the contaminating bacteria form enterotoxins during growth. Diarrhoea, abdominal cramps, nausea and vomiting begin 1–16 h after ingestion of toxin. There is no fever and recovery is usually complete 48–64 h later. Occasional deaths occur, particularly in the elderly. Accounts of food poisoning incidents make dramatic reading[11,33] and equally dramatic film plots. The micro-organisms most commonly involved are *Staphylococcus aureus*, *Clostridium perfringens* (type A) and *Bacillus cereus*. The pre-formed enterotoxins of *S. aureus* (heat stable), *C. perfringens* (heat labile) and *B. cereus* (heat labile) reverse net absorption of fluid and electrolytes in the small intestine[1]. Their inactivation by proteases may account for rapid recovery. *S. aureus* and *C. perfringens* also produce cytotoxins[1,22]. Although *Clostridium botulinum* causes 'food-poisoning', the symptoms are those of a neuroparalytic intoxication.

Non-specific bacterial degradation of protein in some meats can also result in food poisoning, e.g. 'scombroid poisoning' associated with ingestion of dark meat fish[44].

Toxins formed at luminal surfaces

Although the toxins concerned may be similar, disease due to toxins produced in the gut lumen is usually much more severe and protracted than disease due to ingestion of preformed toxins. Sources of infection are similar, i.e. contaminated foods or fluids. Proliferation in the gut is usually dependent upon the ability of the micro-organism to adhere to epithelial cell surface. This ability is in turn dependent upon two genetically determined properties, i.e. the possession by the bacterium of 'adhesive' antigenic groupings and the presence of appropriate receptor sites on the gut epithelial cell of the host. 'Adhesive' antigens reside on filamentous surface appendages of the bacterial cell (fimbriae), are probably plasmid associated and bind very strongly and irreversibly to the small intestinal epithelial cell of the host[5, 22, 34]. Receptor sites on the surface of the host epithelial cell are genetically determined (at least in pigs) and inherited in a simple mendelian manner.

In certain circumstances, e.g. in pre-existing disease that interferes with anti-bacterial mechanisms of the small intestine, organisms that do not possess 'adhesive' antigens may proliferate in the gut lumen. In this way, diarrhoea associated with gastrectomy, blind-loop syndrome and tropical sprue may be due to growth of a variety of toxin producing organisms not normally able to colonize the small intestine.

ENTEROTOXINS

Enterotoxins that alter the biochemical functions of the gut epithelial cell, without causing detectable structural damage are produced by *V. cholerae*[15], enterotoxigenic *E. coli* (ETEC)[15, 37], non-cholera *Vibrio* spp[21], *Klebsiella* spp., *Enterobacter* spp., *Citrobacter* spp., *Serratia* spp., *Pseudomonas* spp., *Aeromonas* spp. and *Edwardsiella tarda*[26]. The capacity to produce some enterotoxins is genetically controlled by DNA in transferable plasmids[37, 39].

The best defined of the enterotoxins is cholera toxin. It binds rapidly and irreversibly to the gut cell and stimulates cellular adenylate cyclase[15]. This results in sustained secretion of isotonic fluid that is maximal in the upper small bowel and persists for the duration of the life span in the affected cells.

Fluid loss can occur at the rate of 5 per cent of body weight per hour. The heat labile enterotoxin of *E. coli* (LT) resembles cholera toxin closely, both antigenically and in its mode of action, but appears to bind less avidly. The rate of fluid loss is 10–100-fold less than in cholera. Heat labile enterotoxins produced by other bacteria listed above are not yet well defined but some are thought to have a similar mode of action[21, 43].

A heat stable enterotoxin (ST) of low molecular weight that is apparently non-antigenic is also produced by *E. coli*[37]. The bowel responds to this toxin by immediate accumulation of fluid in the lumen, but the duration of this action is short lived compared with LT toxin.

CYTOTOXINS

Cytotoxins have been described in cultures of *Klebsiella pneumoniae*, *Enterobacter cloacae* and *E. coli* isolated from patients with tropical sprue[24] and in cultures of *Aeromonas hydrophila* isolated from patients with acute diarrhoea[43]. Little is known of their chemical nature, mode of action or site of activity. Cytotoxins producing gross structural damage are released by *C. perfringens* type C, *C. difficile* and *Vibrio parahaemolyticus*. Colonization of small intestine of malnourished patients by cyotoxic *C. perfringens* type C[27] produces a severe haemorrhagic necrotising enterocolitis with intramural collection of gas, bloody diarrhoea, severe abdominal pain, shock and sometimes death. *C. difficile* has recently been recognized as a major cause of colitis. It is probable that it is present in small numbers in the large intestine and is encouraged to multiply when the normal flora is suppressed by antimicrobial therapy.

The resulting clinical syndrome varies from 'annoying diarrhoea' to abdominal cramps, diarrhoea, tenderness, fever and leucocytosis 4–10 days after initiation of microbial treatment. Toxigenic *C. difficile* produce a cytotoxic exotoxin that is not absorbed to give detectable blood levels, and is rapidly toxic in small dose (1.4 mg) in cell culture. Ultrastructural studies show rapid changes in cell membranes[26]. It has been suggested that *C. difficile* may be a previously unrecognized cause of sporadic diarrhoea in children and adults but its frequent concomitant isolation with other established enteropathogens makes its causative significance still doubtful[14]. Some *S. aureus* strains also produce a cytotoxic exotoxin that results in mucosal damage[25]. These strains were associated with pseudomembranous colitis from 1950 to 1960 and may have been the most important cause of this disease when chloramphenicol and tetracycline were more widely used[8].

Vibrio parahaemolyticus is primarily a marine organism that lives in the sediment of coastal and estuarine waters during winter and colonizes fish and other marine life as the temperature rises during late spring. It is the commonest cause of food poisoning in Japan in summer and is associated with consumption of raw or processed sea products. It is distributed widely in warm coastal waters throughout the world and has been associated with epidemics in Australia, and USA. The organisms multiply rapidly in the gut lumen. In general the strains that are pathogenic produce a β-haemolysin, and an unrelated cytotoxin. In man, the organisms does not usually spread beyond the gut and illness is self-limiting, lasting only a few days[2].

ADHERENCE TO EPITHELIAL SURFACES – POSSIBLE TOXIN

One of the major current enigmas in research on aetiological agents of acute gastroenteritis is the importance of enteropathogenic *E. coli* (EPEC) that do not produce LT or ST enterotoxin or invade epithelial cells. These strains include the 'classical' enteropathogenic strains first described as causes of epidemics among newborn babies in hospital nurseries during the years 1945–1960. The serogroups considered to be enteropathogens are represented in polyvalent and monovalent sera now commercially available to type strains of coliforms. Controversy surrounds the belief that identification of serogroup is of any value in diagnosis, particularly in sporadic cases of diarrhoea[17]. Challenge doses containing 10^{10} EPEC per ml produce diarrhoea in adult volunteers and some strains produce dilatation of the rabbit ileal loop or increase secretion in perfused rat jejunum. The nature of this 'toxin' has still to be identified. Recent research on a strain of *E. coli* isolated from rabbits (RDEC-1) indicates that at least one strain of *E. coli* exists that does not produce LT or ST enterotoxins but can adhere to the mucosal surface, destroy the apical cytoplasm of the epithelial cell and produce severe diarrhoea[7]. A disease with similar histopathology has recently been reported in a human infant[42]. Diarrhoea due to *E. coli* RDEC-1 may be a model of disease due to 'classical' EPEC serotypes.

Attachment of *Giardia* trophozoites to the microvilli of columnar epithelial cells of the proximal small intestine has been demonstrated in a spectacular fashion by scanning electron microscopy[32]. Trophozoites rarely penetrate, but lodge in mucus covering the epithelial cells, or wedge into furrows, particularly at the bases of villi.

Adhesion to the surface of epithelial cells is effected by suction, and may occur by recognition of receptors in the proximal intestine. Disease in man is due to *Giardia lamblia*, and infection may be associated with the possession of blood group phenotype A[4]. The mechanism by which *Giardia* produces acute diarrhoea is not known but could be a toxin. Infection is widespread throughout the world and is endemic in most communities. Epidemics, usually due to contamination of drinking water, have been reported. Ingestion of cysts is followed by stimulation to trophozoite formation when acid is encountered during passage through the stomach[30].

Invasive infections

Invasive organisms attach and then manoeuvre themselves into the interior of the epithelial cell. The exact nature of the invasive process is unknown. In experimental infection, the pathogen first makes contact with the epithelium. The brush border is locally destroyed, and the bacteria are engulfed by an invagination of the cell membrane so that they are contained within vacuoles in the cell cytoplasm[16, 22]. The process by which viruses invade the cell is probably very similar. Micro-organisms do not act as inert particles during this process since non-viable virulent bacteria and viable avirulent bacteria do not penetrate epithelial cells. Following penetration and multiplication, a complex series of events occurs that results in fluid loss, inflammation, ulceration, cramps, tenesmus and fever. The proportion with which any or all of these symptoms occur depends mainly on the level of the gut most affected. Faecal fluid losses can approach those in classical cholera when the site of invasion is the proximal small intestine, e.g. in rotavirus infections, or some *Salmonella* infections. However most invasive pathogens (*Salmonella* spp., *Shigella* spp., *Campylobacter* spp., invasive *E. coli*, *Yersinia enterocolitica*, or amoeba) primarily infect ileum or colon.

The magnitude of fluid losses at these levels of the gut roughly correlates with the severity of the invasive process. Faecal fluid losses may be relatively small, but there can be much pain and fever accompanying the inflammation, and ulceration can result in the passage of multiple stools of small volume containing blood, pus and mucus.

Virus diarrhoea

Rotaviruses are a major cause of acute sporadic diarrhoea in young children requiring admission to hospital throughout the world. Norwalk agent and related agents (possibly caliciviruses) cause acute diarrhoea and vomiting that is comparatively mild and self-limiting[6]. Other 'candidate' viruses have been described including coronaviruses, adenoviruses and a heterogenous collection of small viruses (28–33 nm). Rotaviruses, and possibly other enteric viruses, infect only the mature epithelial cells lining the villi of the small intestine. They are probably 'uncoated' by proteolytic enzymes in the gut lumen and attach to receptors on the epithelial cell surface that may be β-galactosidases. Multiplication in the columnar cell results in lysis of the cell and liberation of virus particles into the gut lumen.

There is widespread denudation of the luminal surface of the upper portion of villi. These are eventually covered by immature crypt cells that are no longer vulnerable to infection. The initial loss of absorptive cells and their replacement by crypt cells that secrete fluid and electrolytes is the probable basis for fluid losses. There is no evidence of toxic damage to the gut during viral infection. Changes in intestinal villus structure are also seen in acute stages of hepatitis and of measles. Measles can cause severe enteritis in malnourished children[9].

Toxin-associated infections

Invasion of epithelial cells by bacteria is not sufficient to cause disease. The pathogens must also be able to multiply and release potent cytotoxins, enterotoxins or endotoxins with a broad range of local and systemic effects.

SUPERFICIAL INFECTIONS

Infection with *Shigella* spp., invasive *E. coli* and parasites (*Entamoeba histolytica*, *Balantidium coli*) is histologically superficial, even though sometimes associated with extensive necrosis and ulceration. The small intestine plays a role in shigellosis. Patients initially present with fever and watery diarrhoea perhaps due to an enterotoxin and the organisms are found in the small intestinal fluid in large numbers. Within a few days they disappear and the colon becomes the target organ[15]. *Sh. dysenteriae* and *Sh. flexneri* both produce enterotoxins that may stimulate cyclic AMP but perhaps not via the adenylate cyclase pathway. They and *Sh. sonnei* produce cytotoxins. *Sh. dysenteriae* also produces a neurotoxin. Shigellosis is essentially restricted to man as host, although some non-human primates are natural hosts. Faecal-oral person-to-person transmission is the natural route of infection. Waterborne outbreaks are not uncommon. The inoculating dose is small, and even in healthy adults, disease can be produced by ingestion of 1–100 bacteria/ml. Invasive *E. coli* belong to restricted serogroups. They may be rare as a cause of disease in man, although few surveys include appropriate techniques for their identification[16].

DISPERSED INFECTIONS

Salmonella spp.,[19,26] *Campylobacter* spp.[20,26] and *Yersinia enterocolitica*[29] also invade ileal and colonic mucosa, and produce inflammation, congestion, oedema, but do not generally produce much local destruction of tissue. Their target is the lamina propria and beyond that the lymphoid tissue either gut associated or at a distance. Understanding of the pathophysiology of diarrhoea in these infections is still limited.

In experimental infections with *S. typhimurium* the extent of the mucosal reaction is important in relation to amount of fluid secreted. It is possible that a large area of inflammation leads to release of local hormones, e.g., vasoactive intestinal peptide that alters intestinal secretion[18]. The involvement of 'enterotoxins' may also be a prerequisite in production of diarrhoea. Salmonellae evoke fluid secretion in the rabbit ileum. This toxin acting on the small intestine is probably the cause of profuse watery diarrhoea sometimes observed in this disease.

Infection with *Salmonella typhi* follows a similar course initially to other *Salmonella* infections but there is secondary spread via the blood stream after proliferation in liver and spleen and other reticulo-endothelial tissue. Diarrhoea occurs in the second week of infection and may dominate the picture, particularly in children. Infection with *Salmonella* spp. (more than 1700 types) is a zoonosis and sources of infection for man are from contaminated food, particularly poultry, powdered egg and milk products. Person-to-person spread can occur.

Since 1970 severe outbreaks of *Salmonella* spp. have been observed due to multi-resistant strains. In areas of South America there has been a radical shift in morbidity and mortality due to this organism. Antibiotic resistant strains are now widespread in calves in the United Kingdom and these might presage widespread outbreaks there and in other countries. Reliable virulence tests are a priority of research in order to understand the pathogenesis and to develop specific prophylaxis.

Campylobacter spp. have recently been incriminated as an important cause of gastroenteritis throughout the world in all age groups. The mode of infection is by ingestion, and as few as 500 organisms taken by mouth have produced symptoms. These usually last 2–3 days, but may persist for 3–6 weeks.

The disease is a zoonosis and sources of infection include poultry, pork, pet dogs, raw milk and contaminated water. Infection can be transmitted from person to person. Disease is most common in very young children and in adults older than 50. In adults a major debilitating illness is often also present (e.g. inflammatory bowel disease, alcoholism, immunosuppression for cancer). The organism is invasive, but does not appear to possess a cytotoxin nor an identifiable enterotoxin. There is little focal epithelial cell destruction and inflammatory invasion. Strains of varying pathogenicity for man may exist.

Much still needs to be learnt about incidence and pathogenic mechanisms of infection with *Y. enterocolitica*. A toxin similar to *E. coli* ST enterotoxin may be produced during growth within the gut mucosa. The invasion property may be temperature sensitive and favoured by low ambient temperatures. Perhaps this explains the high incidence of *Y. enterocolitica* in cold climates. (e.g. Canada, Scandinavia) The illness is characterized by persistent diarrhoea and abdominal pain and prolonged excretion of the organism. The character of the disease depends on the age of the patient. Infants characteristically show diarrhoea with fever. Older children usually develop acute lesions of the terminal ileum or acute mesenteric lymphadenitis resembling appendicitis, while adults may present with enteritis and fever and frequently arthritis. The aged often have no symptoms or develop septicaemia. Source of the infection is sometimes food, particularly milk, and it is found contaminating natural water[29].

Other candidate enteropathogens

Comprehensive surveys encompassing all the above pathogens still fail to identify an aetiological agent in 20–40 per cent of patients. It is worth considering whether 'new' enteropathogens described in veterinary medicine should be sought in man, for example, *Treponema* spp. produce catarrhal inflammation, oedema and occasional haemorrhage in the caecum and colon of mice and pigs[23]. *Cryptosporidium* (members of the enteric coccidia group) occur in many animal species, and are extracellular parasites that adhere to the brush borders of enterocytes. Oocysts have been observed in calves with diarrhoea and have experimentally induced diarrhoea in lambs[41]. Infection with *Cryptosporidium* has also been reported in man[40] in association with severe enterocolitis. Recently, a pandemic of diarrhoea due to parvovirus infection has caused high mortality in young dogs. Although many viruses that cause severe gastroenteritis in farm animals do not seem to have a counterpart in humans, the apparent evolution of this 'new' pathogen in dogs, should keep us alert to the possibility of similarly evolving pathogens in man.

Microbial synergism

Large gaps exist in our information about and understanding of synergism in human infections. Mixed infections with more than one enteric pathogen are observed in 2–3 per cent of patients with acute diarrhoea although the percentage of mixed infections in developing countries is not clear. Mixed infections of enteric bacterial pathogens and parasites are extremely likely. Decreased gastric secretion observed during infection with some intestinal parasites could reduce the dose of bacteria required to establish infection. Synergism resulting in severe gastroenteritis in mice has been observed between *Nematospiroides dubius* and enteropathogenic *E. coli.* Intestinal bacteria may serve as a source of virulence factors for amoeba *in vivo*[28]. Acute gastroenteritis in children is sometimes associated with overgrowth of *Candida albicans* in stomach and upper small intestine that could exacerbate existing damage to brush border enzymes[3].

DEFENSE MECHANISMS OF THE GUT

In order to preserve the integrity of the gut the body calls upon defence mechanisms that are as diverse as the pathogens it encounters.

Non-specific mechanisms

The first major barrier lies in the ability of the stomach to secrete acid and to lower the pH of gastric contents below 4.0. This low pH either rapidly kills most bacteria, or reduces the number of viable organisms below the threshold dose of infectivity. Neutralization of gastric acidity either chemically (sodium bicarbonate), surgically (gastrectomy) or as the result of disease (e.g. pernicious anaemia) increases the risk of bacterial infection of the gut. The second major barrier against ingested micro-organisms lies in maintenance of normal motor and physiological activities of the small intestine. Continual secretion of fluid into the villus crypt washes bacteria and other particles into the lumen of the gut where they are swept away by normal peristalsis. Mucus secreted on to the villus surface may contain antibodies or antibacterial substances against micro-organisms. Neutrophils that migrate through villus epithelium may act as phagocytes or release antibacterial substances on disintegration. The importance of digestive enzymes as a barrier to colonization varies. The absence of biliary and pancreatic secretion is not accompanied by bacterial overgrowth. Trypsin probably encourages infection of epithelial cells by rotaviruses but protects the epithelium from bacterial toxins susceptible to the action of proteases (e.g. *C. perfringens* type C. toxin).

The third major barrier against colonization by an enteric pathogen is the normal resident microflora. This does not participate in the defence of healthy stomach and small intestine where there is no resident flora but is a major defence mechanism in the large intestine. The healthy large intestine contains an abundant and complex microflora. This resists intrusion by competing for nutrients and space on the mucosal surface, by producing toxic metabolites and by maintaining a low oxidation-reduction potential.

Interference with the normal balance of flora in large intestine, for example during antibiotic therapy, can encourage multiplication of opportunistic pathogens and result in acute diarrhoea.

This normal microflora has a less proprietary hold in the ileum where the flow of intestinal contents is slowed and blood supply is reduced. This makes the ileum a vulnerable point of attack, with a heavy reliance on local cellular defence mechanisms in Peyer's patches.

Specific immune mechanisms

The gut is challenged throughout life by many foreign macromolecules presenting at the luminal surface, and possesses complex mechanisms for rejection of potentially harmful micro-organisms. Uncommitted lymphocytes, the majority of which are destined to produce secretory antibodies (IgA or IgM) are present in lamina propria or in gut associated lymphoid tissue. Stimulation of B and T cell division in the presence of a foreign antigen is followed by departure of the cells via mesenteric lymph nodes, thoracic duct, and blood stream and their return to line the gut in the lamina propria. Activated cells produce specific IgM and IgA antibodies that are secreted through the epithelial cells on to the surface of the gut after 4–8 days. Secretory immunoglobulins are effective by complexing with antigen in the gut lumen, neutralizing toxins, preventing viral attachment to host target cells and facilitating rapid elimination from the alimentary tract by agglutination and bacteriostasis[36]. Effective synthesis and secretion of antibodies occurs even in the presence of maternal antibodies. T cells act more directly by recognizing the changes in cell membranes coded by replicating viruses. They destroy the infected cell, often before the virus completes its replicative cycle. The specific interaction between T cells and viral antigens also attracts macrophages that ingest and destroy viruses. Selective deficiencies of B cells are not usually associated with increased incidence of gut infections, with the exception of *G. lamblia*. However patients with T cell deficiencies often develop intractable diarrhoea associated with persistent infection of the gut with viruses and/or *Monilia*.

The nature of the secondary immune response in humans is ill-understood. Protection far outlasts the presence of detectable specific antibodies in gut washings, e.g. significant protection against *V. cholera* enterotoxin lasts at least 8 months after effective local immunization[35]. Much research is still required into duration of immunity after infection with a particular pathogen. It seems likely that this research needs to be based on prospective longitudinal studies in man.

FUTURE STRATEGIES

Research in the field of acute diarrhoeal disease is entering an exciting decade. Important advances in therapy, diagnosis and prophylaxis could reduce morbidity and mortality, at least in childhood. With active encouragement from the World Health Organization, programmes of education in oral rehydration are being undertaken in many developing countries. Disease and death due to diarrhoea has been estimated to take toll of 500×10^6 children annually in these countries. Rational, effective therapy with antidiarrhoeal agents that do not alter intestinal motility but are directed at the prostaglandin or adenylate cyclase systems may prove of value. If not, then agents that act earlier in the pathological sequence, e.g. inhibit binding of toxins or absorb toxins in the gut lumen may prove to be effective, at least in prophylaxis of 'traveller's diarrhoea'.

Antibiotics used in therapy of bacterial infection have proved to be a two-edged sword. Since 1970 there have been outbreaks of disease due to antibiotic resistant strains of *Salmonella* spp.[10,13] and *Shigella* spp. that have sometimes spread widely throughout Central and South America, and the Indian and African continents. The outbreaks were characterized by severity of symptoms, with high morbidity and mortality. There is a need for surveillance laboratories in developing countries to participate in epidemiological studies of resistance-plasmid characterization. Diagnosis of bacterial infections in the gut is being transformed by the appreciation that pathogenicity is determined by possession of transferable plasmids that code for invasiveness or toxin production or other 'aggressive' mechanisms. Techniques derived from molecular biology are already in use to detect enterotoxigenic strains of *E. coli* by DNA colony hybridization[31]. These techniques allow direct detection of virulent strains in stools from patients with acute diarrhoea. A corollary of this knowledge is the exciting possibility that strains of bacteria (e.g. *V. cholera*) could be rendered non-toxigenic without affecting their ability to colonize the gut. Such strains could be potential live oral vaccines.

CONCLUSION

During the past decade there has been a renaissance of research interest in acute diarrhoea: aetiology, pathophysiology, host-microbe interactions and therapy. An aetiological agent can now be identified in 70–80 per cent of patients. Acute diarrhoea remains one of the most common diseases encountered throughout life. Together with malnutrition, it leaves residual underdevelopment that may be life-long and contribute to the cycle of underproduction and poverty in developing countries.

Laboratory research on mechanisms of fluid loss and fluid replacement can now be widely applied to treatment of acute diarrhoea and should markedly reduce mortality in childhood regardless of aetiological agents.

Morbidity due to acute diarrhoea will be reduced by raising the standards of public health and hygiene throughout the world. Even then, rotaviruses and enteric bacterial pathogens will remain a major threat to life in early childhood and in old age. Advances in therapy and in oral vaccination will still be necessary to control death and distress caused by this disease.

References

1 BANWELL, J. G. and SHERR, H. Effect of bacterial enterotoxins on the gastrointestinal tract. *Gastroenterology*, **65,** 467–497 (1973)

2 BARKER, Jr. W. H. and GANGAROSA, E. J. Food poisoning due to *Vibrio parahaemolyticus. Annual Review of Medicine*, **25,** 75–81 (1974)

3 BARNES, G. L., BISHOP, R. F. and TOWNLEY, R. R. W. Microbial flora and disaccharidase depression in infantile gastroenteritis. *Acta Paediatrica Scandinavica*, **63,** 423–426 (1974)

4 BARNES, G. L. and KAY, R. Blood-groups in giardiasis. *Lancet*, **1,** 808 (1977)

5 BEACHEY, E. H. Bacterial adherence: adhesin-receptor interactions mediating the attachment of bacteria to mucosal surfaces. *Journal of Infectious Diseases*, **143,** 325–345 (1981)

6 BLACKLOW, N. R. and CUKOR, G. Viral gastroenteritis. *New England Journal of Medicine*, **304,** 397–406 (1981)

7 CANTEY, J. R., LUSHBAUGH, W. B. and INMAN, L. R. Attachment of bacteria to intestinal epithelial cells in diarrhea caused by *Escherichia coli* strain RDEC-1 in the rabbit: stages and role of capsule. *Journal of Infectious Diseases*, **143,** 219–230 (1981)

8 DEARING, W. H., BAGGENSTOSS, A. H. and WEED, L. A. Studies on the relationship of *Staphylococcus aureus* to pseudomembranous enterocolitis and to post-antibiotic enteritis. *Gastroenterology*, **38,** 441–451 (1960)

9 DOSSETOR, J. F. B. and WHITTLE, H. C. Protein-losing enteropathy and malabsorption in acute measles enteritis. *British Medical Journal*, **2,** 592–593 (1975)

10 EDITORIAL. Salmonellosis – an unhappy turn of events. *Lancet*, **1,** 1009–1010 (1979)

11 EISENBERG, M. S., GAARSLEV, K., BROWN, W., HOROWITZ, M. and HILL, D. Staphylococcal food poisoning aboard a commercial aircraft. *Lancet*, **2,** 595–598 (1975)

12 ELLIOTT, K. and KNIGHT, J. (Eds) *Acute Diarrhoea in Childhood*. (Ciba Foundation Symposium 42) Amsterdam, Elsevier (1976)

13 FALKOW, S. *Infectious Multiple Drug Resistance*, 253–273. London, Pion (1975)

14 FALSEN, E., KAIJSER, B., NEHLS, L., NYGREN, B. and SVEDHEM, A. *Clostridium difficile* in relation to enteric bacterial pathogens. *Journal of Clinical Microbiology*, **12,** 297–300 (1980)

15 FIELD, M., FORDTRAN, J. S. and SCHULTZ, S. G. (Eds) *Secretory Diarrhea*. Bethesda, American Physiological Society (1980)

16 FORMAL, S. B. and HORNICK, R. B. Invasive *Escherichia coli. Journal of Infectious Diseases*, **137,** 641–644 (1978)

17 GANGAROSA, E. J. and MERSON, M. H. Epidemiologic assessment of the relevance of the so-called enteropathogenic serogroups of *Escherichia coli* in diarrhea. *New England Journal of Medicine*, **296,** 1210–1213 (1977)

18 GIANNELLA, R. A. Importance of the intestinal inflammatory reaction in *Salmonella*-mediated intestinal secretion. *Infection and Immunity*, **23,** 140–145 (1979)

19 GIANNELLA, R. A., FORMAL, S. B., DAMMIN, G. J. and COLLINS, H. Pathogenesis of salmonellosis: studies of fluid secretion, mucosal invasion, and morphologic reaction in the rabbit ileum. *Journal of Clinical Investigation*, **52,** 441–453 (1973)

20 GUERRANT, R. L., LAHITA, R. G., WINN, Jr. W. C. and ROBERTS, R. B. Campylobacteriosis in man: pathogenic mechanisms and review of 91 bloodstream infections. *American Journal of Medicine*, **65,** 584–592 (1978)

21 HUGHES, J. M., HOLLIS, D. G., GANGAROSA, E. J. and WEAVER, R. E. Non-cholera Vibrio infections in the United States: clinical, epidemiologic, and laboratory features. *Annals of Internal Medicine*, **88,** 602–606 (1978)

22 JANOWITZ, H. D. and SACHAR, D. B. (Eds) *Frontiers of Knowledge in the Diarrheal Diseases*. New Jersey, Projects in Health Inc. (1979)

23 JOENS, L. A. and GLOCK, R. D. Experimental infection in mice with *Treponema hyodysenteriae. Infection and Immunity*, **25,** 757–760 (1979)

24 KLIPSTEIN, F. A. and SCHENK, E. A. Enterotoxigenic intestinal bacteria in tropical sprue. II. Effect of the bacteria and their enterotoxins on intestinal structure. *Gastroenterology*, **68,** 642–655 (1975)

25 LAMANNA, C. and CARR, C. J. The botulinal, tetanal, and enterostaphylococcal toxins: a review. *Clinical Pharmacology and Therapeutics*, **8,** 286–332 (1967)

26 LAMBERT, H. P. (Ed) Infections of the GI tract. In *Clinics in Gastroenterology*, **8,** 3. Philadelphia, Saunders (1979)

27 LAWRENCE, G. and WALKER, P. D. Pathogenesis of enteritis necroticans in Papua New Guinea. *Lancet*, **1,** 125–126 (1976)

28 MACKOWIAK, P. Microbial synergism in human infections. *New England Journal of Medicine*, **298,** 21–26; 83–87 (1978)

29 MARKS, M. I., PAI, C. H., LAFLEUR, L., LACKMAN, L. and HAMMERBERG, O. *Yersinia enterocolitica* gastroenteritis: a prospective study of clinical, bacteriologic and epidemiologic features. *Journal of Pediatrics*, **96,** 26–31 (1980)

30 MEYER, E. A. and JARROLL, E. L. Giardiasis. *American Journal of Epidemiology*, **111,** 1–12 (1980)

31 MOSELEY, S. L., HUQ, I., ALIM, A. R. M. A., SO, M., SAMADPOUR-MOTALEBI, M. and FALKOW, S. Detection of enterotoxigenic *Escherichia coli* by DNA colony hybridization. *Journal of Infectious Diseases*, **142,** 892–898 (1980)

32 OWEN, R. L., NEMANIC, P. C. and STEVENS, D. P. Ultrastructural observations on giardiasis in a murine model. I. Intestinal distribution, attachment, and relationship to the immune system of *Giardia muris*. *Gastroenterology*, **76,** 757–769 (1979)

33 PEFFERS, A. S. R., BAILEY, J., BARROW, G. I. and HOBBS, B. C. *Vibrio parahaemolyticus* gastroenteritis and international air travel. *Lancet*, **1,** 143–145 (1973)

34 PETERSON, P. K. and QUIE, P. G. Bacterial surface components and the pathogenesis of infectious diseases. *Annual Review of Medicine*, **32,** 29–43 (1981)

35 PIERCE, N. F., CRAY, Jr. W. C. and ENGEL, P. F. Antitoxic immunity to cholera in dogs immunized orally with cholera toxin. *Infection and Immunity*, **27,** 632–637 (1980)

36 PORTER, R. and KNIGHT, J. (Eds) *Immunology of the Gut*. (Ciba Foundation Symposium 46) Amsterdam, Elsevier (1977)

37 SACK, R. B. Enterotoxigenic *Escherichia coli*: identification and characterisation. *Journal of Infectious Diseases*, **142,** 279–286 (1980)

38 SHAW, H. W. In *Familiar Medical Quotations*, edited by M. B. Strauss, 44. Boston, Little Brown (1968)

39 SO, M., CRANDALL, J. F., CROSA, J. H. and FALKOW, S. Extrachromosomal determinants which contribute to bacterial pathogenicity. In *Microbiology, 1974*, edited by D. Schlessinger, 16–26. Washington D.C., American Society for Microbiology (1975)

40 TZIPORI, S., ANGUS, K. W., GRAY, E. W. and CAMPBELL, I. Vomiting and diarrhea associated with cryptosporidial infection. *New England Journal of Medicine*, **303,** 818 (1980)

41 TZIPORI, S., ANGUS, K. W., GRAY, E. W. CAMBELL, I. and CLERIHEW, L. W. Diarrhoea due to *Cryptosporidium* infection in artificially reared lambs. *Journal of Clinical Microbiology*, **14,** 100–105 (1981)

42 ULSHEN, M. H. and ROLLO, J. L. Pathogenesis of *Escherichia coli* gastroenteritis in man – another mechanism. *New England Journal of Medicine*, **302,** 99–101 (1980)

43 WADSTRÖM, T., LJUNGH, A. and WRETLIND, B. Enterotoxin, haemolysin and cytotoxic protein in *Aeromonas hydrophila* from human infections. *Acta Pathologica et Microbiologica Scandinavica*, **84B,** 112–114 (1976)

44 ZIMMER, L., ALTMAN, R. and STARUSZKIEWICZ, W. Scombroid poisoning-New Jersey. *Morbidity and Mortality*, **29,** 106–107 (1980)

19
Response of the small intestine to nutritional deficiencies

C. Richard Fleming and Sidney F. Phillips

INTRODUCTION

Attempts to determine a total surface area for the mucosa of the small intestine are plagued by numerous and doubtful approximations, but any estimate yields an epithelial sheet of major proportions. Using one of these estimates of area, when a turnover time by the epithelium of two to three days is inserted[15], the nutrients calculated to maintain mucosal integrity are impressively large. Thus, it has been estimated that 300 g of cells are shed from the adult human small bowel per day; an amount comprising 95 percent of the cells lost from the entire gut[12]. Specific losses that have been estimated include 20 g of fat and protein each day, much of which is reabsorbed[12]. Little wonder that the small intestine is sensitive to protein-calorie malnutrition. Moreover, as pointed out by Baker[3] intestinal diseases with associated malabsorption are frequent causes of malnutrition, thus establishing a vicious cycle. Further complicating the capacity of the small bowel to respond to generalized malnutrition are the effects of deficiencies of specific nutrients (e.g. vitamin B12, folate, essential fatty acids) on cellular function[22, 28, 31, 46, 64]. In addition, other deficiencies (e.g. vitamin D) can influence particular absorptive properties (e.g. calcium) of the small bowel.

The information we shall review here is tantalizing but often incomplete. One major dilemma is that clinical studies of undernutrition cannot always be clearly grouped by cause – either primary intestinal disease, caloric deprivation or specific deficiencies. Of current interest, and of relevance to the main theme, are the differing effects of enteral and parenteral nutrition on the small bowel. A brief review of this subject comprises the second section of the chapter.

NUTRIENT DEFICIENCIES

Protein-calorie malnutrition

This syndrme often includes diarrhea, raising the possibility of concomitant malabsorption. Included in disturbances attributed to malnutrition *per se* are morphological thinning of the small bowel, loss of brush border disaccharidases, impaired absorption of simple sugars, reduced digestion and absorption of protein and fat, prolonged transit times and bacterial overgrowth of the jejunum[71]. Most clinical observations are of children with kwashiorkor, circumstances that do not always allow for the study of adequate controls. However, data from experimental animals can be used to support a number of conclusions.

Intestinal structure

Morphological changes in jejunal epithelium are well documented in severe clinical malnutrition, and can be reproduced experimentally. Thinning of the mucosa, flattening of epithelial cells and altered appearances of the brush border are accepted as genuine effects by most authors[3, 49, 59, 71]. More severe villous atrophy can be seen, but is considered to be secondary to other factors (e.g. bacterial overgrowth, mucosal damage due to unconjugated bile acids). Accumulation of lipid in epithelial cells has been seen by electron microscopy in association with broadening of villous architecture[69], but abnormalities of generation, migration and maturation of cells are seen only in extreme clinical and experimental examples[8, 71]. Clinical studies from certain geographical regions are complicated in interpretation by what should be considered to be a 'normal' villous architecture[45]; this dilemma has been addressed specifically by Baker[2]. One important consequence of structural changes is altered passive permeability of the mucosa, which could lead to macromolecules gaining access to subepithelial tissues. Thus, rats deprived of protein have been shown to have increased mucosal permeability to ferritin and adenoviruses, raising the possibility of a functional deterioration of intercellular junctions[75].

Brush border enzymes – intestinal absorption

The disaccharidases have received most attention since carbohydrate intolerance, due to disaccharidase deficiency, is important clinically. Thus, much attention has been focused on the control of these enzymes of the microvillous membrane. Moreover, sucrase and maltase activities are augmented when mammals are weaned; and these changes coincide with a decrease in lactase activity (*see* Chapter 1 for additional discussion of these developmental aspects).

Thus, sucrase activity in the jejunum decreases with fasting or when carbohydrate is excluded specifically from the diet[6, 14, 57], and refeeding with sucrose or maltose stimulates a marked and specific increase in enzyme levels. Lactase shows a similar, though much less pronounced, response to lactose withdrawal and refeeding. It has been concluded[38] that there is no clear evidence for the adaptability of lactase to dietary levels of lactose in man. Furthermore, most clinical studies of children with protein-calorie malnutrition are difficult to interpret, since they rely only on oral tolerance tests, clinical responses to test doses of disaccharides and fecal pH to assess digestibility of oligosaccharides. However, James[36] studied eight malnourished Jamaican children using oral loads of test sugars, jejunal perfusion techniques and measurement of brush border enzymes. Disaccharidase levels were reduced in most children, and enzyme activities responded favorably to treatment. Factors other than surface hydrolysis were also thought to be important in determining the level of carbohydrate absorption. Thus, absorption of monosaccharides was often reduced, implying a defect of uptake rather than hydrolysis. Moreover, malnourished children often showed normal rises in blood glucose after oral sugars despite impaired absorption, and diminished peripheral utilization was suggested. Only when mucosal disaccharidases were extremely low was hydrolysis thought to be a rate limiting step. Younoszai's group[22] showed that, in malnourished infant rats, specific activities of lactase, sucrase and maltase were normal, and that a generalized mucosal atrophy was the major factor responsible for low levels of disaccharidase activity.

Because of the use of xylose as a diagnostic test, its absorption has been measured in several groups of malnourished children. Although delayed or diminished urinary clearance of xylose has been reported, there are conflicting results, and not all evidence supports the etiological role for protein malnutrition *per se* in the decreased absorption of xylose reported in undernourished children[3].

Most assessments of nitrogen balance, even in severe malnutrition, suggest that protein absorption is essentially normal[71]. Specific activities of intestinal dipeptidases (gly-pro and val-pro) were reduced to about half those of controls in eight subjects with severe malnutrition and diarrhea[43]. Steatorrhea is better documented[71], and some studies have examined systematically, by conventional fat balance, the effects of supplemental nutrition. Teotia *et al.*[68] found mild steatorrhea (coefficient of fat absorption 80–90 percent) in 20 percent and severe steatorrhea (coefficient less than 80 percent) in 50 percent of 49 patients with protein-calorie malnutrition. Eight patients were retested after nutritional supplementation for periods of four to 15 weeks; all patients absorbed fat better and in five patients, fat absorption returned to the normal range. The etiology of malabsorption is obscure. Viteri and Schneider[71] review the factors contributing to fat malabsorption. They present evidence for the participation of several pathogenic factors:

(1) abnormalities of mucosal structure;
(2) decreased secretion of pancreatic lipase;
(3) impaired micellar solubilization by bile acids; and
(4) bacterial overgrowth.

The presence of bacterial overgrowth could be the important link between these contributing factors, since jejunal deconjugation of bile acids might be expected to contribute to some of the factors listed above.

Disorders of motility and bacterial overgrowth

Evidence for disordered motility is at best circumstantial and consists of reports of gastric distention and slow whole-gut transit in malnourished children[71]. Specific reports of altered segmental transit, intraluminal pressure activities, or smooth muscle function do not appear to be available. On the other hand, Wingate[73] has highlighted the fact that gastric 'hunger contractions' persist during undernutrition, even up to the time of death from starvation!

On the other hand, evidence for microbial contamination of the proximal bowel is somewhat more convincing. In 21 Indonesian children with kwashiorkor, Gracey *et al.*[25] cultured a varied jejunal microflora; in these children and in malnourished Australian aboriginal children[26], *Candida* species were often isolated. Unfortunately, these studies, like most others, do not have post-treatment comparisons; moreover, the establishment of appropriate control values for the jejunal microflora is difficult. Nevertheless, other observations[13,24] support this view. Not surprisingly, fecal material often contains intestinal pathogens including a spectrum of parasites[48].

Secretory IgA was measured in tears, nasal secretions, saliva and duodenal fluid of 10 Indian children with mild and 16 with severe protein-calorie malnutrition; circulating immunoglobulins were also quantified[56]. As others had found, levels of circulating immunoglobulins were normal, but secretory IgA was reduced markedly in the children who were severely malnourished; after treatment 9/16 returned towards normal. Together with disorders of cell mediated immunity[4,62] this abnormality raises the possibility of an increased susceptibility to infection due to immunodeficiency.

Vitamin B12

Serum levels of vitamin B12 are often high in children with protein-calorie malnutrition[70]. Using Schilling tests, which unfortunately employed less than optimal doses of labeled vitamin B12, Alvardo *et al.*[1] demonstrated a significant depression of B12 absorption in Guatemalan children with untreated kwashiorkor. Baker[3] studied 80 children in South India, using more conventional methods, and found a small but significant decrease of B12 absorption in kwashiorkor. In both studies[1,3], dietary supplements of protein increased the degree to which B12 was absorbed. The defects in B12 absorption were not corrected by intrinsic factor, presumably reflecting a primary defect of ileal transport of vitamin B12 or the effects of bacterial overgrowth in the small bowel. No information is available to distinguish between these possibilities, or indeed to suggest that B12 deficiency is important clinically in these patients.

Deficiencies of water soluble vitamins

Distinct from the issues raised by generalized malnutrition are the effects of specific deficiencies on the function of the small intestine. Nevertheless, it must be emphasized that deficiencies of a single nutrient are quite unusual and, in fact, probably never occur, except in the most carefully designed studies in experimental animals. Most information is available on the influence of vitamin B12 deficiency.

In 1967, Foroozan and Trier[22] described the morphology of jejunal biopsies in eight patients with pernicious anemia. Decreased mitosis, shortened villi, megalocytosis of epithelial cells and cellular infiltrates in the lamina propria were observed before treatment with vitamin B12 was instituted; two or more months of treatment reversed all these morphological abnormalities. A number of disorders of absorption associated with deficiency of vitamin B12 have been reported subsequently, notable being the study of Lindenbaum *et al.*[46]. They described impaired jejunal absorption of xylose and reduced ileal absorption of vitamin B12. Though these impairments of absorption are not marked, ileal function is affected more severely, and it was concluded that the small bowel has a metabolic need for vitamin B12. The subject has been reviewed more extensively by Halsted[28].

Abnormalities of intestinal function specific for severe deficiency of folate are less well defined, for the majority of studies have involved alcoholics or patients with tropical sprue. Megaloblastic cell lines and villous changes have been observed clinically[5,32] and similar changes are observed experimentally in rats made deficient in folate[42]. Megaloblastic changes were also produced in rats fed a folate-free diet plus succinylsulfathiazole; these animals also malabsorbed thiamine when folate deficient[34]. Halsted *et al.*[29] studied four hospitalized alcoholic patients, using intraluminal perfusion, and attempted to separate the effects of alcohol *per se* from those of undernutrition and folate deficiency. He concluded that the combination of folate deficiency and alcohol induced a functional abnormality that preceded any structural alterations of the jejunal epithelium.

Pellagra was associated with malabsorption, as assessed by three indices (steatorrhea and/or abnormal Schilling tests and/or decreased xylose absorption), in 22/24 patients from India[50]. Of patients with the most clearcut features of malabsorption, 6/14 recovered partially or completely after treatment with nicotinic acid; however, Halsted[27] drew attention to the additional contribution of protein malnutrition in these patients.

Dogs rendered deficient in niacin develop diarrhea, abnormal villous architecture and a secretory state for electrolytes, glucose and water in the small intestine[52].

Deficiencies of metals and trace elements

Phosphorus

The advent of total parenteral nutrition resulted in many examples of severe hypophosphatemia and led to studies which associated low intracellular stores of ATP and dysfunction of specific organs[21]. Phosphate depletion occurs usually in severe protein-calorie malnutrition when patients are given excessive amounts of parenteral nutrition to which phosphorus has not been added in adequate amounts[63]. A decrease in ATP content of red blood cells, white cells, and platelets results in hemolytic anemia, impaired chemotactic, phagocytic, and bactericidal functions of granulocytes, and shortened platelet survival, respectively[11,76]. Hill *et al.* administered ^{32}P enterally to determine the distribution of phosphorus in rats which were maintained on phosphate-free hyperalimentation or fed a standard diet by mouth[33]. The percentage of ^{32}P recovered from the intestines and liver was significantly less in parenterally fed rats. This reduction of intestinal and hepatic phosphorus during TPN may simply reflect the absence of enteral nutrition and a reduced epithelial cell turnover. Functional and morphological studies of gut function during hypophosphatemia are not available.

Magnesium

Data on small bowel absorption of magnesium in response to magnesium deficiency differ according to techniques of study. Petith and Schedl found that magnesium deficiency in rats, when studied by perfusion of the small intestine *in vivo*, was associated with reduced secretion of magnesium into the bowel lumen; however, absorption did not increase significantly in either the jejunum or ileum[55]. In contrast, Chutkow used ^{28}Mg to show that magnesium deficient animals absorbed 25 percent more magnesium than controls[10], throughout the gut. When rats are depleted of magnesium, active transport of calcium against a concentration gradient from mucosa to serosa is increased[41]. This enhancement of calcium transport is blocked by parathyroidectomy, an observation which is consistent with the hypothesis that magnesium deficiency enhances calcium transfer by stimulating the secretion of parathyroid hormone[51].

Iron

Severe iron deficiency anemia in humans has not caused morphological changes in the small bowel[3]. Xylose absorption/excretion was reduced in 64 percent of iron deficient patients and in general was normalized by the administration of iron supplements[47]. The mechanism of the impaired handling of xylose is unclear. Absorption of fat and vitamin B12 is normal in humans with iron deficiency, although vitamin B12 absorption is frequently impaired in iron deficient rats[3]. Iron absorption is enhanced in patients with iron deficiency[30]. Mice that were made iron deficient by dietary means or venesection displayed increased absorption of iron; mice fed the low iron diet increased iron absorption six fold[20]. Diets deficient in iron have also been associated with the enhanced absorption of cobalt, lead, zinc and manganese.

Zinc

Diarrhea is often mentioned as a clinical manifestation of zinc deficiency; however, this association is certainly not well defined[65]. Many patients said to be zinc deficient have diarrhea from other causes. This could contribute to zinc deficiency, since stool is the major route of zinc excretion. Thus, Wolman *et al.* found a good correlation between zinc content in stools and stool weight[74]. The highest zinc concentrations were found in patients with intact small bowels, 15.2 μg zinc/g of stool, compared with 3.6 μg zinc/g of stool in patients with extensive small bowel resections or high output fistulas. Acrodermatitis enteropathica, a rare familial disease, presents in infancy with diarrhea, failure to thrive, alopecia, and dermatitis. It is associated with low levels of zinc in blood and decreased activities of zinc dependent enzymes. Oral zinc therapy results in dramatic remission of clinical findings, normalization of blood zinc concentrations and a return of the activities of zinc-dependent enzymes. Light microscopy of the small bowel mucosa in acrodermatitis is normal, but electron microscopy reveals abnormal inclusion bodies in the Paneth cells[7]. These inclusion bodies, which disappeared after four months of oral zinc therapy, probably represent proliferation of lysosomes and altered secretory granules. Similar abnormalities in Paneth cells have been reproduced in rats fed a zinc deficient diet[53].

ENTERAL AND PARENTERAL NUTRITION: EFFECTS ON THE SMALL BOWEL

The introduction of nutrients through the lumen of the small intestine offers many advantages. Intestinal hormones are released and biliary, pancreatic, and intestinal secretions are stimulated. Certain of these responses to ingested food influence the morphology of the small bowel in a positive fashion. Thus, gastrin is probably trophic to the small bowel and the pancreas[39]. Exogenous pentagastrin, when administered to rats fed only by parenteral nutrition, prevented the decrease in weight of the small intestine as well as a reduction in disaccharidase activities[40]. Indirect evidence that bile and/or pancreatic secretions have a permissive effect on the morphology of small bowel arose from experiments in rats in which the duodenal segment (containing the papilla of Vater) was transplanted to the ileum after which ileal villi enlarged[72]. However, recent evidence in humans suggests that pancreatic enzymes reduce the activities of brush border enzymes. Pancreatic proteases were shown to significantly decrease disaccharidase activities, both *in vitro* and *in vivo*[61]. Lactase activity in brush border membranes from normal controls was reduced by 26 percent during incubation *in vitro* with trypsin at pH 7.0, and lactase activity was reduced by 75 percent in patients with lactase deficiency. After the *in vivo* addition of pancreatic enzymes, mucosa from patients with pancreatic exocrine insufficiency showed reduced lactase activity; the reduction was 16 percent and 39 percent in patients with normal lactase and in patients with lactase deficiency, respectively.

Complete starvation has profound effects on small bowel morphology and function. Specifically, fasting reduces the turnover of small bowel epithelial cells, small bowel mass, villous size, mitotic index and disaccharidase activities[44]. At least two factors during fasting, absence of oral intake and a negative nitrogen balance, could be responsible for these changes. Most evidence now suggests that intraluminal nutrients and the physiological responses to the ingestion of food, rather than the status of nitrogen balance, are critical for maintaining a normal morphology and function. Thus, rats and dogs that are nourished parenterally and maintained in positive nitrogen balance but which receive no enteral feedings show a reduction in intestinal mass, enzyme activities, and function[18,44]. Levine *et al.* compared rats who received a parenteral nutrition for seven days to rats fed the same solution orally[54]. Gut weight (22 percent), mucosal weight (28 percent), mucosal protein (35 percent), and DNA (25 percent) were decreased in parenterally fed rats. The differences were due primarily to marked changes in the proximal small bowel. Feldman *et al.* evaluated the influence of oral and parenteral nutrition on the adaptation to resection of 50 percent of the small bowel in dogs[18]. Dogs fed intravenously showed no evidence of functional adaptation and mean ileal villous height was reduced; dogs fed orally demonstrated mucosal hyperplasia, an increase in villous height and a corresponding increase in glucose absorption *in vivo*. Eastwood used ^{3}H-thymidine to show that rabbits fed intravenously for 10 days had a significant reduction in epithelial cell renewal in the proximal small intestine when compared to orally fed controls[16].

Composition of enteral nutrition: effects on the small bowel

The response of the small bowel to enteral nutrition appears to differ according to the composition of the diet. A liquid, elemental diet, when fed for two weeks to rats with jejuno-ileal bypass, resulted in compensatory adaptive changes in the residual small bowel in continuity[19]. Since elemental diets are absorbed very rapidly, the distal small bowel may not be challenged with many of these diets. Thus, at a point 30 cm distal to the ligament of Treitz, about 90 percent of carbohydrates had been absorbed from each of three liquid meals which contained sucrose or glucose polymers and which ranged in osmolality from 337 to 696 mmol/kg[58]. Buts *et al.* reported that adaptation failed to occur in the distal gut of rats with a 'short bowel' when they were fed with a chemically defined diet or TPN, whereas rats given an isocaloric macromolecular diet did demonstrate adaptation[9]. Rats fed an elemental diet, Vivonex, for nine days had less increase in gut weight, villous size, and rate of cell turnover when compared to rats fed isocaloric amounts of chow[17]. Thus, elemental and liquid formula diets appear to maintain a normal proximal small bowel whereas the distal small bowel, which is not in direct contact with the liquid diets, shows regression in mass and cell turnover.

Dietary fiber: effects on the small bowel

Dietary fiber may also influence the morphology and function of the small bowel. By light microscopy, the jejunal mucosa of apparently healthy persons from tropical countries shows broad, branched, and fused villi, features that would be considered abnormal in temperate climates[66]. Identical findings were reported in vegetarians in California[54]. Tasman-Jones studied the effect of fiber on the small bowel morphology of weanling rats, animals which are born with finger-like villi. The villous architecture matures into a broad leaf-shaped pattern when animals are fed a normal diet[67]. Rats were fed one of three diets: (1) nutritionally complete but fiber-free; (2) the same diet plus cellulose; or (3) the same diet plus pectin. Animals given no fiber or only cellulose maintained a villous pattern similar to that seen in immature rats whereas the rats fed pectin developed distinct ridging and alterations in the appearance of the mucosa. Thus, the addition of pectin, but not cellulose, allowed for the usual maturation of villi.

Chronic feeding of cellulose and pectin to rats decreased intestinal absorption of glucose[60]. Glucose tolerance is improved in human volunteers and insulin dependent diabetics who receive regular supplements of dietary fiber[23]. The changes seen after chronic administration of fiber are presumably related to functional changes in the small intestine. However, a single meal which is supplemented with cellulose or pectin decreased glucose response to an oral carbohydrate load, probably because of delayed gastric emptying[60] which is thought to be related to the greater viscosity of supplemented meals. Jenkins *et al.* reported that the addition of 15 g of pectin to a 50 g oral glucose load in humans with the dumping syndrome following gastric surgery prevented the occurrence of hypoglycemic symptoms and maintained the blood glucose levels above control values[37]. A trial of 10 g of pectin per day prevented recurrent postprandial hypoglycemic attacks in the most severely affected patient.

In conclusion, the small bowel exhibits major metabolic demands on the body and responds to undernutrition by structural and functional changes. Local effects of foods within the lumen are probably quite important; however, much of the information available currently lacks adequate control observations and can be classified merely as suggestive.

References

1 ALVARADO, J., VARGAS, D., DIAZ, N. and VITERI, F. E. Vitamin B_{12} absorption in protein-calorie malnourished children and during recovery: influence of protein depletion and of diarrhea. *American Journal of Clinical Nutrition*, **26,** 595–599 (1973)

2 BAKER, S. J. Geographical variations in the morphology of the small intestinal mucosa in apparently healthy individuals. *Pathological Microbiology*, **39,** 222–237 (1973)

3 BAKER, S. J. Malnutrition and small intestinal disease. In *Progress in Gastroenterology*, volume III, edited by G. Jerzy Glass, 563–594. New York, Grune and Stratton (1977)

4 BHASKARAM, C. and REDDY, V. Cell mediated immunity in protein-calorie malnutrition. *Journal of Tropical Pediatrics and Environmental Child Health*, **20,** 284–288 (1974)

5 BIANCHI, A., CHIPMAN, D. W., DRESKIN, A. and ROSENSWEIG, N. Nutritional folic acid deficiency with megaloblastic changes in the small bowel epithelium. *New England Journal of Medicine*, **282,** 859–861 (1970)

6 BLAIR, D. B., YAKIMETS, R. W. and TUBA, J. Rat intestinal sucrase. II. The effects of rat age and sex and of diet on sucrase activity. *Canadian Journal of Biochemistry*, **41,** 917–929 (1963)

7 BOHANE, T. D., CUTZ, HAMILTON, J. R. and GALL, D. G. Acrodermatitis enteropathica, zinc, and the Paneth cell. A case report with family studies. *Gastroenterology*, **73,** 587–592 (1977)

8 BROWN, H. O., LEVINE, M. L. and LIPKIN, M. Inhibition of intestinal epithelial cell renewal and migration induced by starvation. *American Journal of Physiology*, **205,** 868–872 (1963)

9 BUTS, J.-P., MORIN, C. L. and LING, V. Influence of dietary components on intestinal adaptation after small bowel resection in rats. *Clinical and Investigative Medicine*, **2,** 59–66 (1979)

10 CHUTKOW, J. G. Effect of magnesium deficiency on location of the intestinal absorption of magnesium in rats. *Proceedings of the Society for Experimental Biology and Medicine*, **123,** 836–840 (1966)

11 CRADDOCK, P. R., YAWATA, Y., VAN SANTEN, L., GILBERSTADT, S., SILVIS, S. and JACOB, H. S. Acquired phagocyte dysfunction: a complication of the hypophosphatemia of parenteral hyperalimentation. *New England Journal of Medicine*, **290,** 1403 –1407 (1974)

12 CROFT, D. N. and COTTON, P. B. Gastrointestinal cell loss in man. *Digestion*, **8,** 144–160 (1973)

13 DAMMIN, G. J. The pathogenesis of acute diarrheal disease in early life. *Bulletin of the World Health Organization*, **31,** 29–32 (1964)

14 DEREN, J. J., BROITMAN, S. A. and ZAMCHECK, N. Effect of diet upon intestinal disaccharidases and disaccharide absorption. *Journal of Clinical Investigation*, **46,** 186–195 (1967)

15 DESCHNER, E. E. and LIPKIN, M. Proliferation of epithelial cells of the gastrointestinal tract in cancer and related diseases. In *Progress in Gastroenterology*, volume III, edited by G. Jerzy Glass, 29–52. New York, Grune and Stratton (1977)

16 EASTWOOD, G. L. Small bowel morphology and epithelial proliferation in intravenously alimented rabbits. *Surgery*, **82,** 613–620 (1977)

17 ECKANAUER, R., SIRCAR, B. and JOHNSON, L.R. Effect of dietary bulk on small intestinal morphology and cell renewal in the rat. *Gastroenterology*, **81,** 781–786 (1981)

18 FELDMAN, E. J., DOWLING, R. H., McNAUGHTON, J. and PETERS, T. J. Effects of oral versus intravenous nutrition on intestinal adaptation after small bowel resection in the dog. *Gastroenterology*, **70,** 712–719 (1976)

19 FENYO, G. and HALLBERG, D. The influence of a chemical diet on the intestinal mucosa after jejuno-ileal bypass in the rat. *Acta Chirurgica Scandinavica*, **142,** 270–274 (1976)

20 GLANAGAN, P. R., HAMILTON, D. L., HAIST, J. and VALBERG, L. S. Interrelationships between iron and lead adsorption in iron-deficient mice. *Gastroenterology*, **77,** 1074–1081 (1979)

21 FLEMING, C. R., McGILL, D. B., HOFFMAN, H. N. and NELSON, R. A. Subject review: total parenteral nutrition. *Mayo Clinic Proceedings*, **51,** 187–199 (1976)

22 FOROOZAN, P. and TRIER, J. S. Mucosa of the small intestine in pernicious anemia. *New England Journal of Medicine*, **277,** 553–581 (1967)

23 GASSULL, M. A., GOFF, D. V., HAISMAN, D. V., HOCKADY, T. D. R., JENKINS, D. J. A., JONES, K., LEEDS, A. R. and WOLEVER, T. M. S. The effect of unavailable carbohydrate jelling agents in reducing the post-prandial glycemia in normal volunteers and diabetics. *Journal of Physiology* (*London*), **259,** 52P–53P (1976)

24 GORBACH, S. L., BANWELL, J. G., JACOBS, B., CHATTERJEE, B. D., MITRA, R. S., SEN, N. N. and MAZUMDER, D. N. G. Tropical sprue and malnutrition in West Bengal. I. Intestinal

microflora and absorption. *American Journal of Clinical Nutrition*, **23,** 1545–1551 (1970)

25 GRACEY, M., STONE, D. E., SUHARJONO and SUNOTO. Isolation of *Candida* species from the gastrointestinal tract in malnourished children. *American Journal of Clinical Nutrition*, **27,** 345–349 (1974)

26 GRACEY, M., SUHARJONO, SUNOTO and STONE, D. E. Microbial contamination of the gut: another feature of malnutrition. *American Journal of Clinical Nutrition*, **26,** 1170–1174 (1973)

27 HALSTED, C. H. Small intestine in pellagra (Letter to editor). *American Journal of Clinical Nutrition*, **26,** 1 (1973)

28 HALSTED, C. H. The small intestine in vitamin B12 and folate deficiency. *Nutrition Reviews*, **33,** 33–37 (1975)

29 HALSTED, C. H., ROBLES, E. A. and MEZEY, E. Intestinal malabsorption in folate deficient alcoholics. *Gastroenterology*, **64,** 526–532 (1973)

30 HEINRICH, H. C. Intestinal iron absorption in man. In *Iron Deficiency*, edited by L. Hallberg, H. G. Harwerth and A. Vannotti, 213–294. New York, Academic Press (1970)

31 HERBERT, V., ZALUSKY, R. and DAVIDSON, C. S. Correlation of folate deficiency with alcoholism and associated macrocytosis, anemia and liver disease. *Annals of Internal Medicine*, **38,** 977–988 (1963)

32 HERMOS, J. A., ADAMS, W. H., LIU, Y. K., SULLIVAN, L. W. and TRIER, J. S. Mucosa of the small intestine in folate-deficient alcoholics. *Annals of Internal Medicine*, **76,** 957–965 (1972)

33 HILL, G. L., GUINN, E. J. and DUDRICK, S. J. Phosphorus distribution in hyperalimentation induced hypophosphatemia. *Journal of Surgical Research*, **20,** 527–531 (1976)

34 HOWARD, L., WAGNER, C. and SCHENKER, S. Malabsorption of thiamine in folate deficient rats. *Journal of Nutrition*, **104,** 1024–1032 (1974)

35 JAMBUNATHON, L. R., NEUHOFF, D. and YOUNQSZAI, M. K. Intestinal disaccharidases in malnourished infants rats. *American Journal of Clinical Nutrition*, **34,** 1879–1884 (1981)

36 JAMES, W. P. T. Comparison of three methods used in assessment of carbohydrate absorption in malnourished children. *Archives of Diseases in Childhood*, **47,** 531–536 (1972)

37 JENKINS, D. J., GASSULL, M. A., LEEDS, A. R., MATZ, G., DELAWARI, J. B. and BLENDIS, L. M. Effect of dietary fiber on complications of gastric surgery: prevention of postprandial hypoglycemia by pectin. *Gastroenterology*, **72,** 215–217 (1977)

38 JOHNSON, J. J. The regional and ethnic distribution of lactose malabsorption. In *Lactose Digestion*, edited by D. M. Paige and T. M. Bayless, 11–22. Baltimore, The Johns Hopkins University Press (1981)

39 JOHNSON, L. R., COPELAND, E. M., DUDRICK, S. J., LICHTENBERGER, L. M. and CASTRO, G. A. Structural and hormonal alterations in the gastrointestinal tract of parenterally fed rats. *Gastroenterology*, **68,** 1177–1183 (1975)

40 JOHNSON, L. R., LICHTENBERGER, L. M., COPELAND, E. M., DUDRICK, S. J. and CASTRO, G. A. Action of gastrin on gastrointestinal structure and function. *Gastroenterology*, **68,** 1184–1192 (1975)

41 KESSNER, D. M. and EPSTEIN, F. H. Effect of magnesium deficiency on gastrointestinal transfer of calcium. *Proceedings of the Society for Experimental Biology and Medicine*, **122,** 721–725 (1966)

42 KLIPSTEIN, F. A., LIFTON, S. D. and SCHENK, E. A. Folate deficiency of the intestinal mucosa. *American Journal of Clinical Nutrition*, **26,** 728–737 (1973)

43 KUMAR, V., GHAI, O. P. and CHASE, H. P. Intestinal dipeptide hydrolase activities in undernourished children. *Archives of Diseases in Childhood*, **46,** 801–804 (1971)

44 LEVINE, G. M., DEREN, J. J., STEIGER, E. and ZINNO, R. Role of oral intake in maintenance of gut mass and disaccharide activity. *Gastroenterology*, **67,** 975–982 (1974)

45 LINDENBAUM, J., GERSON, C. D. and KENT, T. H. Recovery of small intestinal structure and function after residence in the tropics. 1. Studies in Peace Corps volunteers. *Annals of Internal Medicine*, **74,** 218–222 (1971)

46 LINDENBAUM, J., PEZZIMENTI, J. F. and SHEA, H. Small intestinal function in vitamin B12 deficiency. *Annals of Internal Medicine*, **80,** 326–331 (1974)

47 MAGOTRA, M. L., TANDON, B. N. and SARAYA, J. R. Small bowels in iron deficiency anemia. *Indian Journal of Medical Research*, **59,** 1788–1795 (1971)

48 MATA, L. J., JIMINEZ, F., CORDON, M., ROSALES, R., PRERA, E., SCHNEIDER, R. E. and VITERI, F. Gastrointestinal flora of children with protein-calorie malnutrition. *American Journal of Clinical Nutrition*, **25,** 1118–1126 (1972)

49 MAYORAL, L. G., TRIPATHY, K., BOLANOS, O., LOTERO, H., DUQUE, E., GARCIA, F. T. and GHITIS, J. Intestinal, functional and morphological abnormalities in severely protein-malnourished adults. *American Journal of Clinical Nutrition*, **25,** 1084–1091 (1972)

50 MEHTA, S. K., KAUR, S., AVASTHI, G., WEG, N. N. and CHHUTTANI, P. N. Small intestinal deficit in pellagra. *American Journal of Clinical Nutrition*, **25,** 545–549 (1972)

51 MOREHEAD, R. M. and KESSNER, D. M. Effects of magnesium deficiency and parathyroidectomy on gastrointestinal calcium transport in the rat. *American Journal of Physiology*, **217,** 1608–1613 (1969)

52 NELSON, R. A., CODE, C. F. and BROWN, A. L. Jr. Sorption of water and electrolytes, and mucosal structure, in niacin deficiency. *Gastroenterology*, **42,** 26–35 (1962)

53 OTTO, H. F. and WEITZ, H. Elektronenmickroskopische Untersuchungen an Paneth-Zellin der Ratte unter zinkarmer. *Beitrage zur Pathologie*, **145,** 336–349 (1972)

54 OWEN, R. L. and BRANDBORG, L. L. Jejunal morphologic consequences of vegetarian diet in humans. *Gastroenterology*, **72,** A-88/1111 (1977)

55 PETITH, M. M. and SCHEDL, H. P. Effects of magnesium deficiency on duodenal and ileal magnesium absorption and secretion. *Digestive Diseases and Sciences*, **23,** 1–5 (1978)

56 REDDY, V., RAGHURAMULU, N. and BHECKARAM, C. Secretory IgA in protein-calorie malnutrition. *Archives of Diseases in Childhood*, **51,** 871–874 (1976)

57 ROSENSWEIG, N. S. and HERMAN, R. H. Control of jejunal sucrase and maltase activity by dietary sucrose or fructose in man. *Journal of Clinical Investigation*, **47,** 2253–2263 (1968)

58 RUPPIN, H., BAR-MEIR, S., SOERGEL, K. H. and WOOD, C. M. Effects of liquid formula diets on proximal gastrointestinal function. *Digestive Diseases and Sciences*, **26,** 202–207 (1981)

59 SCHNEIDER, R. E. and VITERI, F. E. Morphological aspects of the duodeno-jejunal mucosa in protein-calorie malnourished children and during recovery. *American Journal of Clinical Nutrition*, **25,** 1092–1102 (1972)

60 SCHWARTZ, S. E. and LEVINE, G. D. Effects of dietary fiber on intestinal glucose absorption and glucose tolerance in rats. *Gastroenterology*, **79,** 833–836 (1980)

61 SEETHARAM, B., PERRILLO, R. and ALPERS, D. H. Effect of pancreatic proteases on intestinal lactase activity. *Gastroenterology*, **79,** 827–832 (1980)

62 SELVERAJ, R. J. and BHAT, S. K. Metabolic and bactericidal activities of leukocytes in protein-calorie malnutrition. *American Journal of Clinical Nutrition*, **25,** 166–172 (1972)

63 SILVIS, S. E. and PARAGAS, P. D. Jr. Paresthesias, weakness, seizures and hypophosphatemia in patients receiving hyperalimentation. *Gastroenterology*, **62,** 513–520 (1972)

64 SNIPES, R. L. The effect of essential fatty acid deficiency on the ultrastructure and functional capacity of the jejunal epithelium. *Laboratory Investigation*, **18,** 179–189 (1968)

65 SOLOMONS, N. W. Zinc and copper in human nutrition. In *Nutrition in the 1980's: Constraints on our Knowledge*, 97–127. New York, Alan R. Liss, Inc. (1981)

66 TASMAN-JONES, C. Effects of dietary fiber on the structure and function of the small intestine. In *Medical Aspects of Dietary Fiber*, edited by G. A. Shiller and R. M. Kay, 67–74. New York, Plenum Press (1980)

67 TASMAN-JONES, C., OWEN, R. L. and JONES, A. L. Semipurified dietary fiber and small-bowel morphology in rats. *Digestive Diseases and Sciences*, **27,** 519–524 (1982)

68 TEOTIA, M., TEOTIA, S. P. S., SHARMA, N. L. and KUNWAR, K. B. Fat absorption studies in kwashiorkor. *Indian Journal of Medical Research*, **60,** 620–627 (1972)

69 THERON, J. J., WITTMAN, W. and PRINSLOO, J. G. The fine structure of the jejunum in kwashiorkor. *Experimental and Molecular Pathology*, **14,** 184–188 (1971)

70 VITERI, F. E., ALVARADO, J., LUTHRINGUR, D. G. and WOOD, R. P. Hematological changes in protein-calorie malnutrition. *Vitamins and Hormones*, **26,** 573–577 (1968)

71 VITERI, F. E. and SCHNEIDER, R. E. Gastrointestinal alterations in protein-calorie malnutrition. *Medical Clinics of North America*, **58,** 1487–1505 (1974)

72 WESER. E., HELLER, R. and TAWIL, T. Stimulation of mucosal growth in the rat ileum by bile and pancreatic secretions after jejunal resection. *Gastroenterology*, **73,** 524–529 (1977)

73 WINGATE, D. L. Backwards and forwards with the migrating complex. *Digestive Diseases and Sciences*, **26,** 641–666 (1981)

74 WOLMAN, S. L., ANDERSON, G. H., MARLISS, E. B. and JEEJEEBHOY, K. N. Zinc in total parenteral nutrition: requirements and metabolic effects. *Gastroenterology*, **76,** 458–467 (1979)

75 WORTHINGTON, B. S. and SYROTUCK, J. Intestinal permeability to large particles in normal and protein-deficient adult rats. *Journal of Nutrition*, **106,** 20–32 (1976)

76 YAWATA, Y., HEBBEL, R. P., SILVIS, S., HOWE, R. and JACOB, H. Blood cell abnormalities complicating the hypophosphatemia of hyperalimentation: erythrocyte and platelet ATP deficiency associated with hemolytic anemia and bleeding in hyperalimented dogs. *Journal of Laboratory and Clinical Medicine*, **84,** 643–653 (1974)

Index

Abetalipoprotinaemia, 21
Acarbose, 99
Acid fast organisms in inflammatory bowel disease, 305–306
Acid phosphatase, 11, 45
Acrodermatitis enteropathica, 26, 338
Actin, 21
Aeromonas spp., 321
Aganglionosis, 110, 112
Alimentary allergy, 255–256
Alkaline α-glucosidase, 46
Alkaline phosphatase, 10, 43, 44, 46
  in coeliac disease, 52–54
  in isolated epithelial cells, 59
  in organ culture, neonatal intestine, 65
Allergen challenge, eosinophilia in, 254
Allergic gastroenteropathy, 256–257
Allergic granulomatous angiitis *see* Churg-Strauss syndrome
Allergy,
  definition, 249
  types, 250
Allochthonous micro-organisms, 143
Alpha chain disease, 174–202
  age distribution, 183
  associated diseases, 189
  biochemistry, 185
  clinical features, 184
  endoscopy, 185
  enterocytes in, 21
  faecal fat excretion, 188
  geographical distribution, 183
  haematology, 185
  immunochemical studies, 187
  immunoelectrophoresis, 186–187
  immunohistochemistry, 181
  immunoperoxidase staining, 181
  intestinal function 187–188
Alpha chain disease (*cont.*)
  intestinal fungi, 188
  intestinal parasites, 188
  intraepithelial lymphocytes in, 29, 177
  lymphomas associated, 178
  macrophages in, 33, 177
  malignant neoplasia in, 189–190
  mediterranean type lymphoma and, 191–192
  natural history, 189
  pathogenesis, 190–191
  pathology, 175–181
    electron microscopic appearances, 180–181
    light microscopic appearances, 177–180
    macroscopic appearances, 175–176
  plasma cells in, 31, 177
  protein studies, 185–187
  radiology, 184
  sex distribution, 183
  structural studies, 187
  treatment, 192–194
  xylose absorption, 188
Amino acids, development of absorption, 5
Anaphylactic transfusion reactions, 83
Animal transmission studies, 303–305
  in mice, 304
  in rabbits, 305
Antibodies,
  ferritin-labelled, 49
  interference with adhesions, 157
Antibody-dependent helminthotoxic mechanisms, 169
Anticholingeric (and related) drugs, 137–138
Antigen,
  adhesive, 320–321
  uptake by intact mucosal surfaces, 76–77

Appendix, 29
APUD cells, 24
Argentaffin cells, 24
Argyrophil cells, 24
Arteritis, giant cell, 227, 241–242
Arylsulfatase, 11
Ascaris sp., 163
Aspirin, as prostaglandin synthetase inhibitor, 256
Asthma, exercise-induced, 253
Atopy, 249–264
  basophil cells in, 252–253, 253–254
  classification, 250–254
  definition, 250
  eosinophil cells in, 254
  foods and, 255–256
  gastroenteropathy and, 256–257
  mast cells in, 252–253, 253–254
  mucosa as portal of entry for allergens, 252
  sensitization 251–252
  status, 251
Auerbach's plexus, development of, 2
Autochthonous micro-organisms, 142

B cells, 74–76 *passim*
  in specific immune mechanisms, 327–328
Bacillus cereus, 320
Bacillus subtilis, occupational exposure to enzymes, 251
Bacterial content of intestine, 142–143
  neonatal, 143–148
Balantidium coli, 324
Basal lamina, 22
Basophils,
  in atopy, 252–253, 253–254
  in intestinal parasitism, 168, 169
Beaufray's zonal rotor, 41
Behçet's syndrome, 227, 240–241
Bile acids, 6
Bile salts, fetal and neonatal, 6
Bombesin, 266 (table)
Bone marrow transplantation, 203, 204
  syngeneic, 217
Botulinus toxin, uptake, 76
Bovine serum albumin, 5, 76
Brain-gut peptides, 125
Breast milk, bile-salt stimulated lipase, 12
Bronchial carcinoma, and endocrine cholera, 268
Brooke ileostomy, 295
Brunner's glands, 24
Brush (striated) border, 20, 21, 43, 44, 48
Brush (striated) border enzymes,
  intestinal absorption, 333–334
  lactase action on, 338
  pancreatic enzymes action on, 338
Buerger's disease (thromboangiitis obliterans), 227, 242

Calcitonin, 272
Calcium ion flux, 253
Caliviruses, 323
Calmodulin, 253
Campylobacter spp., 323, 324, 325
Candida albicans, 326, 335
Canine colitis, 303
Canine granulomatous enteritis, 303
Carcinoid syndrome, 112, 272–273
Carcinoid tumours, 112, 272
Castor oil, 284–285
Catalase, 43
Cellular immunity, and intestinal microbial population, 151–252
Cestodes, larval, 166
Chagas' disease, 110, 112, 136
Chelating agents, in intestinal cell culture, 59
Cholecystokinin, 98 (table), 135, 266 (table)
Cholera, 157
Cholera toxin, 62, 321
Cholesterol synthesis, 61
Cholinergic (and related) drugs, 137
Cholinesterases, nematode, 163
Chronic idiopathic intestinal pseudo-obstruction, 285–286
Chronic intermittent stomal obstruction, 296
Churg-Strauss syndrome, 227, 231, 234–235
Citrobacter spp., 321
Clostridial infection, 147, 148
  human, 149–150
  of sheep, 149
Clostridium botulinum, 320
Clostridium difficile, 306, 310, 321–322
  colitis due to toxin, 215
  enterotoxin, 284
Clostridium perfringens, 150, 321
  type A enterotoxin, 284
  type C, 147, 149–150, 321
Coccidia, 215
Codeine, 273
Coeliac disease,
  alkaline phosphatase distribution in, 52–54
  atopy not a mechanism, 257
  basal lamina in, 22
  enterochromaffin cells, duodenal, 24

Coeliac disease (*cont.*)
  enterocytes in, 21
  enteroglucagon in, 106
  gluten challenge, 34, 35
  gluten withdrawal treatment, 53–54
  insulin and polypeptide response reduced, 99
  intraepithelial lymphocytes in, 29
  macrophages in, 31
  organ culture, small intestine, 62–63
  Paneth cell in, 27
  plasma cells in, 31
^{59}Co-cyanocobalamin, 7
Colloidal gold, 49
Colonization resistance, 215
Colostrum, mucosal growth factor, 12
Congenital heart defects, clostridial infection, 148
Continent ileostomy, 295–296
Cortisol, fetal development, 9
Coryneform organisms, Gram-positive, 306
Crohn's disease, 234, 242, 253
  atopy and, 257
  infectious agents/inducers of cytotoxicity in, 302–318
  isolation of organisms, 305–307
  pathogenesis hypothesis, 311 (figure)
  VIPergic neurons in, 110
Crypt cells, 23
Cryptosporidium, 215, 326
Cutaneous basophil hypersensitivity, 253
Cystic fibrosis, 106, 252
Cytochalasin B, 61–62
Cytodifferentiation, 2–4
Cytomegalovirus, 205, 215, 307
Cytopathic agents, transmissable, 310
Cytosol calcium, 253
Cytotoxicity in Crohn's disease and ulcerative colitis,
  infectious agents, 310–311
  mechanisms of tissue damage, 309–310
  possible inducing agents, 307–311
  suggestions for progress, 313–314
  unanswered questions, 312–313
  verification of data, 312–313
Cytotoxins, 320, 321–322
  for colon, ileum, chick embryo cells, 310, 311

Defence mechanisms of intestine, 326–328
  non-specific, 326–327
  specific immune, 327–328
Dexamethasone, 65
Dextran, 49
Diabetes mellitus, intestinal motility in, 287
Diarrheagenic bacteria, motor patterns induced by, 283–284
Diarrhoea,
  acute, 319–331
    invasive infections, 323–326
    motility patterns, 283
    non-invasive (external) infections, 320–323
  annoying, 322
  virus, 323, 324
Dietary fibre, 339–340
Digitonin, 46–48
Dipeptidases, jejunal, 43
Disaccharidase deficiency, 333
Domperidone, 137
Dumping syndrome, 103, 294
Duodenal resection 294
Dystrophia myotonica, 287

Eczema, atopic, 252
Edwardsiella tarda, 321
Egg, allergic reaction to, 251
Eimeria spp., 163 (table), 164, 168 (table), 168
  IgE antibody to, 166
  IgG antibody to, 166
Electroenterogram, 121, 121–122, 126
Endocrine cholera, 268–271
  colon, 270
  humoral mediators, 268–269
  pathophysiology of diarrhoea, 269–271
  small intestine, 270
  treatment of diarrhoea, 271
  upper digestive secretions, 270
Endocrine diarrhoea, 265–268
Endocrine functions, small intestine disorders and, 97–118
Endocytic vacuoles, 52
Endoskeleton, 52
Enkephalin, 269
Entamoeba histolytica, 324
Enteral nutrition, 338–339
  composition, 339
Enterobacter cloacae, 321
Enterobacter spp., 321
Enterochromaffin cells, 24
Enterocyte, 20–22, 58
  biochemical anatomy, 40–57
  brush (striated) border, 20, 21, 43, 44, 48 (*see also* Brush (striated) border enzymes)
  in disease, 21

Enterocyte (*cont.*)
organelles, 43–44
distribution of, control jejunal biopsies, 43
pathology, 52–54
separation by density differences, 41–43
separation by size differences, 51–52
Enteroendocrine cells, 2, 24–56
Enteroglucagon, 98 (table), 98, 104–107
chemistry, 105
clinical significance, 106–107
distribution, 106
physiology, 106
release, 106
Enteroglucagon-producing tumour, 106
Enterokinase, 10
Enteropeptidase, 10
Enterotoxins, 320, 321
Enzymes, development of, 7–12
Eosinophil(s), 168, 169, 254
Eosinophil chemotactic factor (ECF-A), 253, 254
Eosinophilia, 254
Eosinophilic gastroenteritis, 257
Eosinophilic oesophagitis, 257
Epithelial cells, 2
culture, 59
Epithelial growth factor (EGF), 62, 65
Escherichia coli, 77, 142, 310
adherence to epithelial surfaces, 322–323
attachment mechanisms, 157
in Crohn's disease and ulcerative colitis, 306
elimination from Thiry-Vella loop, 151–155
enteropathogenic, (EPEC), 322
enterotoxigenic (ETEC), 321, 328
enterotoxin, 321
infection of babies, 148
invasive, 323, 324
in neonatal intestine, 144–148 *passim*
RDEC-1, 322
in tropical sprue, 321
Essential fatty acids deficiency, 332
Essential mixed cryoglobulinaemia, 241
Exotoxins, 320

Familial visceral myopathy, 285–286
Familial visceral neuropathy, 285–286
Fasting, 338
Fat malabsorption, 334
Feline infectious enteritis, 303
Feline infectious peritonitis, 302
Ferritin, 49
Fetal small intestine, 1–12 *passim*, 65–66
Fibre, dietary, 339–340
Fluorescent assay procedures, 44
Fluorescent enzyme substrates, 44–49
Folate deficiency, 332, 336
Food allergens, 255–256
Formazan, 49
Fructose, 62
^{3}H-Fucose glycoprotein, 63
Fucosidosis, 63

β-Galactosidase, 11
Galactosyl transferase, 52
Gall bladder, fetal, 6
GALT *see* Gut associated lymphoid tissue
Ganglioneuroblastoma, 110, 268
Ganglioneuroma, 268
Gastric inhibitory polypeptide (GIP), 98 (table), 98–100, 266 (table)
actions, 99
chemistry, 98
in endocrine cholera, 269, 270
localization, 99
physiology, 99
release, 99
Gastrin, 135, 266 (table), 266
Gastroenteritis, 325, 326
in farm animals, 326
Giant cell arteritis, 227, 241–242
Giardia lamblia, 188, 215, 323
Giardia muris, 162, 163 (table), 164
IgA antibody to, 165
Giardia trophozoites, 322–323
Glicentin, 105
Glucagon, 138, 266 (table)
Glucagonoma, pancreatic, 273
N-acetyl-β-Glucosaminidase, 11, 43, 46, 47, 49
Glucose, absorption development, 4–5
Glucose-6-phosphatase, 49
α-Glucosidase, 11, 43, 44–45, 49
development, 7–8
β-Glucosidase, 11
β-Glucuronidase, 11
Glutamate dehydrogenase, 43, 46
γ-Glutamyl transferase, 47
Gluten-sensitive enteropathy, 63
mast cells in, 34
Goblet cells, 2, 20, 23, 167
Golgi apparatus, 21, 24, 26, 31, 52
Graft-versus-host disease (GVHD), 203–219
acute, 205, 205–208
chronic, 205, 217–218

Graft-versus-host disease)
  conditioning therapy, 203–204
  differential diagnosis, 214–215
  endoscopy, 212
  grading system, 213
  graft-versus-host reactions, 204–205
  histology, 212–213
  intestinal immunodeficiency in, 213–214
  intestinal structure and function, 218
  malabsorption, 214
  marrow transplantation technique, 204
  natural history, 216
  pathogenesis, 216–217
  radiology, 208
Granulocytes *see* Polymorphonuclear leucocytes
Granulomatous inflammation of intestine in ruminants, 303
Guar, 99
Gut associated lymphoid tissue (GALT), 29–31, 73, 91
  'antigen-driven' clonal expansion, 75
  cell populations, 74–75
  immunization and, 75
  'homing' and other migratory patterns, 75–76
Gut-luminal derived antigens, 75

Habitats, in ecosystems, 142
Haemorrhagic necrotic enteritis, 147–148
Heavy chain diseases, 174
Helminthiasis *see* Intestinal parasites
Henoch-Schönlein purpura, 237–238
Hepatitis B infection, 310
Hereditary hollow visceral myopathy, 285–286
  duodenal motility, 286
Hirschsprung's disease, 110, 112, 308 (table)
Histamine, 252, 253, 254, 272
HLA-B8 negative/positive patients, gluten induced damage *in vitro*, 63
Homeostasis, intestinal, Paneth cell in, 27
Hormonal diarrhoea, 265–279
Host responses to intestinal parasitic infections, 93–94
Human protein hypersensitiveness, 250
Hydrocortisone, 65
5-Hydroxytryptamine (serotonin), 24, 123, 252, 266 (table), 272
Hyperthyroidism, 136, 273, 288
Hypothyroidism, 136, 288

IgA, 5, 75, 81–82
  in human colostrum, 5, 84
  intestinal parasites and, 165
  low level, 252
  in malnutrition, 335
  in milk, 76, 84
  origins, 83–84, 86–87
  subclasses, 83
  transport, 85, 86
IgA cells, 74
IgD, 74, 81
IgE, 81, 84–85
  in atopy, 250–251, 251–252, 253
    radioallergosorbent test (RAST), 250
  intestinal parasites and, 166, 254
IgG, 5, 81–82, 84–84, 85
  parasite-specific antibodies, 166–167
IgG-STS (short term sensitizing) antibody, 250–251
IgM, 85, 86
Ileal-anal anastomosis, 297
Ileal resection, 294
Ileostomy, 295–296
  Brooke, 295
  continent, 295
  obstructing device, 296
  sodium cromoglycate treatment, 258
Immune mechanisms, 73–96
Immunization, and gut-associated lymphoid cells, 75
Immunoblasts, 31
Immunocytes, 73
Immunoglobin, in Paneth cell, 26
Immunoproliferative small intestinal disease, 174
Incretin, 99
Infancy, sudden death in, 82
Infection of adult intestine, 148–150
Infectious agents in acute diarrhoea, 319–331 (*see also* Diarrhoea; Toxins; *and specific organisms*)
Inflammation, chronic, mast/basophil cells in, 253
Inflammatory bowel disease in animals, 302–303
  atopy and, 257
Insulin, 65
Interactions among micro-organisms and host, 142–161
  controlling mechanisms, 151–156
Intercellular junctional complexes, 52
Interdigestive myoelectric complexes (IMC), 280, 292, 293, 297, 298
Interstitial cells of Cajal, 121

Intestinal bypass, 295
Intestinal denervation, 297–298
  transplantation of small intestine, 297–298
  vagotomy, 297
Intestinal epithelium, protective function, 170
Intestinal flora, postnatal development, 12
Intestinal hurry, 294
Intestinal lymphoma, 174–175
Intestinal obstruction, 137
Intestinal pacemaker (setter), 122–123, 293
Intestinal pacing, 299–300
Intestinal parasites, 162–173
  accessory cell responses, 168–169
  antibodies, 165–167
  antigens, 163
  enteric immune responses, 164–169
  IgE and, 166
  lymphoid cell responses, 167–168
  protective functions of intestinal epithelium, 170
  rapid expulsion, 164, 169
  resistance against, 164
  vaccination against, 163
Intestinal pseudo-obstruction, 285
Intestinal resection, 294
Intestinal structure, and nutrient deficiencies, 333
Intestinal transection 293
Intestinal transplantation, 297–298
Intraepithelial lymphocytes, 29, 29–30, 73, 74
Intraluminal pressure change, 127–128
Invasive infections, 323
In vitro studies, intestinal mucosa, 58–72
  everted sac technique, 58
  ex vivo vascular perfusion, 58
  future applications, 66–67
  isolated intestinal cell structure, 58, 59
  organ culture, 58, 59–66 (*see also* Organ culture)
Iron deficiency, 337
Irritable bowel, 135
Isomaltase, development of, 7–8
Isospora belli, 215
Isospora natalensis, 215

J chain, 81, 82–83, 85
Jejunoileal autotransplants, canine, 298
Jejunoileal bypass, 99, 104
Jejunum,
  autotransplants, 297–298
  biopsy, after cow's milk ingestion, 256
Jejunum (*cont.*)
  dipeptidases in, 43
  haemorrhagic necrotic enteritis, 147–148
  necrotising enteritis (pig-bel), 149
  oligopeptidases, higher, in, 43
  organelles from biopsies, 43
  resection 294
  tripeptidases in, 43

K (capsular) antigens, 144–146 *passim*, 148
K-cell, 309, 310
Kallikrein, 254, 272
Klebsiella pneumoniae, 321
Klebsiella spp., 321
Kock pouch, 295–296
Kulchitscky cell, 24
Kwashiorkor, 21, 335

β-Lactalbumin, 5
Lactase, 4, 9–10, 33–34
Lactate dehydrogenase, 43
Lacteals, 34
Lactobacillus acidophilus, 13
Lactobacillus bifidus, 12–13
Lactoferrin, 13, 152, 154–155, 157
Lactose, 4, 13
  intolerance, 9–10
  tolerance tests, 9
Lamina propria, 29–35
Lamina proprial lymphocytes, 73, 74, 327
Laxatives and motility patterns, 284–285
Leucine amino peptidase, 59
Leukotrienes, 253
Lipase, in human breast milk, 12
Lipid(s), 6–7, 12
Lipid factors, 253
Lipoprotein synthesis, 61
Lung, antibacterial defence mechanisms, 159
Lymphatics, intestinal (lacteals), 34
Lymphocytes,
  development in small intestine, 2–4
  in intestinal parasitism, 168
  in lamina propria, 30, 327
Lymphokines, 254
Lymphomas of gastro-intestinal tract, 31, 174
Lymphopoesis, 2
Lymphoreticular tissue, 29–31
Lysosomal enzymes, 10–12
Lysosome hydrolases, 63
Lysozyme, 13, 2627

M cells, 26, 31
  in fetal small intestine, 4
Macrophages, 31–33, 75
Magnesium deficiency, 337
Malabsorptive states, enterocytes in, 21
Malate dehydrogenase, 49
Malnutrition, 333–334
  bacterial overgrowth, 335
  disorders of motility, 335
Maltase, development of, 7–8
Mammary gland (bovine), antibacterial defence mechanisms, 157
Marrow transplantation, 203, 204
  syngeneic, 217
Mast cells, 26, 33, 74
  in atopy, 252–253, 253–254
  in intestinal parasitism, 168–169
Mastocytosis, 267–268
Measles enteritis, 324
Meconium, 2, 6
Meconium corpuscles, 5
Mediterranean abdominal lymphoma, 174, 191–192
Meissner's plexus, development of, 2
Metal deficiencies, 336–338
Metoclopramide, 137
Mice,
  bacterial colonization of small intestine, 157
  transmission studies, 304
Middle Eastern lymphoma, 174
Migrating action potential complex (MAPC), 283–284
Migrating motor (myoelectric) complex (MMC), 129, 133, 134, 280–282
  in bacterial overgrowth, 281
  in diabetic gastroparesis, 282
  disorders of, 281–286
  feeding effect on, 282
  in postoperative ileus, 281–282
  in postvagotomy gastroparesis, 282
  Q-complex, 282
Milk intolerance, 9–10
Mitochondria, 49
Mononuclear phagocytic cells, 31–33,75
Morphogenesis of intestine, 1–2
Motilin, 24, 98 (table), 100–102, 134
  actions, 101
  chemistry, 100
  clinical significance, 102
  localization, 100
  physiology, 101
  release, 101
Motility index, 280
Motility of small intestine, 119–141
  abnormal, 135–137
  in Chagas disease, 136
  in chronic idiopathic intestinal obstruction, 285–286
  in chronic pseudo-obstruction, 285–286
  comparative physiology, 125
  contractile activity, 127
  control mechanisms, 132–135
    endocrine, 134–135
    neural, 133
  in diabetes mellitus, 136
  in diarrhoea, 283
  disorders, 280–291
  electromyography, 126–127
  fasting motor activity, 129
  intraluminal pressure change, 127–128
  laxatives, effects of, 284–285
  in malnutrition, 335
  methods of investigation, 125–126
  motilin, action of, 134
  neuropeptide regulation, 125
  normal, 128–132
  in obstruction, acute/subacute, 137
  opioids, action on, 135
  in paralytic ileus, 135
  peptides, action on, 125, 134–135
  in porphyria, 136
  postprandial activity, 129–132
  radiological investigation, 128
  radionuclide scanning, 128
  in scleroderma, 136
  in Shay-Drager syndrome, 136
  somatostatin, action of, 134
  surgical aspects, 293–301
  therapy of disorders, 137–138
  in thyroid disease, 136
Mucin, 24
Mucosal-associated lymphoid tissues, 73
Mucosal (secretory) immune system, 87–93
  absorption inhibition of nonviable antigens, 89–90
  antibacterial activity, 88–89
  antitoxin activity, 88–89
  antiviral activity, 87–88
  local cell-mediated immunity, 90
  oral tolerance, 90–93
Mucus, 23–24
Muscle of small intestine, 120, 120–123
  different from myocardium, 121
  electrophysiology, 120–123
    basic electrical rhythm, 122
  pacemaker (setter), 122–123, 293
  spontaneous rhythmic depolarization, 121

Mycobacterium johne, 303
Mycobacterium kansasii, 306
Mycoplasma hyorhinis, 309

N cells, 102
Necrotising enterocolitis, 321
Neisseria gonorrhoeae, 83
Neisseria meningitidis, 83
Nematoda dubius, 167
Nematospiroides dubius, 326
Neonatal small intestine, 4–13 *passim*, 64–65, 143–148
Nerves of intestinal muscle, 120, 123
Neuropeptides, 125
Neurotensin, 98 (table), 102–104, 266 (table), 269
  chemistry, 102
  clinical significance, 103–104
  distribution, 102
  dumping syndrome and, 104
  in pancreatic tumours, 104
  physiology, 103
  release, 102
Neutrophil(s), 152–153, 155, 157
Neutrophil chemotactic factor (NCF), 253
Niacin deficiency, in dogs, 336
Niches, in ecosystems, 142
Nifedipine, 253
Nippostrongylus brasiliensis, 163 (table), 164, 168 (table)
  IgA antibody to, 165
  IgG antibody to, 166
  mast cell responses, 169
  trapping in mucus, 170
Nonadrenergic noncholinergic innervation of smooth muscle, 123
Nonmyelinated nerve fibres, in lamina propria, 35
Norwalk agents,323
5′-Nucleotidase, 43
Null cells, 74
Nutritional deficiencies, small intestine response, 332–344
Nuts, sensitivity to, 254

O (bactericidal) antibodies, 145
O antigens, 145
Oligopeptidases, higher, 43
Organ culture, small intestine, 58, 59–66
  adult, 59–63
    methods, 59–60
    results, 60–61
Organ culture, small intestine (*cont.*)
  diseased intestine, 62–63
  fetal, 65–66
  fetal calf serum absence from culture system, 64
  human, 59, 62
  in vitro response, nutrients, hormones, drugs, 61–62
  neonatal, 63–65
Organelles, *see* Enterocyte, organelles

P antigens, 148
Pacemaker (setter), intestinal, 122–123, 293
Palatinase, development of, 7–8
Pancreas,
  endocrine tumour, 268
  glucogonoma, 268
  hyperplasia, 268
  neurotensin in tumours, 104
  vasoactive intestinal polypeptide-producing tumour, 104
Pancreatic cholera, 268
Paneth cell, 23, 26–27, 338
Paralytic ileus, 135
Parenteral nutrition, 338–339
Parvovirus infection in dogs, 326
Peanuts, sensitivity to, 254
Pellagra, 336
Pentagastrin, 62
Peptidases,
  development, 10
  digitonin effect on, 48
  in jejunum, 43
Peristalsis type II, 283
Pernicious anaemia, jejunal biopsies, 336
Peyer's patches (PP), 2, 26, 29, 74–75
  in endocrine cholera, 269
  in intestinal parasitism, 167
Phagocytic vacuoles, granules in, 152, 157
D-Phenylalanine, 45
L-Phenylalanine, 45
PHI, 112
Phosphorus deficiency, 336–337
Pig-bel, 149
Pinocytotic vesicles, 5
Plasmablasts, 30, 31
Plasma cells, 30, 31, 251
Plasmids, 144–145
Plasminogen activator of neutrophil proteases, 254
Platelet activating factor, 252–253
Platinum salts, occupational exposure to, 251

Polyarteritis, 227, 231
  microscopic, 231, 235–236
  nodosa, 227, 231, 232–234
Polymorphonuclear leucocytes (granulocytes), 152–153, 155
  in intestinal parasitism, 168
  in specific immune reactions, 157 (*see also* Basophils; Eosinophils; Neutrophils)
Porphyria, 136
Postnatal intestinal development, 12–13
Postoperative ileus, 292–293
  migratory motor complex and, 281
Primary upper small intestinal lymphoma, 174
Proctitis, sodium cromoglycate for, 258
Proglucagon, 105
Prostaglandin(s), 253, 254, 256, 266 (table)
  in carcinoid syndrome, 272–273
  in endocrine cholera, 269
  in thyroid medullary carcinoma, 272
Prostaglandin synthetase inhibitors, 256
Protein, development of absorption, 5
Protein-caloric malnutrition, 333–335
  nitrogen balance, 334
Prototheca, 303
Pseudofronts, 283
Pseudomonas spp., 321
Pseudomonas-like bacteria, cell wall defective, 305, 306
Pseudo-obstruction, chronic, 135
Pyrophosphate, 49
PYY, 112

Q-complex, 282

Rabbits, transmission studies in, 304–305
Radioallergosorbent test (RAST), 250
Radiotelemetric pressure capsules, 128
Reagin, 250
Repetitive bursts of action potentials (RBAP), 283–284
Reversed intestinal segments, 298
Rheumatoid arthritis, 227, 240
Ricinoleic acid, 284
RNA viruses, in Crohn's disease, 307
Rotaviruses, 323–324
Round worms, 149
Russell bodies, 31

Salmonella spp., 76–77, 323, 324, 325
  antibody resistant, 328
Salmonella typhi, 76, 325
Salmonella typhimurium, 284, 324
Scanning electron microscope, 19–20
Schistosoma mansoni, 94
Scleroderma, 287
Scombroid poisoning, 320
Secretin, 98 (table), 125, 266 (table)
Secretory component, 81, 82
  deficiency
Serine protease, 169
Serotonin (5-hydroxytryptamine), 24, 123, 252, 266 (table), 272
Serratica spp., 321
Sezary syndrome, 31
Shay-Drager syndrome, 136
Sheep, effects of diet change, 149
Shigella dysenteriae, 324
  enterotoxin, 284
Shigella flexneri, 324
Shigella sonnei, 324
Shigella spp., 323, 324
  antibiotic resistant, 328
Shigellosis, 324
Shuttle vesicles, 52
Single-step gradient centrifugation, 50
Slow-reacting substance of anaphylaxis (SRS-A), 253, 254
Smooth muscle, in lamina propria, 34–35
Sodium cromoglycate, 252, 253, 256, 257–258
Solitary lymphoid follicles, 73, 75
Somatostatin, 134
Somatostatinoma, 273
Staphylococcus aureus, 320, 322
Starvation, complete, 338
Steatorrhoea, 334
Strain gauge transducer, 127, 128
Streptococcus faecalis, 142
Streptococcus mutans, 76, 89
Striated border *see* Brush (striated) border; Brush (striated) border enzymes
Subcellular fractionation techniques, 40–54
  affinity chromatography, 40
  centrifugation, 40
  free flow electrophoresis, 40
  further considerations, 52
  gel filtration, 40
  two phase partition, 40
  of whole homogenates, 50
Substance P, 98 (table), 110–112, 266 (table)
  chemistry, 110
  clinical significance, 112
  distribution, 110
  physiology, 110–112
Succinate dehydrogenase, 49

Sucrase, 4
  activity decrease, 333
  development, 4, 7–8
Sucrose, development of absorption, 4
Sucrose density gradient centrifugation, single step, disadvantages of, 45–46
Sugars,
  deficiency, 333–334
  development of absorption, 4–5
Surface areas of small intestine, 332
Sweet potato, 149–150
Synergism, microbial, 326
Systemic lupus erythematosus, 227, 238–240
Systemic mastocytosis, 253

T cells, 74–76 *passim*, 251, 310
  deficiency, 217
  malignancy, 31
  in specific immune mechanisms, 327–328
Taenia taeniaformis, 163
Takayasu's arteritis, 241
Theliolymphocytes, 29
Thelphyllin, 62
Thiry-Vella loop, 133, 134, 151–152
Thromboangiitis obliterans, 227, 242
^{3}H-Thymidine, 339
Thymus, 164, 165
Thyrocalcitonin, 266 (table), 272
Thyroid gland,
  diseases of, 136, 273, 288
  medullary carcinoma, 272
Thyroxine, 65
Tissue factors, low/middle molecular weight, non-viable, 308
Toxin(s),
  cyto-, 320, 321–322
  entero-, 320, 321
  exo-, 320
  formed at luminal surface, 320–321
  pre-formed in food, 320
Toxin-associated infections, 324–325
  dispersed, 324–325
  superficial, 324
β-Toxin, clostridial, 147, 149, 150
ε-Toxin, clostridial, 149
Trace element deficiency, 336–338
Transcobalamin, 7
Transmission electron microscope (TEM), 19–20
  in gastrointestinal tumour pathology, 19
  in infectious gastroenteritis, 19
Transplantation of small intestine, 297–298
Transport processes, development of, 4–7
Treponema spp., 326
Trichinella spiralis, 163 (table), 163
  expulsion, 164, 168 (table), 169, 170
  IgE synthesis suppression, 166
Trichostrongylus colubriformis, 163 (table), 168 (table), 169
Tripeptidases, 43
Triton WR 1339, 49
Tropical malabsorption, enteroglucagon in, 106
Tropical sprue,
  cytotoxins, 321
  enterocytes in, 21
  insulin and polypeptide responses reduced, 99
  intraepithelial lymphocytes in, 29
  plasma cells in, 31
Tuberculin reaction, mast cells in, 253
Tuft cell, 28
Two phase counter-current partition, 40

Ulcerative colitis, 110
  atopy and, 257
  infectious agents/cytotoxicity inducers, 302–318
  isolation of organisms, 305–307
  pathogenesis hypothesis, 311 (figure)
  sodium cromoglycate for, 258
  of swine, 303
Ulcerative enteritis of birds, 303
Ulcerative ileojejunitis, 63
Ultrastructure of small intestine, 19–39

Vagotomy, 297
Vasculitis, 227–248
  aetiology, 229
  classification, 231
  clinical features, 231
  complicating other diseases, 238–241
  pathogenesis, 229–230
  pathology, 230
  treatment, 231
Vasoactive intestinal polypeptide (VIP), 98 (table), 98, 266 (table), 324
  actions, 109
  chemistry, 107
  clinical significance, 109–110
  distribution, 107–109
  in endocrine cholera, 268–269
  physiology, 109
Verapamil, 253
Verner-Morrison syndrome, 109
Vibrio cholerae, 321, 328
Vibrio parahaemolyticus, 321, 322

Vibrio spp., non-cholera, 321
Villous epithelium, 20–22
  atrophy, 34–35, 333
  columnar absorptive cell *see* Enterocyte
  enzymatic activities along axis, 59
  microvilli, 20–21
  striated border, 20–21
VIPoma tumour, 110
Virus diarrhoea, 323–324
Vitamin B12, 7, 62
  absorption in α-chain disease, 188
    in iron deficiency, 337
  deficiency,332, 335
Vitamin D deficiency, 332
Vitamin D3, 62
Vitamins, water soluble, deficiencies of, 335–336

WDHA syndrome, 268
Wegener's granulomatosis, 227, 231, 236–237
Whipple's disease, 31, 33

Xylose absorption test, 188, 334, 336

Yersinia enterocolitica, 323, 324,325

Zinc,
  deficiency, 337–338
  metabolism and Paneth cell, 26
Zollinger-Ellison syndrome, 266–268
Zonal rotor, 51–52
Zoonoses, 325